# The Fundamentals of Stereoelectro-encephalography

# The Fundamentals of Stereoelectro-encephalography

*Edited by*

PATRICK CHAUVEL, MD
Epilepsy Center, Neurological Institute, Cleveland Clinic,
Cleveland, OH, United States

AILEEN MCGONIGAL, MBCHB, PHD
Department of Neurosciences, Mater Misericordiae Hospital
Brisbane, QLD, Australia

Mater Research Institute, Faculty of Medicine, University of Queensland
Brisbane, QLD, Australia

Queensland Brain Institute, University of Queensland
Brisbane, QLD, Australia

GUY M. MCKHANN II, MD
Department of Neurosurgery, Columbia University,
New York, NY, United States

JORGE ÁLVARO GONZÁLEZ-MARTÍNEZ, MD, PHD
University of Pittsburgh Medical Center, Epilepsy & Movement Disorders Program
University of Pittsburgh Epilepsy Center, Cortical Systems Laboratory, UPMC Presbyterian
Pittsburgh, PA, United States

ELSEVIER

THE FUNDAMENTALS OF STEREOELECTROENCEPHALOGRAPHY ISBN: 978-0-443-10877-8


*Publisher:* Patrick Manley Jr
*Acquisitions Editor:* Mary Hegeler, Melanie Tucker
*Editorial Project Manager:* Sara Pianavilla
*Production Project Manager:* Selvaraj Raviraj
*Cover Designer:* Mark Rogers

3251 Riverport Lane
St. Louis, Missouri 63043

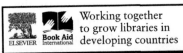

# Contributors

**Melissa M. Asmar, MD, MSc**
Department of Neurology and Comprehensive Epilepsy Center
University of California
Davis, CA, United States

**Thandar Aung, MD, MS**
Department of Neurology
University of Pittsburgh
Pittsburgh, PA, United States

**Patrick Chauvel, MD**
Epilepsy Center
Neurological Institute
Cleveland Clinic
Cleveland, OH, United States

**Daniel L. Drane, PhD, ABPP(CN)**
Department of Neurology
University of Washington School of Medicine
Seattle, WA, United States

Departments of Neurology and Pediatrics
Emory University School of Medicine
Atlanta, GA, United States

**Jay R. Gavvala, MD, MSCI**
Texas Institute for Restorative Neurotechnologies
Department of Neurology
McGovern Medical School
University of Texas Health Science Center at Houston
Houston, TX, United States

**Jorge Álvaro González-Martínez, MD, PhD**
Department of Neurosurgery
Epilepsy Center
University of Pittsburgh Medical Center
Pittsburgh, PA, United States

**Ammar Kheder, MD**
Children's Healthcare of Atlanta
Atlanta, GA, United States

Division of Pediatric Neurosciences
Helen DeVos Children's Hospital
Grand Rapids, MI, United States

Michigan State University College of Human Medicine
Grand Rapids, MI, United States

Pediatric Institute and Department of Neurology
Emory University School of Medicine
Atlanta, GA, United States

**Aileen McGonigal, MBChB, PhD**
Department of Neurosciences
Mater Misericordiae Hospital
Brisbane, QLD, Australia

Mater Research Institute
Faculty of Medicine
University of Queensland
Brisbane, QLD, Australia

Queensland Brain Institute
University of Queensland
Brisbane, QLD, Australia

**Guy M. McKhann II, MD**
Department of Neurosurgery
Columbia University
New York, NY, United States

**John C. Mosher, PhD**
Texas Institute for Restorative Neurotechnologies
Department of Neurology
McGovern Medical School
University of Texas Health Science Center at Houston
Houston, TX, United States

**Nigel P. Pedersen, MBBS, FAES, FANA**
Center for Neuroscience
University of California
Davis, CA, United States

Department of Neurology and Comprehensive Epilepsy Center
University of California
Davis, CA, United States

Programs in Neuroscience
Psychology
Biomedical Engineering
University of California
Davis, CA, United States

**Jean Régis, MD**
Aix-Marseille University
Department of Functional and Stereotactic Neurosurgery
Timone Hospital
Marseille, France

**Hussam Shaker, MD**
Epilepsy Center
Trinity Health Hauenstein Center
Grand Rapids, MI, United States

**Stephen Thompson, MD**
Faculty of Health Sciences
McMaster University
Hamilton, ON, Canada

**Agnès Trébuchon, MD, PhD**
APHM
Timone Hospital
Clinical Neurophysiology
Marseille, France

INSERM UMR1106
Institut des Neurosciences des Systèmes
Aix-Marseille Université
Faculté de Médecine Timone
Marseille, France

Service de Neurophysiologie Clinique
Hôpital de la Timone
Marseille, France

**Teja Mannepali, PhD**
Texas Institute for Restorative Neurotechnologies,
Department of Neurology
McGovern Medical School
University of Texas Health Science Center at Houston
Houston, TX, United States

# Preface

Stereoelectroencephalography or SEEG, designed in the middle of the last century, is a method for presurgical investigation of epilepsy. Its visionary inventors in Hospital Sainte-Anne, Paris, developed SEEG over a 30-year period, before expanding to a few centers in France, Switzerland, and Italy. Such a slow spread is not only explained by the fact that the technical (surgical and electrophysiological) facilities were only available in a few centers at that time, but also because of recognition of the level of multidisciplinary expertise that was required. This multidisciplinary expertise was carefully nurtured and transmitted from one expert team to another via an ongoing process of teaching, apprenticeship, and senior mentoring. Some 60 years later, the same requirements are mandatory. Nowadays, if the financial resources in developed countries can easily solve the technical needs, the question of the academic multidisciplinary competence, and apprenticeship process for SEEG training, remains a real preoccupation. This is a growing problem, especially since SEEG practice is expanding very fast in very large continents such as North America or Asia.

This volume is a first step to draw attention and bring basic information to adult and pediatric neurologists and neurosurgeons interested in starting an epilepsy surgery program using SEEG. It is a compendium resulting from a course held over several years in the United States, organized by the four coeditors of this book.

The tripod of SEEG is anatomy, electrophysiology, and semiology. These three components form an essential basis of knowledge for guiding practice. Anatomy for SEEG is an anatomy of hypotheses and trajectories in the brain's tridimensional space, taking into account both its structural and functional (connectivity) aspects. Its referential system (the Talairach Stereotaxic Space) affords a rational representation of cortical (and subcortical) structures making explicit their topographic relations as well as their network organization. Interpretation of electrophysiology in SEEG departs to some degree from the basic concepts guiding EEG and ECoG recordings. Explicitly, SEEG is not just "depth EEG." Basic background in neurophysiology is necessary to recognize the full spectrum of normal patterns as they vary across different brain regions, and to distinguish these from pathological activities. A grounding in neurophysiology (and some understanding of related biophysics) is also essential to figure out the localization of seizure generators using frequency, latency, cooccurrence, and spatial–temporal dynamics as tools. Electrical stimulation is an integral part of the SEEG method, with the main goal of triggering habitual seizure symptoms and signs, which also contributes to understanding of the relation of epileptogenic zone to brain function. Clinical semiology is the key to understanding the nature of the neural systems involved in seizures and their temporal organization. Semiology is the driver behind the entire method from video-EEG to surgery and is the clinical ground truth that validates the significance of the anatomy–electrophysiology interrelations. This is why SEEG is a stepwise and comprehensive method whose principles are applicable from the time of the outpatient clinic until the end of the recording. SEEG experience teaches us how to interview a patient about their seizures, and how to read an EEG.

The underlying goal of any SEEG exploration is to investigate therapeutic possibilities for the refractory epileptic seizures of the patient undergoing exploration. Surgical planning is predicated upon the delineation of each explored structure's role in the primary organization of seizures, propagation pathways, and their relation to each other, as well as to underlying cerebral function. The methodology of SEEG is equally well suited to exploring epilepsy with and without radiologically visible lesions, but patient selection and choice of electrode trajectory are the two key aspects that define the success or failure of all SEEG explorations. These aspects may sound simple but are composed of multiple complex decisions, hence the need for careful training and apprenticeship, as well as future research efforts to optimize practice.

SEEG explores an individual epilepsy in a singular brain. Neuropsychology and cognitive neuroscience are part of the SEEG constituent disciplines rather than being only required to establish functional constraints before surgical decision. In SEEG, they also contribute to ictal analysis and to specific behavioral assessment during stimulation. Their advances provide essential information for research progress in the comprehension of clinical semiology. Beyond the individual patient level, meticulous study of group-level SEEG data in terms of semiologic patterns and signal correlates has been an indispensable step in the journey toward more refined understanding of epilepsy as a network disorder.

**Patrick Chauvel, Aileen McGonigal,**
**Guy McKhann, Jorge González-Martínez**
May 2024

# Contents

CHAPTER 1

# Creation and Evolution of SEEG

PATRICK CHAUVEL, MD

Stereoelectroencephalography (SEEG), a stereotaxic approach for exploration of the pharmaco-resistant epilepsies, was created 65 years ago by J Talairach, MB Dell and J Bancaud at Hospital Sainte-Anne, Paris.[1] For the first time ever, it allowed recording of patients' seizures in the three-dimensional brain space. The principles of SEEG, based on establishing anatomo-electro-clinical correlations in the patient's seizures, did not change since 1965. But the technologies for anatomical topography, electrophysiology, clinical observation, and surgery have dramatically evolved. However, it remains a complex investigation and a hard to standardize procedure, since it must always be tailored to the patient's individual case.

After the publication of the "SEEG in Epilepsy" book in 1965 by Bancaud and Talairach and their collaborators,[2] the 70's were marked by multiple papers on semiology and localization, and by three major books: (i) Angiography of Cerebral Cortex by Gabor Szikla,[3] (ii) EEG/SEEG Surface/Depth Correlations by Jean Bancaud,[4] (iii) and the Novel Approach of Epilepsy Surgery by Jean Talairach.[5] Due to a tight collaboration between the research labs of the INSERM Unit 97 "Unite de Recherches sur l'Epilepsie" and the Department of Neurosurgery at Hospital Sainte-Anne, the publications on pathophysiology of focal epilepsies emerged during the 70's and 80's, with papers on temporal[6] and frontal seizures semiology,[7,8] the cingulate gyrus,[9] the role of the frontal cortex in generalized seizures,[10] mechanisms of startle epilepsies,[11] as well as monkey models of motor cortex epilepsies,[12] role of cortical monoaminergic terminals,[13,14] and alteration of amino acids neurotransmitters with iontophoresis and ion-sensitive microelectrodes.[15] In parallel, a new approach in cognitive neurophysiology developed in SEEG on declarative memory[16] and on auditory cortex physiology.[17] The great originality of the clinical/research group structure led to the production of new concepts, like the network hypothesis on the epileptogenic zone, all inspired by the practice of SEEG.

SEEG developed only in Hospital Sainte-Anne, Paris until the mid-70ies. Then Talairach and Bancaud's pupils exported the method: Heinz-Gregor Wieser in Zurich, Guy Bouvier in Hospital Notre Dame, Montreal, and Alain Rougier in Bordeaux. Many neurologists and neurosurgeons from South America visited Sainte-Anne in the 70's and 80's, and some of them stayed longer than a habitual visit as they were political refugees from Chile and Argentina. Osvaldo Betti developed stereotactic radiosurgery with Gabor Szikla then came back to Buenos Aires. Silvia Kochen, a neurologist, after having been a pupil of Bancaud for 2 years, launched an SEEG-based epilepsy surgery program in Buenos Aires. In the 80's, just after Jean Talairach retired, the pioneers' team was decimated by the deaths of Gabor Szikla (stereotaxy surgeon) and Alain Bonis (neurologist). Antonino Musolino and Claudio Munari became in charge of stereotaxy, Suzanne Trottier and Patrick Chauvel in charge of neurological care. Jean-Paul Chodkiewicz succeeded Jean Talairach in 1980, and Patrick Chauvel succeeded Jean Bancaud in 1986.

The group split up in 1990. Claudio Munari moved to Grenoble, France and Patrick Chauvel to Rennes, France. Each developed new EMUs with SEEG. Philippe Kahane, Munari's first resident, was instantly fascinated by SEEG, and Jean-Pierre Vignal, who was in the Sainte-Anne team, accompanied Chauvel. Then, with Munari training Jean Isnard, and Chauvel training Philippe Ryvlin, a new group emerged in Lyon. A few years later, Chauvel moved to Marseille and Munari to Milan. Each of the branches differentiated and enriched the SEEG compendium. Munari worked on new stereotaxic implantation modes like hypothalamic hamartomas[18] and insula oblique trajectories. He actively promoted SEEG-guided epilepsy surgery in children,[19] and carefully studied the relations between lesions and epilepsies.[20] After his premature death, his Niguarda team in Milan led by Giorgio Lo Russo, Laura Tassi and Stefano Francione performed refined correlations with histopathology in malformations of cortical development with Roberto Spreafico and studied the sleep-related frontal seizures with Lino Nobili.[21,22] Chauvel had been interested since the early 80's by semiology

The Fundamentals of Stereoelectroencephalography. https://doi.org/10.1016/B978-0-443-10877-8.00003-6

and physiology of motor seizures then of frontal seizures in general. With his American colleague Antonio Delgado-Escueta who imported the SEEG method to the US, he organized the jubilee celebration for Jean Bancaud in 1987. Gathering the most renowned specialists at that time, they published the first book on frontal lobe seizures and epilepsies in 1992.[23] This book was the first initiative to disentangle the complexity of frontal seizures' semiology and electrophysiology. Then the Chauvel branch initiated a multidisciplinary strategy based on SEEG. It assembled neurologists, neurophysiologists, neuropsychologists, cognitive neuroscientists, and biomedical engineers working as one team. Eric Halgren and Catherine Liegeois-Chauvel were the first to study cognition from intracerebral recording data.[16,17] Jean-Louis Coatrieux and Fabrice Wendling adapted signal processing methods to the SEEG signal and were the first to design computational models to interpret it.[24] This innovative approach was born in Rennes. The same philosophy was applied after Chauvel moved to Marseille (in 1997), where Jean Regis was elaborating a functional surgery program based on stereotaxy. The Institut de Neurosciences des Systemes (INS) reproduced at a bigger scale what had previously been validated in assembling epileptology, neuropsychology, cognitive neurophysiology with basic neurophysiology and applied mathematics. The link between all these disciplines was the SEEG method.

Meanwhile, Ryvlin and Kahane animated a Lyon-Grenoble axis and developed epilepsy imaging and engineering approaches.[25] Jean-Pierre Vignal and Louis Maillard, both pupils of the Chauvels at different times, created a new center in Nancy, France with Herve Vespignani. Luc Valton, who had been trained in Marseille, opened a new center in Toulouse, France, and pursued the same philosophy with Emmanuel Barbeau who collaborated with Liegeois-Chauvel when he was in the same Institute.[26] The way this web grew over time in 10 years is interesting, as it is a team story and a human adventure.

Apart from a few exceptions mentioned above, the School of SEEG remained in Paris for 30 years (1960–90). The initiative of starting a new program and taking responsibility for preparing an electrode implantation map away from the shrine was experienced as scary by first-generation pupils even after they had spent some 20 years with the Master. Jean Bancaud died in 1993. The few French Sainte-Anne alumni felt the need to initiate an annual French master class of epilepsy that they named "Ecole Pratique Jean Bancaud". Their objectives were to keep on exploring together the complexity of the method and to teach the young neurologists on semiology as study of its mechanisms became accessible from analysis of many cases investigated with SEEG. This Ecole is still active today and takes place yearly in France; it took the name of "Ecole Pratique Bancaud-Talairach" after the death of Jean Talairach in 2007.

Hans Luders had got to know the SEEG pioneers in 1987 when he attended Bancaud's jubilee symposium on frontal lobe epilepsies in France. In the early 2000s, there were debates between Cleveland Clinic subdural grids (SDG) defenders and the French SEEG protagonists on the respective accuracies of the two methods for epileptogenic zone localization. Then Luders and his colleagues published data on SDG morbidity and then decided to evaluate the capabilities of SEEG.[27] Invited by Alim Benabid in Grenoble and in Milan after Claudio Munari's death, they got convinced and marked an historic turning point in adopting the method. A few years later, Jorge Gonzalez-Martinez was sent on mission in France and came back after being trained in the stereotaxic method.[28]

Thirty years after Antonio Delgado-Escueta imported Bancaud's concepts at UCLA, Imad Najm invited Patrick Chauvel to join the Cleveland Clinic team. Chauvel retired from Aix-Marseille University Department of Clinical Neurophysiology and Institut de Neurosciences des Systemes and was succeeded by Fabrice Bartolomei and Viktor Jirsa. Catalyzed by the Cleveland Clinic international influence, the last 10 years have seen a worldwide development of SEEG-guided epilepsy surgery. As a side effect of a new French-American functional connectivity, SEEG secondarily spread in Europe outside France and Italy, and around the world (especially China, Taiwan, India and Australia, as well as South America and the Middle East).

The real benefit of such fast expansion of SEEG for epilepsy surgery is difficult to estimate. The method is not straightforward and cannot be standardized. SEEG is not depth EEG (Local Field Potential -LFP- is the signal, connectivity is the framework). A multidisciplinary and close-knit teamwork is required. The body of knowledge that is relevant to perform SEEG is not theoretical and bookish but based on a real apprenticeship and training through mentoring. SEEG requires to think outside of the box, so that the learning curve is steep. Indications for SEEG should critically depend on the team's SEEG experience. This is currently not the case.

The next future will tell whether we are now attending an apotheosis or contemplating the apoptosis of SEEG.

The current difficulties faced by SEEG are due to multiple conceptual and technical/practical pitfalls. They could be summarized in saying that (i) most of the apprentices do not take SEEG as a comprehensive method; (ii) neurologists and neurosurgeons often consider SEEG as a depth version of grids, so that their first preoccupation is "to cover" a maximal volume of brain or to "target deep structures"; (iii) a crucial conceptual leap remains to be made for a correct analysis of the SEEG data.

*SEEG as a comprehensive method.* SEEG doesn't start with electrode implantation. As implantation relies upon precise hypotheses of epileptogenic networks involved, the data for their generation must be collected in phase I. As a team is gaining experience in SEEG, the content of phase I becomes more and more elaborated and the hypotheses more accurate. The master word here is semiology. Semiology is the study of signs. Semiology is not limited to clinical signs but also encompasses electrical and imaging signs. There is a clinical, an electrical and an imaging semiology in epilepsy. A sign is descriptive in nature: it has no absolute value; it always must be "interpreted". In the SEEG method, signs are interpreted through a correlative process: the goal of video-EEG recording of seizures is to establish electrical-clinical correlations; imaging semiology describes the radiological signs of a putative epileptogenic "lesion" and as such it must be anatomically compared to the results of electrical-clinical correlations. Phase I is definitely the most important step in the SEEG method. If you do not get from video-EEG clearly explicit and falsifiable hypotheses in terms of epileptogenic networks, an implantation plan cannot be designed. Unlike SDG where indecision on localization leads to lateralize and to "cover", SEEG can be properly performed only when prior estimate of seizure onset and propagation networks is available. Reaching this level of competency is not immediate. Therefore, there is a learning curve for a team to get expertise in electrical-clinical correlations. An apprentice team should not attempt to do SEEG in non-straightforward cases.

Unlike the two-dimensional SDG, *SEEG is a three-dimensional brain exploration.* Electrode labeling of an electrode as its deep target is a proof of incomprehension of the method. Adjusting electrode *trajectory* is the essential task to be performed before SEEG. A correct estimation of the epileptogenic zone localization can only be achieved by comparison of seizure onset with its early and late propagation: this is the process that allows to define the primary organization of the ictal discharge. If too many electrode contacts are recording white matter or are not optimally placed in propagation areas of the network, SEEG interpretation becomes arbitrary. Electrode implantation plan must take account of three factors: anatomical sampling, volume sampling and eventual surgical landmarks. There are always one or several missing electrode(s). The systematic use of anatomo-electro-clinical correlations allied with direct electrical stimulation is a means of compensating for a suboptimal implantation.[29]

Getting familiar with *SEEG profoundly changes the way that we apprehend epilepsy.* The simplistic notion of focus can no longer be envisaged, as the existence of multi-structural (i.e., amygdala, hippocampus, and entorhinal cortex; or orbitofrontal and anterior cingulate cortex; or insula and cingulate gyrus) epileptogenic zone is a prominent feature. A multi-structural seizure onset generating multi-directional cortico-cortical propagation simultaneously and bilaterally in different lobes is a common observation especially in supra-sylvian and parietal-occipital epilepsies. To identify an epileptogenic zone (i.e., the minimal network capable to synchronize the areas involved at seizure onset thus triggering the patient's seizures) among multiple areas involved in a seizure dynamical state remains a challenge every time. To use too restricted criteria like seizure onset time and relative latencies (a usual practice in SDG) is inadequate in SEEG where frequency patterns prove to be the most accurate marker.[30] However, a still undetermined "epileptic cutoff frequency" is inadequate as a concept, and a sampling issue is always present. The diagnostic situation here can be likened to an inverse problem, where the use of a priori information as a constraint allows to minimize the number of solutions. Given that the available data are multimodal (anatomy, electrical spontaneous or stimulation-triggered activities, current and anamnestic clinical semiology), a clinical reasoning process[31] must be followed to make decisions on surgical strategy.

While SEEG is resetting your conceptualization of epilepsy, it will change your interpretation of EEG. The pioneers early understood that several conditions needed to be met for an epileptiform or an epileptic discharge to be recorded on surface EEG.[4] For instance, the activities from depth sources are not recorded in routine scalp EEG. As a rule, hippocampal or amygdalar activities are not detected if they have not spread to lateral temporal cortex; the same is true for orbitofrontal discharges. However, interictal spikes can be detected from the scalp temporal electrodes if hippocampal and lateral cortex spikes are synchronous, or if the lateral cortex alone is discharging. Ictal fast activities are exceptionally recorded in scalp EEG; this also depends on the geometry of the generators.[32] This consideration is to emphasize that most of the time teams starting with an SEEG program do not understand how much they should invest in the quality of video-EEG. The number of scalp electrodes is insufficient, the montages are inadequate. MEG will never replace EEG, but its intrusion in the presurgical investigations brought new insights on source localization in a world only paying attention to the waveforms.[33]

Current evolution of SEEG is full of paradoxes. It has swiftly proliferated outside of France since the last decade. Epileptologists and neurosurgeons are satisfied with its clinical tolerability by patients. Advances in robotics have simplified the stereotaxic procedure. However, it is too often used as a technique for targeting deep structures rather than as a comprehensive anatomical method to design trajectories of multi-lead electrodes allowing cortical networks exploration. SEEG being presumed less invasive than SDG, neurosurgery is attempting to promote less invasive techniques like laser interstitial thermal therapy or thermocoagulation, as if the size of the epileptogenic zones had decreased with technical evolution. In parallel, video-EEG amplifiers technology has steadily progressed so that hundreds of channels can be managed in smaller size and weight boxes. Higher sampling rates and better digital filters allow good quality recording of infra-slow to high-gamma activity. However, Epilepsy Monitoring Unit architecture and technicians/nurses training are far from being optimal in many centers. Per- and post-ictal semiology assessment is often insufficient. This nonoptimal phase I increases the risk of inadequate electrode implantation plan with too many electrodes in an attempt "to cover" a maximal brain volume like in SDG approach. "Depth grids" are replacing cortical surface grids. Obviously, this situation is a direct consequence of time/productivity increased pressure on hospital personnel by health system economic constraints. From this perspective, SEEG is a complicated and expensive method.

Will technological advances compensate for the workforce problem? Recent advances in signal processing allow a rapid quantification of interictal activities and guided identification of epileptogenic zone. But the medical/scientific training requirements might become an issue in the future. SEEG is not ECoG. A neuroscience/neurophysiology background is mandatory, a specific academic environment is required, so that research programs can be developed in tight relation with the epilepsy team. Its electrophysiology competency will directly benefit from a multidisciplinary environment. Improvement in clinical semiology assessment depends not only on the material conditions above mentioned, but also on the team interest in neuropsychology, behavioral neurology, and cognitive neuroscience in general. In an SEEG-based epilepsy surgery program, the specialized team includes nurses and electrophysiology technicians. Specific teaching must be organized on a permanent basis, with video-EEG and SEEG interpreted together. A solution for improving good practices in the SEEG method would be to reconfigure EMU architecture, for instance from a rectangular to a circular shape with nurse/tech team in the center. This would facilitate rapid and efficacious access to the patient. With the reading rooms in the same space, the neurologists/nurses/technicians interaction would be greatly facilitated. Performance in SEEG-guided epilepsy surgery critically depends on the team learning curve, much more than on technological advances.

A global analysis of the evolution of SEEG shows that its principles and its mode of clinical reasoning have not significantly changed since its creation. Even after major advances in neuroscience, its basic concepts (anatomo-electro-clinical correlations, stimulations procedure, epileptogenic zone, etc.) are not outdated. What its pioneers had early perceived about the nature of epilepsy has now received a scientific basis. "Primary organization" and "multidirectional propagation" of focal seizures are now expressed in terms of neural networks features. Ictal "fast activity" remains a reliable marker of an epileptogenic zone and has now been identified as an abnormal gamma-range oscillation.[34,35] Cognitive neuroscience and electrophysiology have profoundly changed the landscape around SEEG with extension of the indications of explorations and operations as a corollary. The use of "functional mapping" has now invaded SEEG practice. This new custom is a little awkward as the inherent sampling bias of SEEG prevents from real mapping from taking place. In the classical SEEG, functional mapping was performed through ictal anatomo-electro-clinical correlations with special attention to functional impairment. The seizure was used to map the functions.[36] Utilization of stimulation behavioral data for functional surgical outcome prediction is only licit in primary cortices. They are a few synapses away from sensory receptors or muscle effectors with which they are topically hardwired. From a hodological perspective, the relationship between associative cortices and cognitive functioning is far more complex. This is why functional impairment through stimulation is more easily obtained with white matter than "language areas" in SEEG. As cognitive functioning is underpinned by network activity, a disruptive stimulation effect does not necessarily prognosticate a post-surgery functional deficit following ablation of the area stimulated. Development of other techniques, like transient cortical cooling, would be more appropriate for an accurate anticipation of functional outcome.

SEEG has steadily evolved over the last decades. From the 24 channels ink-writing EEG machine acute recordings (SEEG lasted 12 h) at Hospital Sainte-Anne in the 60's to the current 256 channels chronic video-SEEG monitoring, the technique has gradually progressed. From the pneumoencephalography and contrast ventriculography practiced in the stereotaxic frame used for the pre-SEEG "reperage"[37,38] to the structural and functional brain imaging incorporating the Talairach system,[39] the accuracy of electrode localization has tremendously improved. Robotic systems for electrode implantation have also increased anatomical precision and largely contributed to SEEG expansion in simplifying the stereotaxic procedure. SEEG signal processing brings refined markers of the epileptogenic zone while providing valuable insights into the pathophysiology of human focal epilepsies. Video image processing with the help of AI is now able to classify clinical semiology sequences, awaiting for the clinicians to put much effort into it.[40] At last, emphasis on concerted research approaches combining simultaneous surface (EEG-MEG) and depth recording with imaging should eventually open a passage to fully non-invasive presurgical investigations. SEEG is the ideal tool for this transition. A glorious future for SEEG could therefore be its gradual disappearance.

## REFERENCES


1. Bancaud J, Dell MB. Technics and method of stereotaxic functional exploration of the brain structures in man (cortex, subcortex, central gray nuclei). *Rev Neurol (Paris)*. 1959;101:213–227.
2. Bancaud J, Talairach J, Bonis A, et al. La Stéréo-Electroencéphalographie dans l'épilepsie. In: *Informations Neurophysiopathologiques Apportées Par L'investigation Fonctionnelle Stéréotaxique*. Masson & Cie; 1965.
3. Szikla G, Bouvier G, Hori T, Petrov V. *Angiography of the Human Brain Cortex. Atlas of Vascular Patterns and Stereotactic Cortical Localization*. Berlin Heidelberg New York: Springer-Verlag; 1977.
4. Bancaud J, Talairach J, Geier S, Scarabin JM. *EEG et SEEG dans les tumeurs cerebrales et l'epilepsie*. Paris: Edifor; 1973.
5. Talairach J, Bancaud J, Szikla G, Bonis A, Geier S, Vedrenne C. New approach to the neurosurgery of epilepsy. Stereotaxic methodology and therapeutic results. 1. Introduction and history. *Neurochirurgie*. 1974;20(Suppl 1):1–240.
6. Bancaud J. Clinical symptomatology of epileptic seizures of temporal origin. *Rev Neurol*. 1987;143:392–400.
7. Geier S, Bancaud J, Talairach J, Bonis A, Enjelvin M, Hossard-Bouchaud H. Automatisms during frontal lobe epileptic seizures. *Brain J Neurol*. 1976;99:447–458. https://doi.org/10.1093/brain/99.3.447.
8. Geier S, Bancaud J, Talairach J, Bonis A, Szikla G, Enjelvin M. The seizures of frontal lobe epilepsy. A study of clinical manifestations. *Neurology*. 1977;27:951–958. https://doi.org/10.1212/wnl.27.10.951.
9. Talairach J, Bancaud J, Geier S, et al. The cingulate gyrus and human behaviour. *Electroencephalogr Clin Neurophysiol*. 1973;34:45–52. https://doi.org/10.1016/0013-4694(73)90149-1.
10. Bancaud J, Talairach J, Morel P, et al. "Generalized" epileptic seizures elicited by electrical stimulation of the frontal lobe in man. *Electroencephalogr Clin Neurophysiol*. 1974;37:275–282. https://doi.org/10.1016/0013-4694(74)90031-5.
11. Bancaud J, Talairach J, Lamarche M, Bonis A, Trottier S. Neurophysiopathological hypothesis on startle epilepsy in man. *Rev Neurol*. 1975;131:559–571.
12. Chauvel P, Louvel J, Lamarche M. Transcortical reflexes and focal motor epilepsy. *Electroencephalogr Clin Neurophysiol*. 1978;45:309–318. https://doi.org/10.1016/0013-4694(78)90183-9.
13. Chauvel P, Trottier S. Role of noradrenergic ascending system in extinction of epileptic phenomena. *Adv Neurol*. 1986;44:475–487.
14. Trottier S, Lindvall O, Chauvel P, Björklund A. Facilitation of focal cobalt-induced epilepsy after lesions of the noradrenergic locus coeruleus system. *Brain Res*. 1988;454:308–314. https://doi.org/10.1016/0006-8993(88)90831-1.
15. Pumain R, Kurcewicz I, Louvel J. Fast extracellular calcium transients: involvement in epileptic processes. *Science*. 1983;222:177–179. https://doi.org/10.1126/science.6623068.
16. Halgren E, Marinkovic K, Chauvel P. Generators of the late cognitive potentials in auditory and visual oddball tasks. *Electroencephalogr Clin Neurophysiol*. 1998;106:156–164. https://doi.org/10.1016/S0013-4694(97)00119-3.
17. Liegeois-Chauvel C, Musolino A, Chauvel P. Localization of the primary auditory area in man. *Brain*. 1991;114:139–151.
18. Munari C, Kahane P, Francione S, et al. Role of the hypothalamic hamartoma in the genesis of gelastic fits (a video-stereo-EEG study). *Electroencephalogr Clin Neurophysiol*. 1995;95:154–160. https://doi.org/10.1016/0013-4694(95)00063-5.
19. Munari C, Lo Russo G, Minotti L, et al. Presurgical strategies and epilepsy surgery in children: comparison of literature and personal experiences. *Childs Nerv Syst*. 1999;15:149–157. https://doi.org/10.1007/s003810050358.
20. Munari C, Berta E, Francione S, et al. Clinical ictal symptomatology and anatomical lesions: their relationships in severe partial epilepsy. *Epilepsia*. 2000;41:S18–S36. https://doi.org/10.1111/j.1528-1157.2000.tb06043.x.
21. Zucca I, Milesi G, Medici V, et al. Type II focal cortical dysplasia: ex vivo 7T magnetic resonance imaging abnormalities and histopathological comparisons: 7T Imaging in FCD II. *Ann Neurol*. 2016;79:42–58. https://doi.org/10.1002/ana.24541.

22. Gibbs SA, Proserpio P, Francione S, et al. Clinical features of sleep-related hypermotor epilepsy in relation to the seizure-onset zone: a review of 135 surgically treated cases. *Epilepsia*. 2019;60:707–717. https://doi.org/10.1111/epi.14690.
23. Chauvel P, Delgado-Escueta AV, Halgren E, Bancaud J. *Frontal Lobe Seizures and Epilepsies*. Raven Press; 1992.
24. Wendling F, Badier JM, Chauvel P, Coatrieux JL. A method to quantify invariant information in depth-recorded epileptic seizures. *Electroencephalogr Clin Neurophysiol*. 1997;102: 472–485. https://doi.org/10.1016/S0013-4694(96)96633-3.
25. Kujala J, Jung J, Bouvard S, et al. Gamma oscillations in V1 are correlated with GABAA receptor density: a multi-modal MEG and Flumazenil-PET study. *Sci Rep*. 2015;5:16347. https://doi.org/10.1038/srep16347.
26. Barbeau EJ, Chauvel P, Moulin CJA, Regis J, Liégeois-Chauvel C. Hippocampus duality: memory and novelty detection are subserved by distinct mechanisms: hippocampus duality. *Hippocampus*. 2017;27:405–416. https://doi.org/10.1002/hipo.22699.
27. Hamer HM, Morris HH, Mascha EJ, et al. Complications of invasive video-EEG monitoring with subdural grid electrodes. *Neurology*. 2002;58:97–103. https://doi.org/10.1212/WNL.58.1.97.
28. Gonzalez-Martinez J, Bulacio J, Alexopoulos A, Jehi L, Bingaman W, Najm I. Stereoelectroencephalography in the "difficult to localize" refractory focal epilepsy: early experience from a North American epilepsy center: *SEEG in the United States*. *Epilepsia*. 2013;54:323–330. https://doi.org/10.1111/j.1528-1167.2012.03672.x.
29. Chauvel P, Gonzalez-Martinez J, Bulacio J. Presurgical intracranial investigations in epilepsy surgery. In: *Handbook of Clinical Neurology*. Elsevier; 2019:45–71. https://doi.org/10.1016/B978-0-444-64142-7.00040-0.
30. Grinenko O, Li J, Mosher JC, et al. A fingerprint of the epileptogenic zone in human epilepsies. *Brain*. 2018; 141:117–131. https://doi.org/10.1093/brain/awx306.
31. Norman GR, Monteiro SD, Sherbino J, Ilgen JS, Schmidt HG, Mamede S. The causes of errors in clinical reasoning: cognitive biases, knowledge deficits, and dual process thinking. *Acad Med*. 2017;92:23–30. https://doi.org/10.1097/ACM.0000000000001421.
32. Cosandier-Rimélé D, Bartolomei F, Merlet I, Chauvel P, Wendling F. Recording of fast activity at the onset of partial seizures: depth EEG vs. scalp EEG. *Neuroimage*. 2012;59: 3474–3487. https://doi.org/10.1016/j.neuroimage.2011.11.045.
33. Burgess RC. MEG for greater sensitivity and more precise localization in epilepsy. *Neuroimaging Clin*. 2020;30: 145–158. https://doi.org/10.1016/j.nic.2020.02.004.
34. Bartolomei F, Chauvel P, Wendling F. Epileptogenicity of brain structures in human temporal lobe epilepsy: a quantified study from intracerebral EEG. *Brain*. 2008;131: 1818–1830. https://doi.org/10.1093/brain/awn111.
35. Li J, Grinenko O, Mosher JC, Gonzalez-Martinez J, Leahy RM, Chauvel P. Learning to define an electrical biomarker of the epileptogenic zone. *Hum Brain Mapp*. 2020;41:429–441. https://doi.org/10.1002/hbm.24813.
36. Trébuchon A, Chauvel P. Electrical stimulation for seizure induction and functional mapping in stereoelectroencephalography. *J Clin Neurophysiol*. 2016; 33:511–521. https://doi.org/10.1097/WNP.0000000000000313.
37. Talairach J, David M, Tournoux P, Corredor H, Kvasina T. Atlas d'anatomie stereotaxique. In: *Reperage radiologique indirect des noyaux gris centraux, des regions mesencephalo-sous-optique et hypothalamique de l'homme*. Paris: Masson & Cie; 1957.
38. Talairach J, Szikla G, Tournoux P, et al. Atlas d'Anatomie Stereotaxique du Telencephale. In: *Etudes Anatomo-Radiologiques*. Paris: Masson & Cie; 1967.
39. Talairach J, Tournoux P. *Co-planar Stereotaxic Atlas of the Human Brain. 3-Dimensional Proportional System: An Approach to Cerebral Imaging*. Stuttgart: Georg Thieme Verlag; 1988.
40. Hou J-C, Thonnat M, Bartolomei F, McGonigal A. Automated video analysis of emotion and dystonia in epileptic seizures. *Epilepsy Res*. 2022;184:106953. https://doi.org/10.1016/j.eplepsyres.2022.106953.

CHAPTER 2

# Concepts of Cortical Anatomy and Talairach Stereotaxic Space Applied to the SEEG Method

JEAN RÉGIS, MD • JORGE ÁLVARO GONZÁLEZ-MARTÍNEZ, MD, PHD

Stereoelectroencephalography (SEEG) concepts are directed toward the precise identification of the parcel of the cortical ribbon responsible for seizure genesis in patients with drug resistant epilepsy. The phase I preoperative workup (noninvasive phase) based on careful analyses of the electro-clinical and radiological explorations is designed to harvest all information supposed to have "localizing value" of the cortical area (s) generating the ictal discharge. When these "localizing" information are too uncertain to propose an upfront corticectomy but strong enough to propose a coherent hypothesis about the location of the epileptogenic zone (EZ) in the individual anatomy, a phase II can be proposed (SEEG).

How phase I data are translated in terms of anatomical hypotheses and stereotaxic coordinates, how the hypotheses are conceptualized in implantation strategy and how the electroclinical information generated by the SEEG are interpreted, are all aspects that are fundamentally rooted in the understanding of the 3D anatomo-functional organization of the cerebral cortex. In this chapter, we will discuss the fundamentals of cortical anatomy and stereotaxic space applied to the SEEG methodology.

## A BRIEF HISTORY OF CORTICAL ANATOMY

Raised by the debate between equipotentiality and phrenology in the XVIII century[1] the meticulous study of how specific areas of the cerebral cortex are involved in functional specialization took off with the "modern localizationism" of Paul Broca (1824–80), the renowned French surgeon and anatomist. The systematic study of correlation between neurological symptoms and localization of lesions in the brain (the anatomo-clinical method) created the need for detailed morphological study of the cerebral cortex. In 1854 Louis Pierre Gratiolet published "Mémoire des plis cérébraux de l'homme et des primates"[2] and in 1892 Daniel John Cunningham published "Contribution to the surface anatomy of the cerebral hemispheres".[3] These two major comprehensive contributions created a base for further studies of the cerebral cortex and have remained unchallenged until now. The discovery by Fritz & Hitzig in 1870 that electricity could stimulate the brain and that specific parts of the cortex were involved in motor function, with different regions of cortex relating to different parts of the body (somatotopy) led rapidly to neurosurgeons like Wilder Penfield (1891–1976) systematically using cortical electrical stimulation as a tool for functional brain mapping in general neurosurgery and epilepsy surgery.

Thanks to the discovery of X-rays by Wilhem Conrad Röntgen in 1895, Remy and Contremoulin introduced the concept of stereotactic frame and stereotaxic image-guided navigation in 1897.[4] Subsequently, the use of stereotactic methodology for human functional neurosurgery by Spiegel and Wycis started at the end of the 1940's mainly for psychiatric surgery and movement disorders.[5]

The basic concept of stereotaxic neurosurgery was to provide neurosurgeons with a method allowing them to safely navigate in the brain using the "language of numbers" (analytic geometry). The frame allowed the intracranial space of the patients to be represented within an ortho-normed tridimensional Euclidean space with tripolar coordinates defining the position of each point of the patient's intracranial space. The frame at the same time offered a remarkably stable way of fixation of the skull in addition to a reference to the stereotactic space. Numerous frames have been manufactured, usually relying either on the Cartesian

The Fundamentals of Stereoelectroencephalography. https://doi.org/10.1016/B978-0-443-10877-8.00010-3

coordinates or on polar coordinates (or both). Some frames combine Cartesian coordinates and analogic targeting capacities.

## THE STEREOTAXIC APPROACH FOR BRAIN ANATOMY: THE 3-DIMENSIONAL SPACE

In the late 1950's, Jean Talairach and Gerard Guiot went to visit Spiegel and Wycis in Philadelphia and founded stereotactic functional neurosurgery in France. At this time the only types of imaging available were plain X-ray, ventriculography invented by Walter Dandy in 1918 and angiography invented by the Portuguese neurologist Antonio Egas Moniz in 1927, confining neurosurgeons to indirect targeting of the intracerebral targets of functional neurosurgery. However, neurosurgeons had previously rapidly understood that the wide variability of relationship between intracranial targets for functional operations and the bony structures provided by X-rays was far too imprecise to use it as landmarks for trajectories in the brain. The introduction of air ventriculography[6] gave access to the visualization of deep anatomical landmarks like the foramen of Monroe and the pineal gland, used by Spiegel and Wycis as reference structures for the very first stereotactic atlas as early as 1925.

Following the introduction of electroencephalography (EEG) in humans by Hans Berger in 1924, Forster and Altenburger performed the first invasive EEG recording around 5 years later. Then, Wilder Penfield and Herbert Jasper systematically used EEG recording of interictal activities and electrical stimulation of the exposed cortex in awake patients in order to map respectively the epileptic focus around the lesion and surrounding functional areas, in order to guide the resective surgery. Jean Talairach was a meticulous anatomist and the first to use stereotactic methodology for epilepsy. Thanks to the use of stereotactic methodology, Talairach proposed to insert deep electrodes into selected structures, allowing not only recording of interictal activities and mapping of the functional value of the investigated structures but also recording ictal (seizure-related) electrical activity, which was supposed, according to Bancaud, to be a better descriptor of the cortical areas generating seizures, which would be necessary to remove for successful outcome of epilepsy surgery.[7] The first stereoelectroencephalographic recordings using deep electrodes were acute, recording patients while they remained fixed in the stereotactic frame for several hours, waiting for seizures.[8] Then, Talairach and Bancaud moved toward chronic recording with patients keeping their implanted electrodes as long as several weeks.[9] Depending on the pre-SEEG hypotheses the strategy of implantation was shaped based on the range of anatomo-physiological correlations known at this time. This principle of the SEEG methodology challenged the capacity of the neurosurgeons to reach discrete deep critical structures in the pre-CT and pre-MRI era.

Jean Talairach proposed the use of the anterior commissure-posterior commissure (AC-PC) referential system visible on ventriculography, and proportionalization for indirect targeting of deeply seated targets but also cerebral cortex.[10] Talairach published a first atlas summarizing the statistical positions of the main brain structures in the AC-PC reference system in 1957.[11,12] He introduced the teleradiography technique with an X-ray source at more than 4 m from the receptor and orthogonality of the beam to the receptor. Teleradiography has the advantage of the absence of magnification factor and cushion deformity and allows direct calculation within a 3D space without mathematical transformation, thanks to strictly orthogonal X-rays and thus a high geometrical reliability. His homemade stereotactic frame was a very rigid one, designed to host a grid system specially adapted to multiple trajectories of the SEEG approach (Fig. 2.1).

The fundamental concepts of stereotaxic cortical and subcortical localization, as described above, are intrinsically related to the methods associated with Talairach's approach and the distinct utilization of direct and indirect stereotaxic localization methods. As a short explanation, the direct method is applied to the intracranial targets, structures and lesions that are visible on MRI. As a complementary method, indirect targeting localization is required in structures that are not MRI-visible such as, for example, the motor cingulate cortical areas and the entorhinal or perirhinal cortices. Despite the

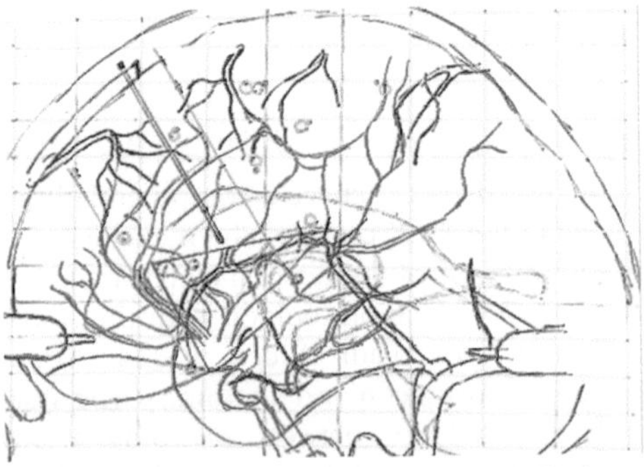

FIG. 2.1 A typical SEEG from the early 1990's based on ventriculography, Talairach atlas ACPC referenced and ventriculography. Note the electrode in the anterior insula and in the thalamus.

significant improvements in imaging modalities, the indirect targeting method and the application of the Talairach stereotaxic space still play an important role in defining important anatomical-functional structures that are not visible with the direct MRI-based methods.

## DEFINITIONS RELATED TO THE TALAIRACH STEREOTAXIC SPACE

For the indirect localization of cortical and subcortical structures, Jean Talairach and colleagues developed a method of stereotaxic localization that is based on precise anatomical landmarks. In the Talairach reference system, three reference lines constitute the basis for the three-dimensional proportional grid system. These three lines are: 1. AC-PC, VAC and the midline:

1. AC-PC line: the reference line passes through the superior edge of the anterior commissure and the posterior edge of the posterior commissure. It follows a path which is parallel to the hypothalamic sulcus, dividing the thalamic from the subthalamic region. The AC-PC line defines the horizontal plane.
2. VAC: this is a vertical line adjacent to the posterior margin of the anterior commissure. This line is the basis of the vertical frontal plane.
3. VPC: this is a vertical line adjacent to the anterior margin of the posterior commissure.
4. Midline: This is the interhemispheric, sagittal plane.

The study of a series of human cadaver hemispheres under formal stereotaxic conditions yielded the concept of the "noyau chirurgical" or surgical nucleus, that portion of the volume of a nucleus possessing the same coordinates in all the hemispheres surveyed. Clearly aware of the importance of stereotaxic neurosurgery for clinical and research, Talairach developed the concept of the "proportional grid system" as the basis of the methodology for the reasoned assembly and comparison of data from successive patients with cerebral hemispheres of individual sizes and proportions.

Distances from these planes and reference points are measured in millimeters. Because of the individuals' variations in height, length and width of human brains, these measurements are only applicable to one individual. This becomes increasingly true with greater distances from the basal lines. For this reason, highly precise millimetric measurements can only be applied to the gray central nuclei.[13,14] To deal with this variability, a three-dimension proportional grid system was created, first proposed in 1967. The three-dimensional proportional grid system takes into consideration the maximal dimensions of the brain in three planes of space and, for this reason, adapting to all brains of all dimensions. This proportional localization system marks off the distances separating the basal lines and the cortical periphery defined by lines through:

The highest point of the parietal cortex.

The most posterior point of the occipital cortex.

The lowest point of the temporal lobe.

The most anterior point of the frontal lobe.

The most lateral point of the parietal-temporal cortex.

The volume defined by these planes are then divided into several different blocks:

Above the AC-PC line in eighths.

Below the AC-PC line in quarters.

Anterior to the VAC line and posterior to VPC line in quarters.

The space between the two perpendiculars erected through the anterior and the posterior commissures is divided into three zones (E1, E2 and E3), and it consistently defines the localization of the motor cortex.

The AC-PC system turned out to be very reliable for deep nuclei and cerebral cortex. Talairach's coworker Gabor Szikla (1928–83) developed a methodology that allowed visualization of the 3D anatomy of the cerebral cortex based on its arterial vasculature. Cortical veins remain at the surface of the cortex and go from gyral crown to gyral crown bridging sulci. On the contrary, the arterial supply dives into sulci creating arterial loops in the sulci (Fig. 2.2).

Based on the atlas of arterial loops in sulci published by Gabor Szikla in 1977, a generation of stereotactic neurosurgeons became able to target specific gyri individually with sub-millimetric precision while avoiding vessels, thanks to stereotactic cerebral angiography.[15] The level of precision and safety of this methodology

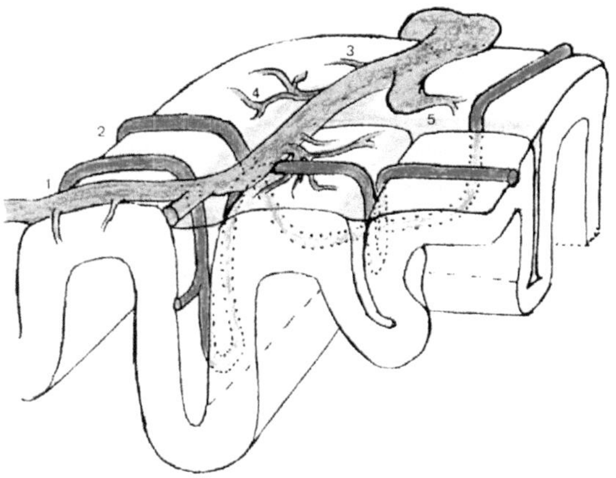


FIG. 2.2 Relationship between veins, arteries and the sulco-gyral 3D relief (Original drawing Jean Régis).

of SEEG implantation, based on in vivo direct visualization of the 3D anatomy of the cerebral cortex long before the CT-scan & MRI era is quite incredible (Fig. 2.3). Then in the 1970's, Talairach, Bancaud and coworkers provided the epilepsy surgery community with a completely new approach of investigation for drug resistant epilepsies.[16]

## THE TALAIRACH STEREOTAXIC SPACE APPLIED TO SEEG METHODOLOGY

The application of the proportional Talairach stereotaxic space provides a normalized method that can be applied across different subjects, allowing statistical studies and group analysis, because each individual case can be reduced to a common scale. For example, in the frontal lobe, the primary somatomotor cortical area (Brodmann area 4) contributes to the formation of the pyramidal tract and is intrinsically connected with areas six and 5, sending efferent fibers to the thalamus, lenticular nucleus, substantial nigra and zona incerta. From an anatomical point of view, area four is located at the depth of the central sulcus and not accessible through the dorsolateral aspect of the hemisphere. From a stereotaxic point of view, area four is almost completely located within the stereotactic space between the VAC and VPC.

Area six is known to be involved in motor functions and extrapyramidal syndromes and it contributes to the corticospinal tract. In the mesial surface, it is located between the VAC and VPC. From an anatomical-functional aspect, this area corresponds to the supplementary motor areas.

Area eight represents a large portion of the frontal eye field for voluntary conjugate movements of the eyes. It is connected by long association bundles with other cortical regions, in particular the occipital lobe, and by projection fibers with the brain stem and the oculomotor nerves. In the dorsal lateral surface area eight is located anterior to the VAC, where the frontal eye fields (FEF) cortical area is located. Areas 9 and 10 belong to the pre-frontal area, mainly connecting with the thalamic dorso-medial nucleus.

### Patterns of SEEG Explorations

After the authors have discussed some anatomical and stereotaxic landmarks associated with SEEG explorations, we will demonstrate how the theoretical parts are applied to the SEEG implantation strategies, particularly focused on anterior temporal exploration based on Talairach stereotaxic coordinates.

To report a schematic and didactic method of implantation, the authors divided the temporal lobe into four anatomical-functional regions. We report only the orthogonally oriented trajectories due to the consistency of implantation and the adequate exploration of the mesial and lateral compartments in the temporal lobe using the Talairach stereotaxic space.

#### *The temporal pole*

In humans, the temporal pole is located ventral to the sylvian fissure, at the rostral tip of the temporal lobe, in the most rostral part of the middle cranial fossa. Rostrally, the temporal pole is in contact with the dura that is adjacent to the sphenoid greater wing. The caudal limits are not well defined, with no clear

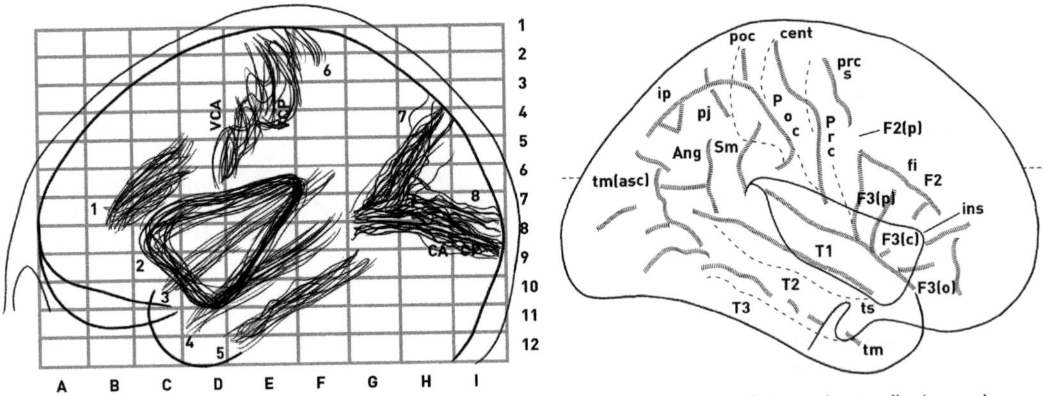


FIG. 2.3 On the left panel, the indirect localization based on the AC-PC based coordinate system demonstrates the remaining variability and the proportionalization in the stereotactic space. On the right panel, the analysis of the arterial loop provides high precision targeting of cortical structures at the individual patient level.

anatomical separation from other portions of the temporal lobe. Its caudal boundary can be arbitrarily defined as the virtual plane defined by the limitans sulcus of the insula, in continuation with the limen insulae.

From a cytoarchitectonic aspect, the temporal pole contains two areas. The most dorsal aspect, in proximity with the Sylvian fissure, was classified as Area 38 by Brodmann in 1909 and as temporopolar area TG by Von Economo and Koskinas in 1929. This area is mostly constituted of agranular cortex, similar to the most ventral and rostral aspects of the insula cortex and the most posterior aspect of the orbitofrontal cortex. From a structural aspect, these areas are highly connected through the uncinate fascicle (Fig. 2.4). From the Talairach coordinates aspect, the temporal pole is located anterior to the VAC and ventral to the AC-PC line, more precisely at the C10 coordinate in the dorsal aspect and D12 in the ventral aspect (Fig. 2.4, panels B and C). The electrode trajectory located in the dorsal aspect of the temporal pole (C10) explores the dorsal lateral and mesial surface (the sylvian surface) of the superior temporal gyrus. Eventually, if vascularity allows, the trajectory can be extended through the sylvian cistern to also explore the most rostral and ventral aspects of the limen insulae, and the more posterior aspect of the orbito-frontal cortex, in the BA25. This trajectory allows the exploration of three different cortical regions (the temporal pole, the limen insulae, and the caudal aspect of the orbito-frontal surface), all corresponding to agranular paralimbic cortex.

## The central core

The central core of the temporal lobe corresponds to Brodmann area 21 in the dorsal lateral aspects. BA 21 is located in the rostral aspect of the middle temporal gyrus, lying posterior to the boundaries of the temporal pole (BA 38) and anterior to BA 37, which lies at the posterior limits of the temporal lobe. Dorsally it is limited by the superior temporal sulcus, a deep and well-defined sulcus, which is mostly an uninterrupted sulcus and extends from the temporal pole to the temporal parietal transition. Ventrally, the middle temporal gyrus is separated from the inferior temporal gyrus by the combination of several small and discontinuous sulci, that, in combination, form the so-called inferior temporal sulcus. The projection of BA 21 into the mesial planes corresponds to the temporal horn of the lateral ventricle, the amygdala and the head of hippocampus, and the anterior and posterior mesial surface of the uncus.

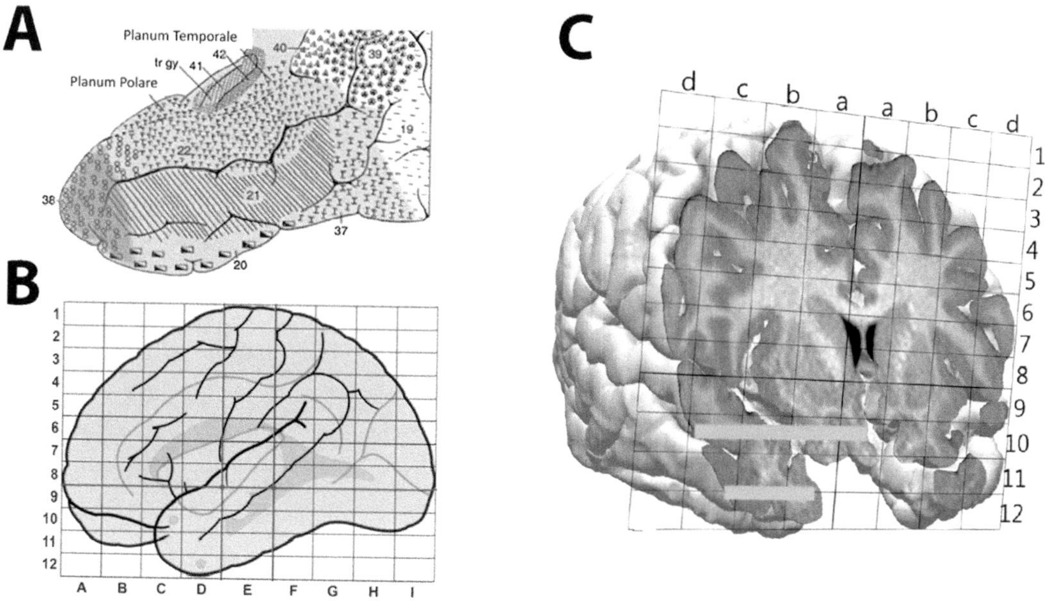


FIG. 2.4 Implantation in the temporal pole compartment. Panel A depicts the different cytoarchitectonic areas that correspond to the temporal neocortical areas, including BA38. Panel B depicts the representation of two orthogonal electrode trajectories (*green dots*) in the Talairach stereotaxic frame. Panel C depicts the representation of the two temporal pole electrode trajectories in relation to the 3D cortical and subcortical anatomy (*green bars*).

From a stereotaxic coordinate perspective, the structures located in the central core of the temporal lobe are located between the VAC and the VPC planes on sagittal orientation, precisely in column E of the Talairach coordinate system. Electrodes implanted in an orthogonal orientation, immediately posterior to VAC, at the most anterior areas of E10, will explore the anterior uncus and the amygdaloid complex in the mesial contacts and the dorsal lateral neocortex (BA 21) in the lateral contacts. In the more lateral contacts, the trajectory trespasses the depths of the rostral aspect of the superior temporal sulcus and the crown of the middle temporal gyrus. The amygdaloid complex is in proximity with VAC, centered approximately at 5 mm posterior or anterior to the vertical line. The anterior uncus is located at the mesial projection of the amygdaloid complex, with the dorsal aspect corresponding to the piriform cortex.

Immediately ventral and posterior to the "amygdala trajectory", at E10, is the so-called hippocampus trajectory. The hippocampus electrodes explore the more caudal aspect of the uncus, transpassing the head of the hippocampus to finally end at the dorso-lateral aspect of the middle temporal gyrus (Broadman area 21). Immediately ventral to the hippocampus trajectory, in the E column, is the anterior basal temporal electrode that will explore the anterior basal parahippocampal area where the entorhinal and perirhinal cortices are located (Brodmann area 28), in the most mesial aspect of the trajectory. More laterally, the trajectory will pass by the anterior fusiform cortex and the basal and lateral aspects of the temporo-occipital sulcus and inferior temporal gyrus (Brodmann area 20) (Fig. 2.5).

In addition to these trajectories, depending on the hypotheses of implantation, the planum polare and temporale of the superior temporal gyrus can be explored with orthogonally oriented electrodes. Here, the trajectories can be extended through the Sylvian fissure to also explore the ventral aspects of the insula cortex, more precisely the anterior and posterior

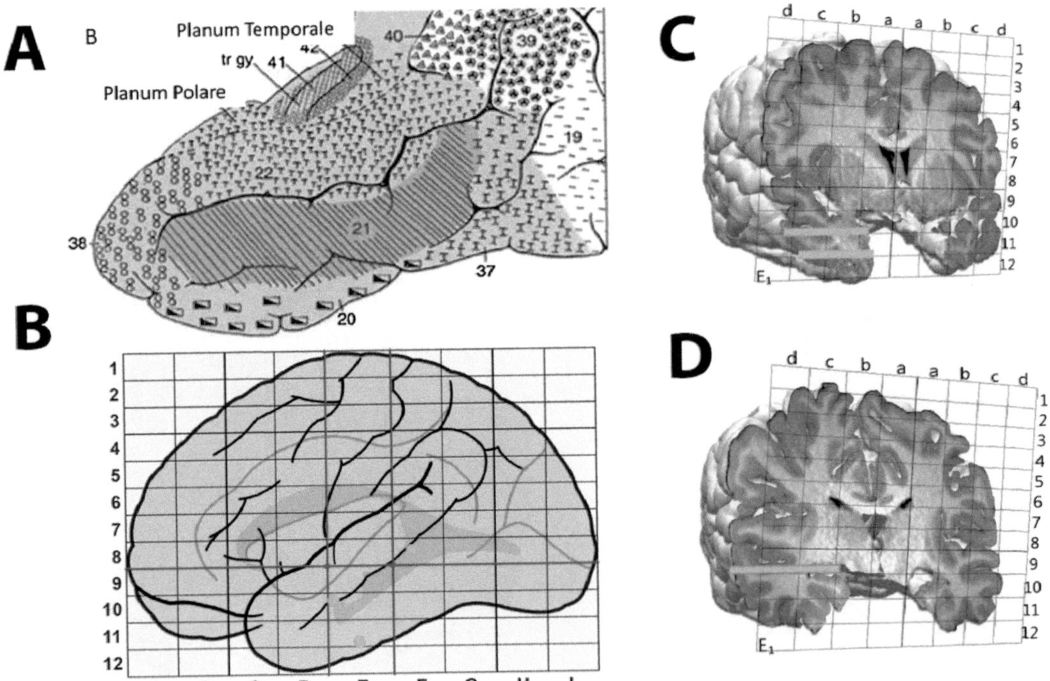


FIG. 2.5 Trajectories sampling the central compartment in the temporal lobe. Panel A depicts the different cytoarchitectonic areas that correspond to the dorsolateral temporal neocortical areas, including BA21 and 20. Panel B depicts the representation of four orthogonal electrode trajectories (*green dots*) in the Talairach stereotaxic frame. Panel C depicts the representation of the two central core trajectories in relation to the 3D cortical and subcortical anatomy, indicating the trajectory aiming to the amygdaloid nucleus and the entorhinal cortex. Panel D depicts the representation of the orthogonal electrode aiming the hippocampal formation.

portions of the posterior long gyrus of the insula. The planum polare trajectory is normally positioned at the D9 coordinate and the planum temporale trajectory is normally positioned at the E7 coordinate.

Lastly, the posterior aspect of the temporal lobe, including the dorsal lateral and basal surfaces, are explored with two electrode trajectories which are both located posterior to the VPC line. The "tail of the hippocampus" trajectory is positioned at the F8 coordinate, exploring from mesial to lateral, the posterior aspect of the parahippocampal gyrus, the tail of the hippocampus, and the depths of the caudal superior temporal sulcus, an important multi-model associative cortex located at the transition between the temporal, parietal, and occipital lobe. The posterior basal temporal trajectory is normally positioned at the F10 coordinate. This electrode trajectory trespasses several important basal temporal cortical and subcortical structures responsible for cognitive and language function related to the ventral stream, such as the basal temporal language area, the face and place recognition areas, in the mid fusiform and posterior parahippocampus gyrus. From mesial to lateral, the trajectory explores the posterior aspect of the collateral fissure, the fusiform gyrus, the occipital-temporal sulcus and finally the more basal and dorso-lateral aspects of the inferior temporal gyrus, almost at the transition with the occipital lobe. Electrodes implanted in this area can be oriented in orthogonal position, always posterior to the VPC line.

## THE CYTOARCHITECTONIC VERSUS THE STRUCTURAL MORPHOLOGY

In the 1980's, neuroscience was giving a lot of value to cellular exploration of the brain functioning but had lost interest for the study of the macroscopic morphological anatomy of the cerebral cortex. At this time, Brodmann cytoarchitectonic maps were the only serious way to "functionally" map the cortex for neuroscientists. However, in the pragmatic neurosurgical field this dogma was poorly operational. First, cytoarchitectonic mapping may be the parcellation of the cortex with the best matching with maps of functional specialization but cytoarchitectonic maps from different anatomists are dramatically different from one to the other (Fig. 2.6).

Second, no imaging modality provides a neurosurgeon with a depiction of the cytoarchitectural mapping of the individual patient he or she is taking care of. Interestingly, with the advent of modern functional brain imaging with PET and functional MRI in the 1990's, a need appeared to identify the location of all these cortical regions of interest, and macro structural anatomy of the cerebral cortex regained interest. Frackowiak developed statistical parametric mapping (SPM) which addressed this issue using Talairach 3D space and largely contributed to popularizing the atlases published by Talairach. [17] Finally, the claim that there is no relationship between sulco-gyral anatomy and "functional mapping" mainly came from groups without access to methods enabling to decrypt the tremendous complexity of the 3D cerebral cortex and properly address this issue.[18–20]

## THE FUNCTIONAL LIMITING VALUE OF THE SULCO-GYRAL ANATOMY

It is of utmost importance during SEEG planning and interpretation to be able to identify anatomo-functionally relevant units that are meaningful in terms of possible homologies with data from the literature or from other patients. However, the 3D complexity of the cerebral cortex in humans is paramount due to one of the highest gyration indexes of all the species. An observation of the cortex from outside demonstrates a large interindividual variability of the traces created by the sulcal limits between gyri (Fig. 2.7).

The atlas from Ono is a comprehensive description of these variations of surface aspects of sulci. [21] Some sulcal structures can be represented depending on the individual by one or two sulci, such as the central sulcus (Fig. 2.8) or by one or up to six like the precentral sulcus, not to mention smaller sulcal structures that are even more variable. The study of the classical depiction of the cerebral cortex anatomy is rapidly leading to the evidence that the classical strategy of labeling sulci and gyri is erroneous and unsuited to describing cortical anatomy with consistency among individuals.

### Stability of the Cortical Sulcifunctional Relationship: The Racoon Homunculus Model

Welker has studied the somatotopy of the sensori-motor cortex of the racoon in conjunction with its sulco-gyral anatomy and its variability between individuals. 22 The sulco-gyral surface drawings are described as different between individuals, sulci being present or absent with six roughly different patterns. The authors observe that the inconstant sulci are always located in between somatotopically distinct areas and that a model integrating all the inconstant sulci fits the different somatotopic segments in all individuals (Fig. 2.9).

### Human Ventral Temporal Cortex Example

Weiner et al. have studied the functional limiting value of the mid-fusiform sulcus, separating the fusiform gyrus into lateral and mesial parts, which plays a pivotal

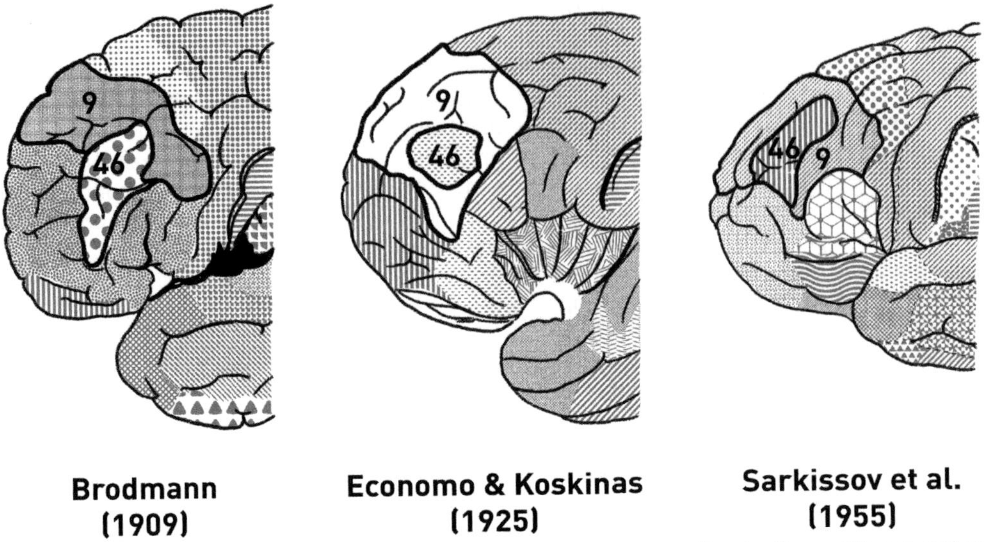


FIG. 2.6 Cytoarchitectonic maps of the left lateral frontal lobe according to three different authors demonstrating very significant differences in the boundaries of these areas.

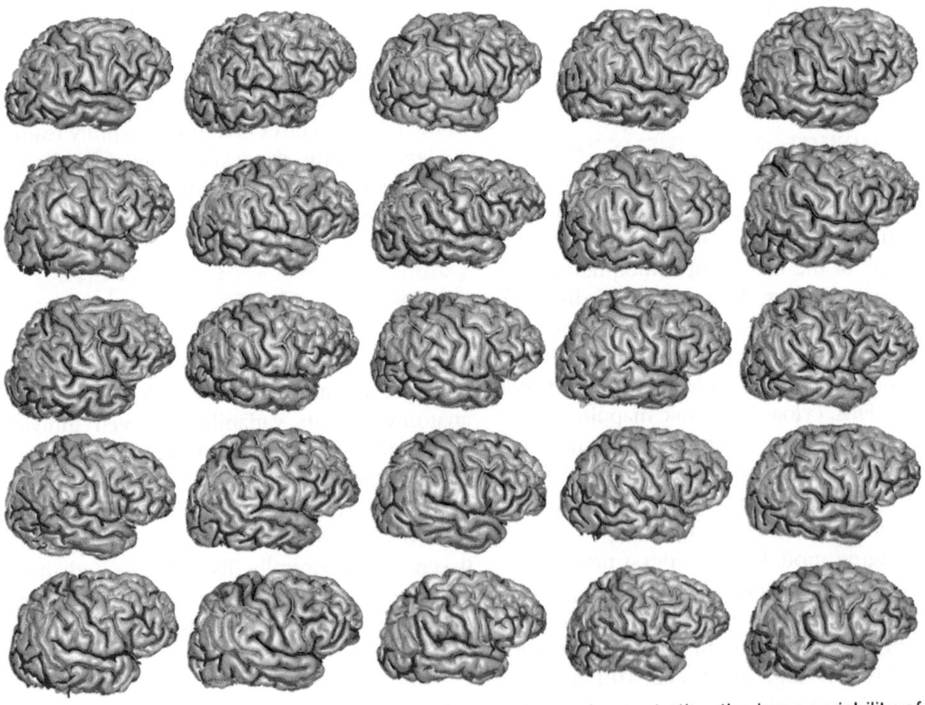

FIG. 2.7 Identification of the main sulci in 25 right hemispheres demonstrating the large variability of the surface aspect.

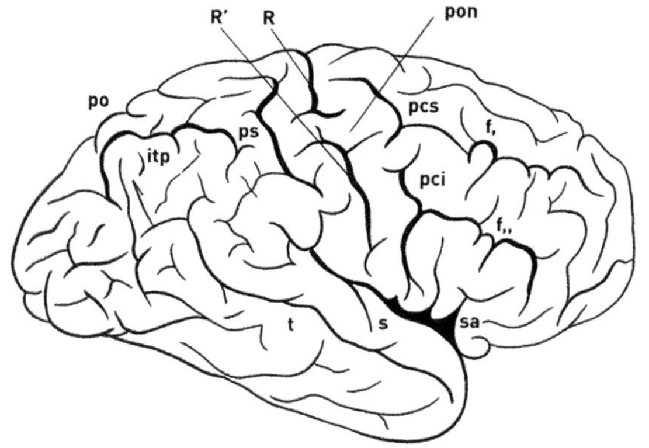


FIG. 2.8 Example of sulci variability. Sernoff's figure describing the postmortem case of a right hemisphere with "2" central sulci.

role in high-level vision.[23] The authors, in a series of 69 subjects, demonstrated that this macroanatomical landmark identifies both cytoarchitectonic and functional divisions of high-level sensory cortex in human. Additionally, they showed that the anterior tip of this sulcus corresponds precisely to the location of a face selective region. This example, among numerous other demonstrations in the modern literature, shows that accurately identified sulci are likely to have a strong functional limiting value.

## Formation of Cortical Foldings

At the beginning of the gyration process (around 6 months) all the normal human in utero cortex has the same surface aspect corresponding to the main sulci (central fissure, calcarine fissure, superior temporal sulcus, inferior frontal sulcus).[24] The sulci visible at this age are what we call the sulcal roots, a term our group coined in 1995.[19] Then, with the ongoing process of expansion of the surface of the cerebral cortex, operculization phenomena appear, with parcels of cortex developing and overlapping the others. Sometimes a complete gyrus can be buried by an operculization process, hiding this gyrus to an external examination of the surface aspect of the cerebral cortex. These gyri are called by Cunningham "Annectant Gyrus" and by Gratiolet "Pli de passage" referring to the white matter included in these buried gyri and enhancing the dual nature of these structures.[20] Such a mechanism of operculization helps to explain the disappearance of the insula from the surface aspect by the development of peri-sylvian opercula. In the end, the final surface aspect from the adult cortex seen from the outside is highly variable in between individuals.

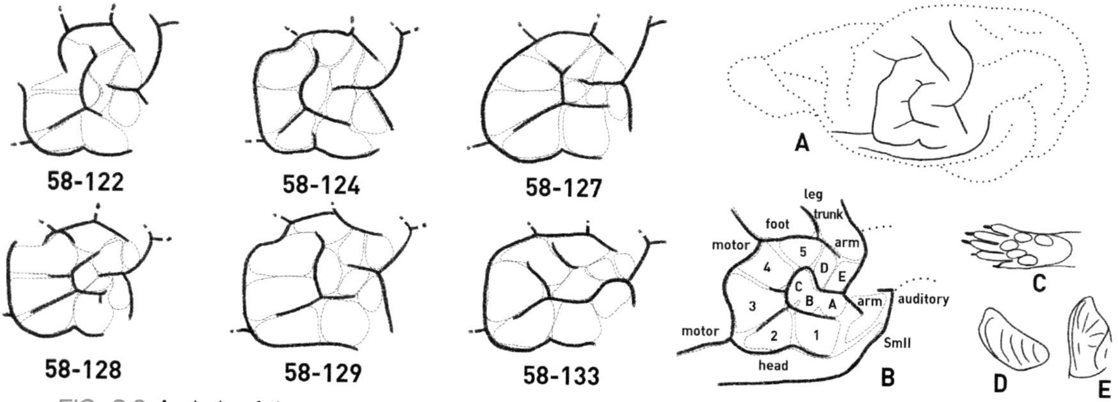


FIG. 2.9 Analysis of the sulco-gyral anatomy of the racoon sensori-motor area investigated by evoked potentials and cortical stimulation demonstrating both the variability of the sulco-gyral patterns and the stability of the relationship between sulcal landmarks and functional maps.

## Depth Versus Surface Sulci Morphological Analyses

Before the beginning of gyration, proto-sulcal and proto-gyral maps already exist. Cells from the embryonic cerebral vesicle themselves carry intrinsic programs from specific cortical regionalization (protomap model # tabula rasa model) according to Pasko Rakic.[25] The cytoarchitectony and connectivity of cortex at the bottom wall and crown of sulci are different and some authors have proposed the tension-based hypothesis[26] suggesting that strongly connected regions will be located on different sides of a gyrus and that sulci may form from region-specific tensions pulling in opposite directions.

In the 1990's, thanks to the development of MRI, powerful computer workstations and the collaboration with the team of Jean François Mangin (expert in morphological mathematics) we have been able to develop a generic model of the development of the cerebral cortex.[20,27–33] Mangin et al. developed methods enabling us to extract from morphological MR 3D objects corresponding to sulci. The pipeline extracts morphological features of each sulcus and its neuronal network compared to those of a cohort of normal subjects. This work shows that sulcal roots corresponding to the deepest part of the main sulci are very stable between individuals and good landmarks for automatic morphological recognition. Then, the best way to make reliable homologies in between cortices from different individuals is to analyze these from their deepest aspects and the poorest approach is to attempt to do it from the surface aspect.

## SULCAL ROOT CONCEPT: A GENERIC MODEL INSTEAD OF A DESCRIPTION OF ENDLESS VARIATIONS

If variations between individuals are structural variations, meaning that some structures exist in some patients but not in others, then a generic model would not be feasible. There are numerous arguments in the literature against structural variability outside of the specific case of congenital malformations. Then the cortical ribbon is supposed to be constituted of a series of structures in a fixed number and relative spatial relationship[34](Fig. 2.10).

### Operational Generic Model of the Human Cerebral Cortex

#### *Application to the cingulate gyrus*

The cingulate gyrus is an important area frequently explored in frontal lobe epilepsies. The surface aspect can be very different between individuals (Fig. 2.11) and between right and left side. In the cingulate gyrus, the distinction between Brodmann areas 24 and 32 is critical because these two areas belong to two different networks, having a very different functional role and connectivity, with area 24 more related to limbic motor manifestations and area 32 related to higher degree of executive motor function. The presence of a marked intracingulate sulcus can create a pseudo-gyrus impression into the mesial wall of the frontal lobe, challenging the distinction between areas 24 (located in proximity with the callosal marginal fissure) and area 32 (located in the vicinity of the cingulate sulcus). However, the superimposition of the sulci with different patterns of surface aspect across different subjects reveals a common structure despite different surface appearances (Fig. 2.11 C–H).

### Developmental Abnormalities Detection

In addition to a better capacity to perform proper homologies, the automatic detection of sulcal roots enables identification of abnormal gyration patterns in epileptic patients, which have been demonstrated to be a frequent marker of the topography of the epileptogenic zone.[35] These abnormal gyration patterns have turned out to be associated with the topography of the epileptogenic zone in a cohort of 12 patients (Fig. 2.12) with frontal lobe epilepsies.[35]

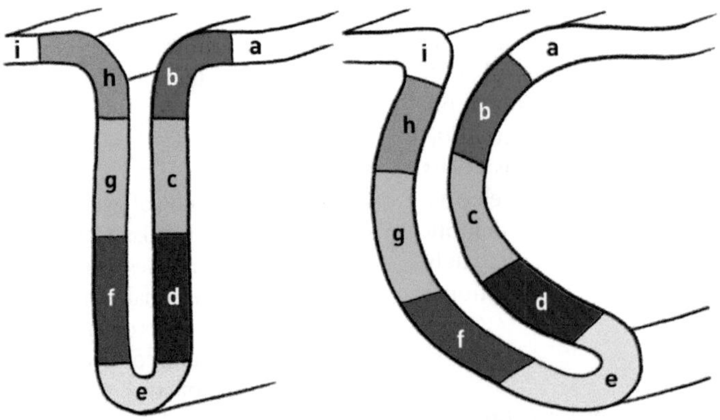


FIG. 2.10 Demonstration of how with a fixed number of maps but a variable representation of these maps in surface dimension, the depth of the sulcus keeps its limiting value when the maps on each side of the sulcal lips are varying.

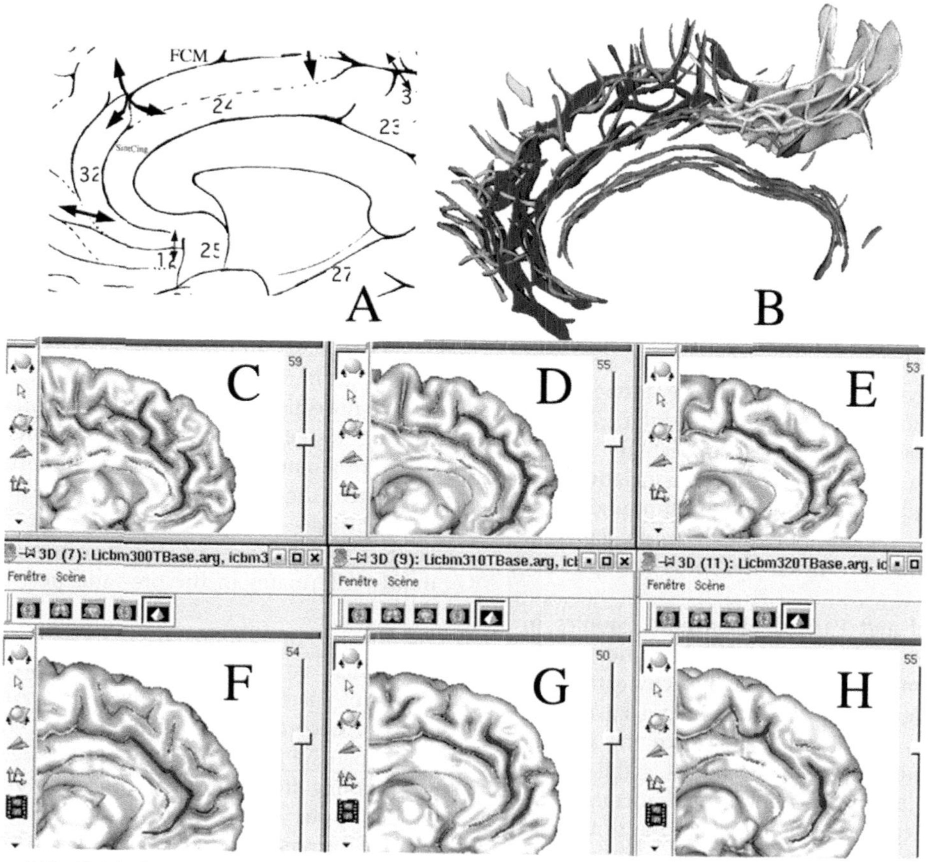


FIG. 2.11 Patterns of cingulate and intra-cingulate sulci, defining Broadman areas 24 and 32.

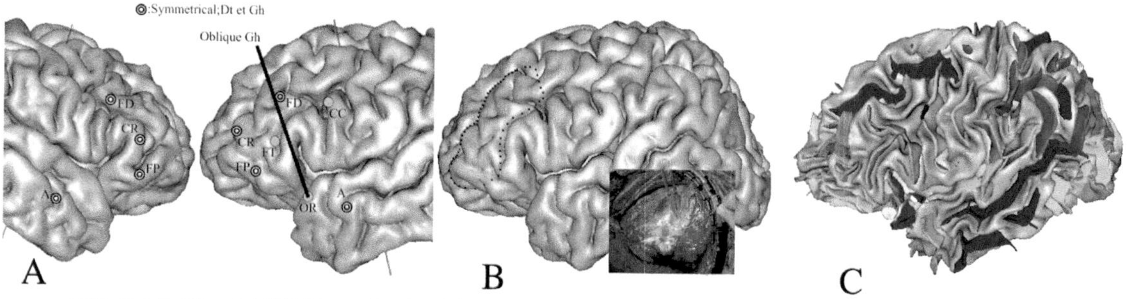


FIG. 2.12 Bifrontal SEEG investigation (A) in young girl with non-lesional severe drug resistant epilepsy. The SEEG demonstrated the organization of the epileptogenic zone around the left intermediate frontal sulcus and the corticectomy led to complete seizure freedom (B). Post processing of the pre-operative MR using "anatomist" pipeline (blindly) showed that only one sulcal structure had a morphological feature outside the normal range, namely the left intermediate frontal sulcus (C).

## THE MERIDIAN PARALLEL GYRAL CONNECTIVITY MODEL

### Structural Connectivity Applied to SEEG

The identification of epileptogenic networks and propagation network is critical in epilepsy explorations. It is likely that white matter connectivity is different from individual to individual and that the pathological network is also likely to be patient specific. The fingerprinting of the individual connectome is still in its infancy.[36–39] It is also rational to propose sulco-gyral recognition based on individual connectome identification and whole brain functional parcellation of the cortex based on individual connectomes.[40]

Levels of gyri connectivity can be intracortical, subcortical, sub-gyral, lobar or capsular. Among neocortical areas, the levels of connectivity can be associated with primary, secondary, associative sensory, motor, multimodal associative or limbic and paralimbic areas. Clearly, all these areas represent different patterns of connectivity. Some examples are as follows:

A. The Frontal and Parietal Operculum: Studies in monkeys have demonstrated that some specific functional maps have specific connectivity favoring specific distant maps. The supramarginal gyrus and Brodmann's area 44 (operculum of the inferior frontal gyrus) have this kind of relationship, frequently leading to record simultaneous intracranial epileptiform activity when one of them is the primary source generator of the activity. On the contrary, the triangular part of the inferior frontal gyrus (BA 45) has a different spectrum of connection with auditory and visual cortices, the somatosensory associative areas, the superior temporal sulcus multimodal areas and paralimbic areas.
B. The Central Sulcus and the Intraparietal Cortex: The principal sulcus and the intraparietal sulcus have been demonstrated in monkeys to have a majority of long-distance connections as opposed to the surrounding areas respectively in the frontal lobe and parietal lobe. The involvement of these structures may account for interlobar distant propagation in some patient seizures. Hence, homologies of these structures within human cortex is not straight forward. The principal sulcus of monkeys corresponds to Brodmann areas 46 and 9/46, which corresponds to the intermediate frontal sulcus in humans.[41] The intraparietal sulcus of monkey separates area five and 7, which are areas separated by the superior postcentral sulcus in humans.
C. The Parietal Operculum with Pre-Motor Cortical Areas: The second most connected area to the secondary somatosensory areas is the pre-motor cortical areas.[42–44] Thus, when the involvement of the parietal operculum in the epileptogenic zone is suspected, it makes sense to discuss adding an electrode in area 4/6.

The identification of epileptogenic networks and propagation network is critical in epilepsy investigation. Archi, paleo, meso and neo-cortices have obviously different status in brain hodology:

A. The archi-cortical and paleo-cortical cortices: According to Petrides and colleagues, isocortical maps originated from two primary primordial structures: the archicortical (hippocampal) and paleocortical (olfactory and insular cortex). Further progression of the two evolutionary trends culminates in the pre- and post-rolandic areas.
B. The Insular fan: From the basal allocortical core of the insula[45] to the sylvian operculum, we observe waves of increasing cytoarchitectonic complexity until an isocortical appearance.
C. The Cingulate fan: At the level of the cingulate gyrus, starting from the indusium griseum (dorsal hippocampus remnant) to the cingulate gyrus, similar waves of increased cytoarchitectonic complexity are observed, ending with an isocortical structure.
D. The neocortical gyral crossing: Consequently, the cortex can be modeled as organized between two limbic poles (the hippocampal and olfactory insular one) with intermediate mesocortical zones of gradual complexity separating the isocortical equator from the limbic pole. The evolutionary cytoarchitectural and modality specific trends are organized according to the meridian axes and the somatotopic trend is organized according to the parallel axes. This schematic simplification has the advantage of enhancing two predominant orthogonal subcortical axes of connectivity likely to be frequently used by contiguity seizure propagation. This level of regional connectivity is to be accounted as complementary to the interlobar specific highways and specific functional connectivity among different Broadman areas (Fig. 2.13).

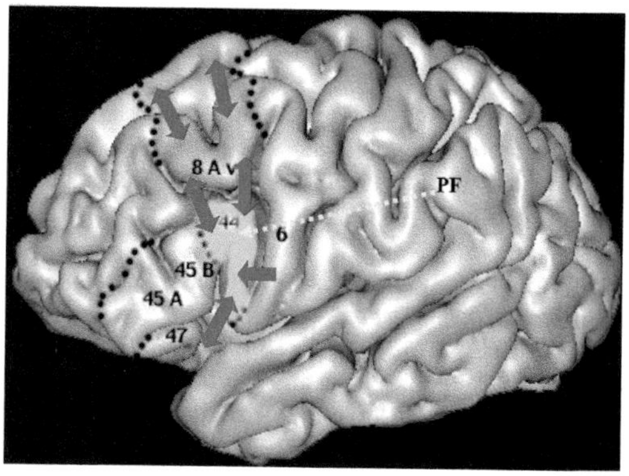


FIG. 2.13 The two levels of organization of connectivity for the left area 44 in orthogonal patterns.

## CONCLUSIONS

In SEEG, the fundamental concepts of stereotaxic cortical and subcortical localization are intrinsically related to the methods associated with Talairach's approach and the distinct utilization of direct and indirect stereotaxic localization methods. An optimal understanding of cortical functional anatomy, structural connectivity, and stereotaxic coordinates is essential to obtain an adequate implantation and SEEG guided resections. The direct method is applied to the intracranial targets, structures and lesions that are visible on MRI. As a complementary method, indirect targeting localization is required in exploring structures from which function cannot be determined by anatomical landmarks. such as, for example, the motor cingulate cortical areas and the entorhinal or perirhinal cortices. Despite significant improvements in imaging modalities, the indirect targeting methods (utilizing the Talairach coordinate system) still play an important role in defining important anatomical-functional structures that are not visible with the direct MRI-based methods. Three-dimensional functional-anatomical knowledge is the most important aspect related to the surgical management of medically refractory epilepsy, SEEG related or not.

## REFERENCES


1. Jastrow J. Localization of function in the cortex of the brain. *Science*. 1886;8:398–399.
2. *Gratiolet: Mémoire sur les plis cérébraux de l'homme et des primates*. 1854. Paris.
3. Cunningham DJ, Horsley V. *Contribution to the Surface Anatomy of the Cerebral Hemispheres*. Dublin: Royal Irish Academy; 1892.
4. Remy C, Contremoulin G. The use of the X-rays for anatomical researches. *Nature*. 1897;1411.
5. Spiegel EA, Wycis HT, Marks M, Lee AJ. Stereotaxic apparatus for operations on the human brain. *Science*. 1947; 106:349–350.
6. Dandy WE. Ventriculography following the injection of air into the cerebral ventricles. *Ann Surg*. 1918;68:5–11.
7. Talairach J, Bancaud J. Lesion, "irritative" zone and epileptogenic focus. *Confin Neurol*. 1966;27:91–94.
8. Talairach J, Szikla G. Application of stereotactic concepts to the surgery of epilepsy. *Acta Neurochir Suppl*. 1980;30:35–54.
9. Talairach J, Bancaud J, Bonis A, Tournoux P, Szikla G, Morel P. [Functional stereotaxic investigations in epilepsy. Methodological remarks concerning a case]. *Rev Neurol (Paris)*. 1961;105:119–130.
10. Talairach J, Szikla G, Bonis A, Tournoux P, Bancaud J, Mempel E. Functional stereotaxic exploration of epilepsy. *Presse Med*. 1962;70:1399–1402. contd.
11. Talairach J, Szikla G, Tournoux P, Prosalentis A, Bordas-Ferrier M. *Atlas d'Anatomie Stéréotaxique du Télencéphale*. Paris: Masson; 1967.
12. Talairach J, Tournoux P. *Co-planar Stereotaxic Atlas of the Human Brain*. New York: Thieme medical; 1988.
13. Talairach J. *Atlas d'anatomie stéréotaxique: repérage radiologique indirect des noyaux gris centraux des régions mésencéphalo-sous-optique et hypothalamique de l'homme*. 1957 **(No Title)**.
14. Talairach J, David M, Tournoux P, Corredor H, Kvasina T, Atlas d'Anatomie Stéréotaxique. *Repérage Radiologique indirect des Noyaux Gris Centraux des Régions Mésencephalosousoptique et Hypothalamique de l'Homme*. Paris: Masson & Cie; 1957.
15. Szikla G, Bouvier G, Hori T, Petrov V. *Angiography of the Human Brain Cortex*. Springer-Verlag; 1977.
16. Talairach J, Bancaud J, Szikla G, Bonis A, Geler S, Vedrenne C. Approche nouvelle de la neurochirurgie de l'epilepsie. Méthodologie stéréotaxique et résultats thérapeutiques. *Neurochirurgie*. 1974;20:92–98.
17. Friston KJ, Frith CD, Liddle PF, Frackowiak RS. Comparing functional (PET) images: the assessment of significant change. *J Cereb Blood Flow Metab*. 1991;11:690–699.
18. Régis J. Anatomie sulcale profonde et cartographie fonctionnelle du cortex cérébral. In: *Marseille: Université D'Aix Marseille II*. 1994:272.
19. Regis J, Mangin JF, Frouin V, Sastre F, Peragut JC, Samson Y. Generic model for the localization of the cerebral cortex and preoperative multimodal integration in epilepsy surgery. *Stereotact Funct Neurosurg*. 1995;65:72–80.
20. Regis J, Mangin JF, Ochiai T, et al. Sulcal root generic model: a hypothesis to overcome the variability of the human cortex folding patterns. *Neurol Med -Chir*. 2005;45: 1–17.
21. Ono M, Kubik S, Abernathey C. *Atlas of the Cerebral Sulci*. Stuttgart: georg Thieme Verlag; 1990.
22. Welker WI, Seidenstein S. Somatic sensory representation in the cerebral cortex of the raccoon. *J.Comp.Neurol*. 1959;111:469–501.

23. Weiner KS, Golarai G, Caspers J, et al. The mid-fusiform sulcus: a landmark identifying both cytoarchitectonic and functional divisions of human ventral temporal cortex. *Neuroimage*. 2014;84:453–465.
24. Studholme C, Rousseau F. Quantifying and modelling tissue maturation in the living human fetal brain. *Int J Dev Neurosci*. 2014;32:3–10.
25. Rakic P. Neurobiology. Neurocreationism–making new cortical maps. *Science*. 2001;294:1011–1012.
26. Van Essen DC. A tension-based theory of morphogenesis and compact wiring in the central nervous system. *Nature*. 1997;385:313–318.
27. Cachia A, Mangin JF, Riviere D, et al. A generic framework for the parcellation of the cortical surface into gyri using geodesic Voronoi diagrams. *Med Image Anal*. 2003;7: 403–416.
28. Mangin J, Frouin V, Bloch I, Regis J, Samson Y, Lopez-Krahe J. 3D visualization of the cortical sulcal topography. In: *8th Conf. On Computer Assisted Radiology*. Winston Salem; 1994:179–184.
29. Mangin J, Frouin V, Regis J, Bloch I, Belin P, Samson Y. Towards better management of cortical anatomy in multimodal multi-individual brain studies. *Phys Med*. 1996; 12-S1:103–107.
30. Mangin J, Régis J, Bloch I, Frouin V, Samson Y, Lopez-Krahe J. A Markovian random field based random graph modelling the human cortical topography. *CVR Med'95 905 of LNCS*. 1995:177–183.
31. Mangin JF, Riviere D, Cachia A, et al. A framework to study the cortical folding patterns. *Neuroimage*. 2004;23(Suppl 1):S129–S138.
32. Ochiai T, Grimault S, Scavarda D, et al. Sulcal pattern and morphology of the superior temporal sulcus. *Neuroimage*. 2004;22:706–719.
33. Riviere D, Mangin JF, Papadopoulos-Orfanos D, Martinez JM, Frouin V, Regis J. Automatic recognition of cortical sulci of the human brain using a congregation of neural networks. *Med Image Anal*. 2002;6:77–92.
34. Bartolomei F, Khalil M, Wendling F, et al. Sulcal root generic model: a hypothesis to overcome the variability of the human cortex folding patterns. *Epilepsia*. 2005;46: 677–687. https://doi.org/10.1111/j.1528-1167.2005.43804.x.
35. Régis J, Tamura M, Park MC, et al. Subclinical abnormal gyration pattern, a potential anatomic marker of epileptogenic zone in patients with magnetic resonance imaging-negative frontal lobe epilepsy. *Neurosurgery*. 2011;69: 80–93. discussion 93-84.
36. Jirsa VK. Connectivity and dynamics of neural information processing. *Neuroinformatics*. 2004;2:183–204. https://doi.org/10.1385/NI:1382:1382:1183.
37. Jirsa VK, Proix T, Perdikis D, et al. The Virtual Epileptic Patient: individualized whole-brain models of epilepsy spread. *Neuroimage*. 2017;145:377–388.
38. Jirsa VK, Sporns O, Breakspear M, Deco G, McIntosh AR. Towards the virtual brain: network modeling of the intact and the damaged brain. *Arch Ital Biol*. 2010;148:189–205.
39. Poupon C, Clark CA, Frouin V, et al. Regularization of diffusion-based direction maps for the tracking of brain white matter fascicles. *Neuroimage*. 2000;12:184–195.
40. Huang H, Vasung L. Gaining insight of fetal brain development with diffusion MRI and histology. *Int J Dev Neurosci*. 2014;32:11–22.
41. Petrides M, Pandya DN. Comparative architectonic analysis of the human and the macaque frontal cortex. In: FBaJ G, ed. *Handbook of Neuropsychology*. Vol 9. Elsevier science; 1994:17–58.
42. Burton H, Carlson M. Second somatic sensory cortical area (SII) in a prosimian primate, Galago crassicaudatus. *J Comp Neurol*. 1986;247:200–220.
43. Donoghue JP, Parham C. Afferent connections of the lateral agranular field of the rat motor cortex. *J Comp Neurol*. 1983;217:390–404.
44. Kawamura K, Otani K. Corticocortical fiber connections in the cat cerebrum: the frontal region. *J Comp Neurol*. 1970; 139:423–448.
45. Mesulam MM, Mufson EJ. Insula of the old world monkey. I. Architectonics in the insulo-orbito-temporal component of the paralimbic brain. *J Comp Neurol*. 1982;212:38–52.

CHAPTER 3

# The Stereotactic Technique in the SEEG Method

JORGE ÁLVARO GONZÁLEZ-MARTÍNEZ, MD, PHD

## INTRODUCTION

*SEEG is a stereotaxic method that embraces a stereotactic technique*

In the SEEG method, as the main goal is to acquire precise anatomical localization of inter-ictal and ictal activities, and to provide reliable seizure electro-clinical correlations, effort should be concentrated on time and space resolution of seizure analyses. A precise SEEG stereotactic technique is essential to accomplish a successful evaluation.[1–9]

An important step in the SEEG method is to define a strategy for electrode placement. The electrode implantation must be designed to question specific hypotheses of localization, as well as checking functional constraints and definition of surgical resection boundaries. The electrode implantation plan will depend on four data categories that better characterize the patient's epileptic seizures[10–12]:

- Ictal data: video-EEG recording of seizures with analysis of electro-clinical correlations, completed by an early injection ictal SPECT, whenever possible.
- Interictal data: interictal electromagnetic activity from video-EEG and MEG or high-resolution EEG; PET; neuropsychological and neurological assessment.
- Structural/morphological data: high resolution and technically adequate MRI (T1 and FLAIR images, reformatted in three different orientations) with image processing when available.
- Functional data provided by Wada test and fMRI and MEG studies

A basic principle in the formulation of hypotheses is to maintain independence for each category while deliberating about localization and extension of the hypothetical EZ. The independence among categories will circumvent inherited bias associated with the non-invasive methods. As a practical example, not all the MRI identifiable lesions are equivalent in terms of epileptogenicity and their relevance in the hypothesis build up are very variable. In a case of a lesion suggestive of focal cortical dysplasia whose location on MRI is discordant from seizure semiology, the question directed to SEEG could be about epileptogenicity of the MRI visible lesion and its spatial limits, and the hypotheses being about possible different sizes of EZ. In other types of malformations (like polymicrogyria or nodular heterotopia) the question could be if part of the lesion(s) if any is (are) epileptogenic or contributory to the organization of the seizure patterns. In non-developmental vascular, degenerative lesions or traumatic lesions, as encephalomalacia or hippocampal sclerosis, which epileptogenic networks are the consequence of the lesion(s) (if any) or still related to it. In MRI-negative epilepsies, implantation will mainly rely upon electro-clinical data. Careful and undogmatic attention must be exercise regarding subtle lesions with unclear or incomplete imaging features, as the so-called "pseudo-lesions": normal variants or illusions caused by poor segmentation or low MRI quality that create false MRI interpretations, which can generate erroneous implantation plans and suboptimal guided resections.[10] MRI visible lesions that are not epileptogenic or are related to parts of the epileptogenic zone are perhaps one of the main causes of failure epilepsy surgery.

This chapter is intended to provide guidance and suggestions regarding the technical aspects of the SEEG method. As in any aspect related to SEEG, individual nuances must be considered and carefully incorporated into the SEEG plan. No guidance and suggestions are absolute.

The Fundamentals of Stereoelectroencephalography. https://doi.org/10.1016/B978-0-443-10877-8.00002-4

## PLANNING ELECTRODE IMPLANTATIONS USING ELECTROCLINICAL CORRELATIONS

*The implantation plan starts with careful and weighted interpretation of non-invasive data. Not all non-invasive data has the same weight when formulating the hypothesis of implantation*

As a general principle, SEEG implantations are design to target key areas of the hypothetical epileptic network, taking into account the cortical volume to be covered. A highly restricted focal implantation will be inefficient and likely excessive because signal information derived from electrodes located in the same gyrus will be roughly similar. Consequently, the (surgical) boundaries of epileptogenic regions are impossible to delineate (because the temporo-spatial ictal dynamics would be impossible to decipher) if some electrodes were not placed remotely in "non-epileptogenic" regions.

Two other important aspects will guide appropriate SEEG implantations: (i) functional "mapping" and (ii) "sentinel" electrodes, to help defining corticectomy limits. The SEEG implantation must be designed to localize the epileptogenic zone, but also to provide the anatomical boundaries of the possible resection.[2–4] The extent of the epileptogenic zone and the interface with possible eloquent cortical areas are equally important goals for the SEEG explorations. For example, in the above cases, if the hypothetical temporal-perisylvian epilepsy is in the dominant hemisphere, some electrodes will be added at the periphery of the core hypothesis electrodes, that is, in the posterior superior temporal and supra-marginal gyri as well as in the posterior inferior frontal gyrus on the one hand, in the anterior and mid-cingulate gyrus on the other hand.

Expressing hypotheses for designing the implantation is a critical step in SEEG method. The main hypothesis of localization must be falsifiable by the others of lower order and vice-versa. The process requires the generation of alternatives hypotheses, making clear in anatomical terms, the diverse interpretations of the multimodal data collected during phase I. Not only the electro-clinical data, but also the imaging and neuropsychological data will be included in the discussion. The optimal way to organize it is to sort out data by their specific place in the epileptogenic process. Therefore, electro-clinical data allied with ictal SPECT depict the ictal state/network whereas EEG/MEG and PET the inter-ictal state, and MRI, EEG and PET the lesional area. So, the hypotheses do not only infer the possible ictal networks but also their relations with MRI or PET images as well. Therefore, electrode implantation implements the whole hypothetical framework in stereotaxic space.

## THE STEREOTACTIC SPACE DEFINED BY TALAIRACH

*The indirect targeting, informed by a pre-defined stereotactic space coordinate system, supplements the direct targeting, which is provided by MR images. Both are complementary and necessary*

Over the years, several brain stereotactic coordinate spaces were developed and applied in different scientific and clinic scenarios. Historically, the Talairach coordinate system has been applied in the SEEG method since the method's inception in the late 50's.[7,13,14]

In the process of designing the plan for a SEEG implantation, the formulation of the implantation hypotheses is translated to an anatomical stereotactic space. This step is extremely important because corresponds to the first stage in the transition between the theoretical phase to the surgical application of the principles of SEEG and generated hypotheses. In this "transition period," a universal and equally understood communication path between surgeons and epileptologists takes place. The stereotactic space, which is defined by stereotactic coordinates, corresponds to the communication path, or the "common language," in this phase of the SEEG planning, translating the electro-clinical correlations to the stereotaxic space. Equally important, the "common language" provided by the stereotaxic space concept allows a direct comparison across subjects, of patterns of intracortical electrical recordings and structural and functional connectivity. Such comparative analysis improves basic knowledge and concepts of neurobiology that will be apply in several neuroscience subfields.

On an individual basis, despite great progression in medical imaging techniques, they still lack adequate localization of functional cortical areas. Sulci and gyri are clearly identified in modern MRI but accurate identification of key anatomo-functional features are rarely achieved without a system of reference. A combination of direct visualization of structures with indirect localization that is based on a reference system is likely the most adequate method to understand and guide the SEEG implantations and its related guided resections.

The three-dimensional proportional system designed by Talairach and colleagues allows for a practical and precise exploration of key cortical structures.[15] At first impression, cerebral sulci and gyri are so variable across individuals that they would be unfit for any possibility of common localization based on universal reference points. However, there are major lines of cortical enfolding that provide the cortex its most general morphology and permits the collection of so-called "normalized" data.

Three reference lines constitute the basis of the Talairach three-dimensional proportional grid system: the AC/PC, the VAC, the VPC and midline:

1. *The AC-PC line:* The line passes through the superior edge of the anterior commissure and the inferior edge of the posterior commissure. It follows a path essentially parallel to the hypothalamic sulcus, separating the thalamic from the subthalamic region.
2. *The VAC (vertical AC) line:* The line is passing through the posterior/ventricular margin of the anterior commissure, orthogonal to the AC-PC plane.
3. *The VPC (vertical PC) line:* The line is passing through the anterior/ventricular margin of the posterior commissure, orthogonal to the AC-PC plane.
4. *The midline:* This is the midline interhemispheric sagittal plane

Because of individual variations in heights, length and width of human brains, these measurements, measure in millimeters, are only applicable to one individual. This become more evident in anatomical areas that are distant from the AC-PC line. Consequently, in order to overcome the limitation, a proportional system is applied. The three-dimensional proportional system is established according to the maximal dimensions of the brain in the three planes of space. The system adapts to brains of all dimensions. The proportional localization system marks off the distances separating the basal lines and the more peripheral cortical areas by the definition of limiting planes, which are defined by the following points of reference.

1. The highest points in the parietal lobes.
2. The most posterior point of the occipital cortex
3. The lowest point of the temporal lobe
4. The most anterior point of the frontal cortex
5. The most lateral point of the parietal-temporal cortex.

The total volume is then divided by horizontal lines, above the AC-PC, in eights, below AC-PC in quarters, anterior to VAC is quarters and posterior to VPC in quarters.

The proportional grid system allows the localization of cortical and subcortical structures with relative precision in all three stereotaxic planes (Fig. 3.1).

## SEEG IMPLANTATION PATTERNS

*The hypothesis of implantation is primordial*

As discussed above, the hypotheses are typically generated during a multidisciplinary patient management conference based on the results of non-invasive tests and the appropriate interpretation of these results. It is important to consider that the SEEG exploration has as the primordial goal, the anatomical localization of the epileptogenic zone, but also its anatomical limits and interface with potential eloquent areas. With this premise in mind, SEEG depth electrodes should sample the anatomical lesion (if identified) and surrounding tissue, the more likely structure(s) of ictal onset, the early and late spread regions, and the possible functional networks (cognitive, sensorial-motor, language, visual, etc) involved in seizure semiology or in the hypothetical surgical resection plan.[16–18]

A three dimensional "conceptualization" of the network is an essential component of the pre-surgical implantation strategy.[12] The conceptualization will consider the three-dimensional aspects of depth electrode recordings, which despite a limited contact size (which is largely compensated by the interpolation process made possible by the electrophysiological methodology: frequencies, spatial and temporal analyses), enable an accurate sampling of the structures along its trajectory, from the entry site to the final impact point. Importantly, the trajectory of the SEEG electrodes is equally important than the target or entry point areas. Consequently, the investigation may include lateral and mesial surfaces of the different lobes, deep-seated cortices as the depths of sulci, insula, posterior areas in the inter-hemispheric cortical surface, etc. The implantation should also consider the different cortical cytoarchitectonic areas involved in seizure organization patterns and their likely connectivity to other cortical and subcortical areas. It is important to emphasize that the implantation strategy is not to map lobes or lobules, but epileptogenic networks, which may involve cortical structures localized in multiple lobes. Furthermore, the exploration should take into consideration possible alternative hypotheses of localization.[8,19,20]

*Excessive number of electrodes must be avoided*

The aim to obtain all the possible information from the SEEG exploration should not be pursued at the expense of an excessive number of electrodes, which will likely increase the morbidity of the implantation. In general, implantations that exceed 15 depth electrodes are rare and the requirement of excessive number of electrodes may indicate a not so well formulated pre-implantation hypothesis framework. In addition, the possible involvement of "eloquent" regions in the ictal discharge requires their judicious coverage, with the two-fold goal to assess their role in the seizure organization and to define the boundaries of a safe surgical resection.

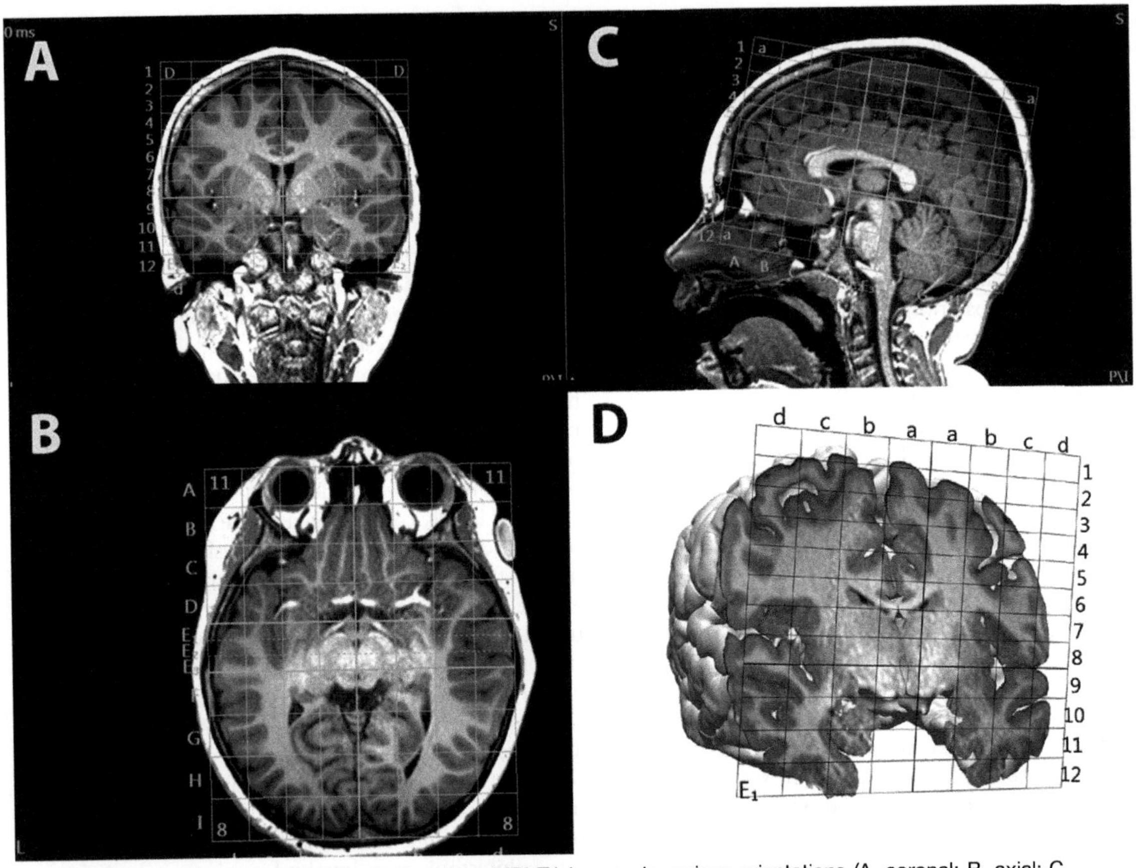


FIG. 3.1 The Talairach stereotactic space. MRI T1 images in various orientations (A, coronal; B, axial; C, sagittal) with the interpolation of the Talairach grid stereotactic grid system. Panel D depicts the 3D MRI T1 digital reconstruction within the stereotactic space.

The SEEG implantation patterns are based on a tailored strategy of exploration. In consequence, standard implantations for specific areas and lobes are difficult to conceptualize since SEEG evaluations are individualized, varying from patient to patient. Consequently, patterns of standard SEEG coverage should be applied with extreme caution and reservation. Nevertheless, a few "typical" patterns of coverage are observed.

1. *Temporal/Limbic explorations.* Cases of temporal lobe epilepsy with consistent anatomo-electro-clinical findings suggesting a mesial temporal/limbic network involvement can be operated on after non-invasive investigation only. In general, the use of invasive monitoring is not necessary when semiological and electrophysiological studies demonstrate typical non-dominant mesial temporal epilepsy and imaging studies demonstrate an undisputable MRI lesion (mesial temporal sclerosis, as an example) that fits the initial localization hypothesis. Nevertheless, extra-operative invasive exploration with SEEG recordings may be required in patients in whom the hypothetical EZs are suspected to involve extra-temporal areas as well, where there is a question regarding the limits of the EZ, laterality is unclear, and when there is a potential interface with functional cortical areas, as posterior primary language areas or memory supportive areas in dominant mesial temporal structures. In these scenarios, the implantation pattern points to disclose a preferential spread of the discharge to the temporo-insular-anterior perisylvian areas, the temporo-insular-orbitofrontal areas, or the posterior temporal, posterior insula, temporo-basal, parietal and posterior cingulate areas. Consequently, sampling of extra-temporal limbic areas must be wide enough to provide information to identify a possible extra-temporal origin of the seizures that could not been anticipated with precision according to non-invasive methods of investigation (Fig. 3.2A)

2. *Perisylvian explorations:* they are very common, in general involving multiple lobes around the anterior perisylvian (frontal, insula and temporal lobes) and the posterior perisylvian areas (Rostral Parietal, insula and caudal temporal areas). The explorations are typically organized, according to the electro-clinical correlations, in onion-ring fashion, centered around the limen insulae, following the patterns of cortical organization, as described by Mesulam and colleagues (REF). The electrodes are in general implanted in orthogonal orientation, in order to sample the multiple architectonic areas involving the opercular and insular regions (Fig. 3.2B).
3. *Frontal-parietal networks explorations:* Due to the large volume of the frontal and parietal lobes, and the complexity of their bidirectional connections, a higher number of electrodes are frequently required for an adequate coverage of this region. In most patients, however, excessive sampling can be avoided, and the implantation to more limited portions of the frontal and parietal lobes can be performed. This can be accomplished by a careful formulation of the pre-implantation hypotheses. The suspicion of orbito-frontal epilepsy, for instance, often requires the investigation of gyrus rectus, the frontal polar areas, the anterior cingulate gyrus and the anterior portions of the temporal lobe (temporal pole). Similarly, seizures that are thought to arise from the mesial surface of the pre-motor cortex are evaluated by targeting at least the rostral and caudal part of the supplementary motor area (SMA), the pre-SMA area, different portions of the cingulate gyrus and sulcus, as well as the primary motor cortex and mesial and dorsal-lateral aspects of the parietal lobe. Consequently, the hypothesis-based sampling often allows localization of the EZ in the frontal and/or parietal lobes, and in some cases may allow the identification of relatively small EZs. Eventually, frontal-parietal network explorations may be bilateral, and sometimes symmetrical, mainly when a mesial frontal-parietal epilepsy is suspected, and the non-invasive methods of investigation failed in lateralizing the epileptogenic process (Fig. 3.2C).

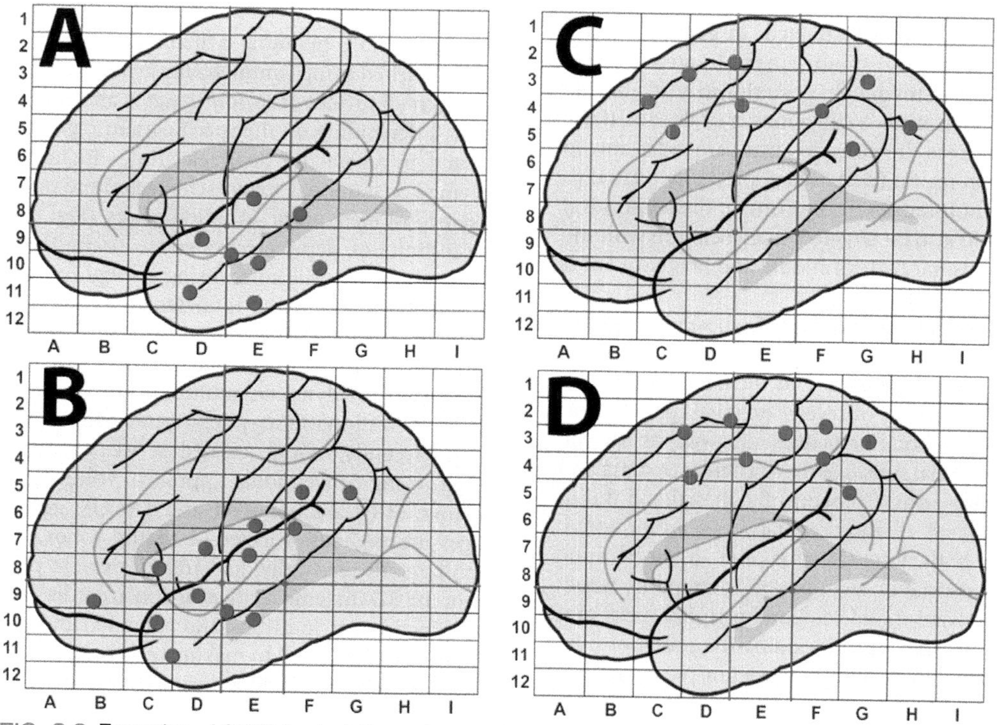


FIG. 3.2 Examples of SEEG implantation schemes. Red dots represent orthogonally planned electrodes, sampling a specific cerebral volume, from dorsal lateral to mesial surfaces. Panel A depicts an example of a temporal-limbic exploration. Panel B depicts an anterior and posterior perisylvian SEEG exploration. Panel C depicts a frontal-parietal exploration. Panel D depicts a Rolandic and perirolandic exploration.

4. *Rolandic and Peri-Rolandic Explorations:* Electrodes in rolandic and peri-rolandic regions are normally placed when there is a need to define the posterior margin of the resection in frontal explorations or the anterior margin in parietal-occipital explorations, or when the EZ may be located in or near rolandic cortex. The main goal here is to evaluate the rolandic participation to the ictal discharge and to obtain a functional mapping by intracerebral electrical stimulation. In this location, depth electrodes are particularly helpful to sample the depth of the central sulcus, as well as the descending and ascending white matter fibers associated with this region. Also, in many instances, it would be important to explore the immediate adjacent frontal and parietal cortical areas in close anatomical and functional association with the rolandic cortex, as the most caudal portions of the superior frontal gyrus, the pre-central sulcus, the caudal portions of the superior frontal gyrus, the post-central sulcus and the most rostral portions of the superior parietal lobule. In addition, the most central aspect of the cingulate gyrus and sulcus (most possible localization of the cingulate motor areas) should also be targeted. In general, in stereotactic terms, the motor cingulate area is likely located just immediately posterior to VAC, but its precise localization is still a matter of debate. If the rolandic areas in consideration are adjacent to the Sylvian region (perisylvian, probably related to the face motor and sensory cortex), the sub-central gyri should also be targeted, in association with the adjacent insular cortex (middle and posterior short insular gyri) (Fig. 3.2D).
5. *Occipital-parietal explorations:* In the posterior regions, placement of electrodes limited to a single lobe is extremely uncommon, due to the frequent simultaneous involvement of several occipital, parietal and posterior temporal structures, as well as to the multidirectional spread of the discharges to supra and infra-sylvian areas. Consequently, mesial and dorsal lateral surfaces of the occipital lobes are explored, covering both infra-calcarine and supra-calcarine areas, in association with posterior temporal, posterior perisylvian, basal temporal-occipital areas and posterior parietal areas including the posterior inferior parietal lobule and the posterior pre-cuneus. In posterior epilepsies, bilateral explorations are generally needed due to rapid contralateral spread of ictal activity. In addition, in many circumstances, the caudal aspect of the frontal lobe (dorsal-lateral and mesial regions) is also explored with "sentinel" electrodes.

## Stereotactic Image Acquisition and The Stereotactic "Repérage"

*The 'repérage,' or spotting, is the last phase before the surgical step of implanting the SEEG electrodes*

By applying an imaging software, the multiplanar MR imaging (volumetric T1, thin cuts—1 mm, and no gaps) are digitally fused with vascular imaging modalities, which may include a CTA and CTV or a stereotactic angiogram. Once the images are digitally fused, the AC-PC points are selected, and the images are reformatted accordingly. With this task, the AC-PC plane, and the correspondent VAC and VPC are defined and the Talairach coordinate grid is digitally projected to the patient's anatomical and vascular images. Additional datasets, such as PET and MEG images can be loaded to the software, allowing multiple imaging fusion for SEEG electrode planning. The stereotactic reperage is usually performed before the implantation, in general the day before (Fig. 3.3).

## SEEG Implantations: Technical Nuances

*Stereotactic accuracy is primordial for the SEEG safety and efficacy*

Once the SEEG planning is finalized, the desired targets are reached using commercially available intracerebral depth electrodes of various lengths and number of contacts, depending on the specific brain regions to be explored. In general, the depth electrodes are implanted applying conventional stereotactic technique or by the assistance of stereotactic robotic devices (Fig. 3.4). In both techniques, depth electrodes are inserted through 2.5 mm diameter drill holes, using orthogonal or oblique orientation, allowing intracranial recording from lateral, intermediate or deep cortical and subcortical structures in a three-dimensional arrangement, thus accounting for the dynamic, multidirectional spatiotemporal organization of the epileptogenic pathways.[6,17,18]

More recently, robotic assisted devices were applied. Similar to the conventional approach, volumetric preoperative MRIs are obtained and DICOM formatted images are digitally transferred to the robot's native planning software. Individual trajectories are planned within the 3D imaging reconstruction according to predetermined target locations and intended trajectories. Trajectories are selected to maximize sampling from superficial and deep cortical and subcortical areas within the pre-selected zones of interest and are oriented orthogonally in the majority of cases to facilitate the anatomo-electrophysiological correlation during the extra-operative recording phase and to avoid possible trajectories shifts due to excessive angled entry points.

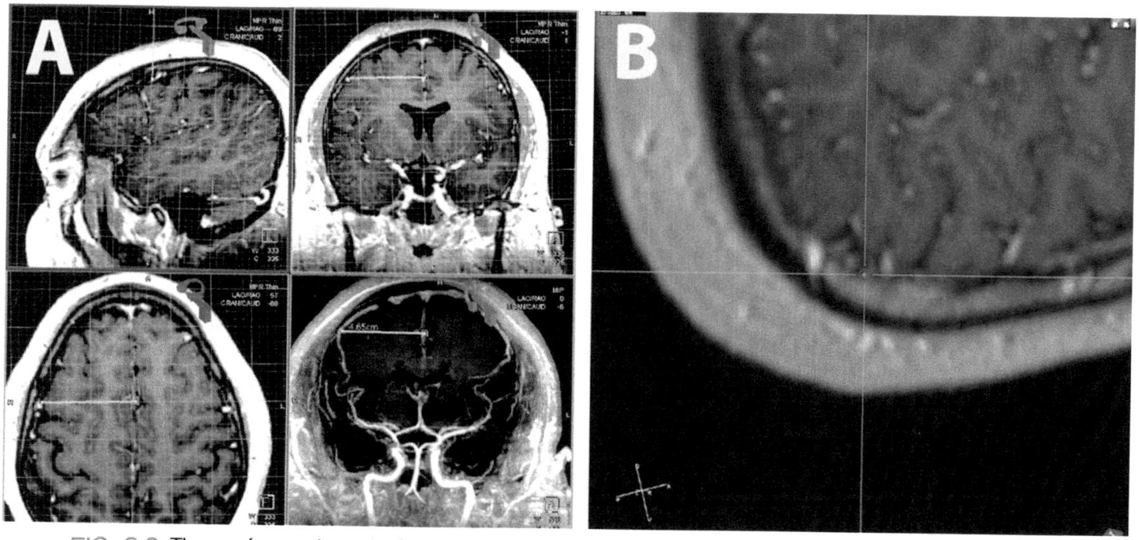

FIG. 3.3 The repérage phase in SEEG planning. Panel A depicts the planning of orthogonally oriented trajectories, now taking into consideration the vascular anatomy by using contrasted MRI sequences. Panel B depicts a close view at the entry point of a specific electrode trajectory, showing an optimal trajectory through an intended avascular path.

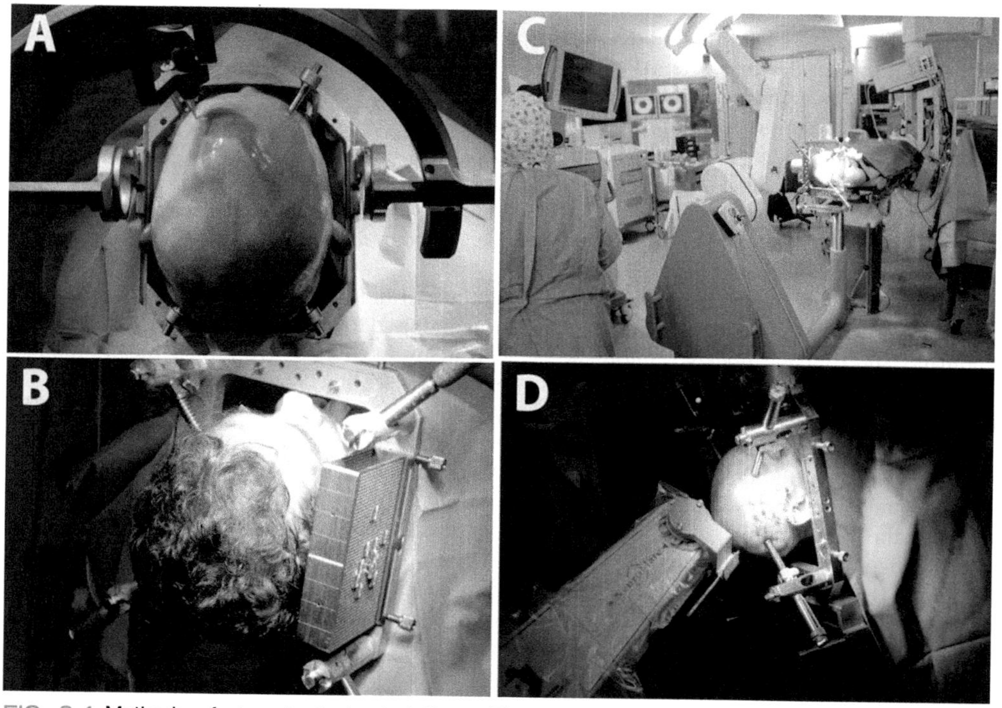

FIG. 3.4 Methods of stereotactic implantations. (A) The Leksell stereotactic frame. (B) The Talairach stereotactic system, with the Talairach frame and the double gird panel. (C) The robotic system neuromate attached to the Talaraich stereotactic system. (D) Close view of an SEEG implantation using the neuromate robot.

Nevertheless, when multiple targets are potentially accessible via a single non-orthogonal trajectory, these multi-target trajectories are selected in order to minimize the number of implanted electrodes per patient.

All trajectories are evaluated for safety and target accuracy in their individual reconstructed planes (axial, sagittal, coronal), and along the reconstructed "probe's eye view." Any trajectory that appeared to compromise vascular structures are adjusted appropriately without affecting the sampling from areas of interest. A set working distance of 150 mm from the drilling platform to the target are initially utilized for each trajectory, but later adjusted to maximally reduce the working distance and, consequently, improve the implantation accuracy. The overall implantation schemas are analyzed using the 3D cranial reconstruction capabilities and internal trajectories are checked to ensure that no trajectory collisions are present. External trajectory positions are examined for any entry sites that would be prohibitively close (less than 1.5 cm distance) at the skin level (Fig. 3.5).

On the day of surgery, patients are placed under general anesthesia. For each patient, the head is placed into a three-point fixation head holder. The robot is then positioned such that the working distance (distance between the base of the robotic arm and the midpoint of the cranium) is approximately 70 cm. The robot is locked into position, and the head holder device is secured to the robot. No additional position adjustments are made to the operating table during the implantation procedure. After positioning and securing the patient to the robot, image registrations are performed. Semi-automatic laser based facial recognition is utilized to register the preoperative volumetric MRI with the patient. The laser is first calibrated using a set distance calibration tool. Preset anatomical facial landmarks are then manually selected with the laser. The areas defined by the manually entered anatomic landmarks subsequently undergo automatic registration using laser based facial surface scanning. Accuracy of the registration process is then confirmed by correlating additional independently chosen surface landmarks with the registered MRI. After successful registration, the planned trajectories' accessibilities are automatically verified by the robot software.

The patients are then prepped and draped in a standard sterile fashion. The robotic working arm is also draped with a sterile plastic cover. A drilling platform, with a 2.5 mm diameter working cannula is secured to the robotic arm. The desired trajectories are selected on the touch screen interface. After trajectory confirmation, the arm movement is initiated using a foot-pedal. The robotic arm automatically locked the drilling platform into a stable position once reaching the calculated position for the selected trajectory. A 2 mm diameter handheld drill (Stryker) is introduced through the platform and used to create a pinhole. Dura is then opened with an insulated dura perforator using monopolar cautery at low settings. A guiding bolt (Ad-Tech, Racine, WI, U.S.A.) is screwed firmly into each pinhole. The distance from drilling platform to the retaining bolt is measured and this value is subtracted from the standardized 150 mm platform to target distance. The resulting difference is recorded for later use as the final length of the electrode to be implanted. This process is repeated for each trajectory. All pinholes and retaining bolts are placed prior to beginning electrode insertion. A small stylet (2 mm in diameter) was then set to the previously recorded electrode distance and passed gently into the parenchyma, guided by the implantation bolt, followed immediately by the insertion of the pre-measured electrode. This process is repeated until all electrodes are placed at appropriate depth and secured tightly.

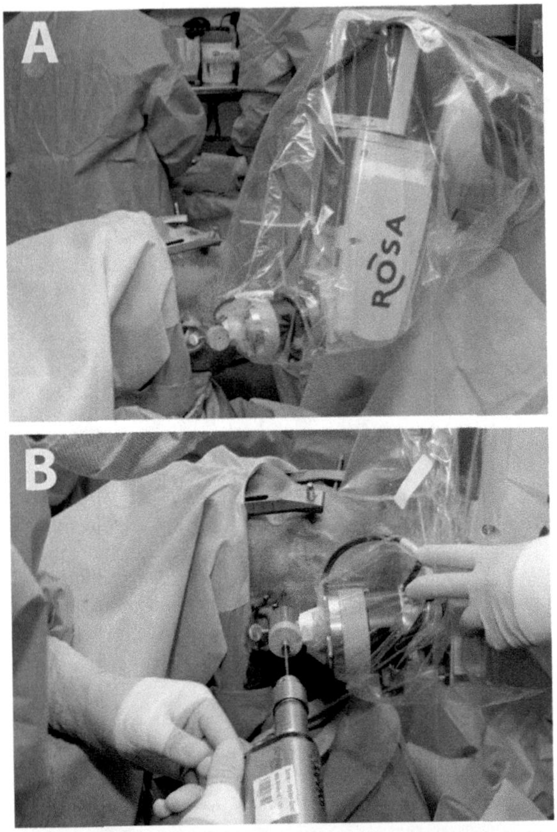


FIG. 3.5 The ROSA implantation system. A. Intraoperative picture depicting the robotic arm aligned to a temporal SEEG trajectory. Panel B is depicting a close view during the implantation of a temporal SEEG electrode, during the drilling step, guided by the robotic arm.

Post-implantation, thin-sliced CT scans are performed after the patient has awoken from anesthesia. The reconstructed images were then fused with the MRI dataset using fusion software. The resulting merged datasets are displayed and reviewed in axial, sagittal and coronal planes allowing verification of the correct placement of the depth electrodes (Fig. 3.6).

After the implantation, a brain image is obtained within the first 24 h (a stereotactic thin cut brain CT). The reasons for the post op images are (1) to identify post-operative radiological complications that might interfere with the post-operative expected course, and (2) to localize the precise anatomical location of the implanted electrodes. In SEEG analyses, the relevant SEEG signals and the correlation of ictal semiology are matched with the anatomical position of each electrode contact from which the signals are obtained.

## SEEG Complications

*When performed with the appropriate technique, SEEG implantations are safe*

Munari et al.[21] reported on their experience with SEEG in 70 patients undergoing a collective total of 712 electrode implantations. Within this cohort, an individualized and tailored surgical resection was performed in 60 patients (85.7%). In their series, specifically relating to SEEG, the authors identified one complication ensuing from the procedure; this entailed the formation of an asymptomatic intracerebral hematoma following the removal of an SEEG electrode (accounting for a morbidity rate of 1.4%, or 0.1% per electrode). More recently, Guenot et al.[22] presented a series of 100 patients collectively undergoing 1118 SEEG electrode implantations for invasive EEG monitoring. Here, SEEG was deemed helpful in 84 patients (84%) by either annulling or confirming (and additionally, in the latter case, guiding) surgical resection of the EZ. Moreover, SEEG confirmed the indication for resection in 14 cases (14%) that were previously disputed based on the non-invasive work-up. These authors reported on five complications (5% of cases), including two electrode site infections (0.2% per electrode), two intracranial electrode fractures (0.2% per electrode) and one intracerebral hematoma resulting in death (accounting for a mortality rate of 1% in the study). In a large series, Cossu et al. reported a morbidity rate of 5.6%, with severe permanent deficits from intracerebral hemorrhage in 1%.[9] In another study, Tanriverdi et al.[23] summarized their experience with a subgroup of 491 refractory epilepsy patients collectively undergoing 2490 intracerebral SEEG electrode implantations and 2943 depth electrode implantations.[23] Based on the authors' experience, they identified four patients (0.8%) with an intracranial hematoma at the electrode site (0.07% per electrode) and nine patients (1.8%) with an infection arising from electrode placement (0.2% per electrode); moreover, they reported no mortalities ensuing directly

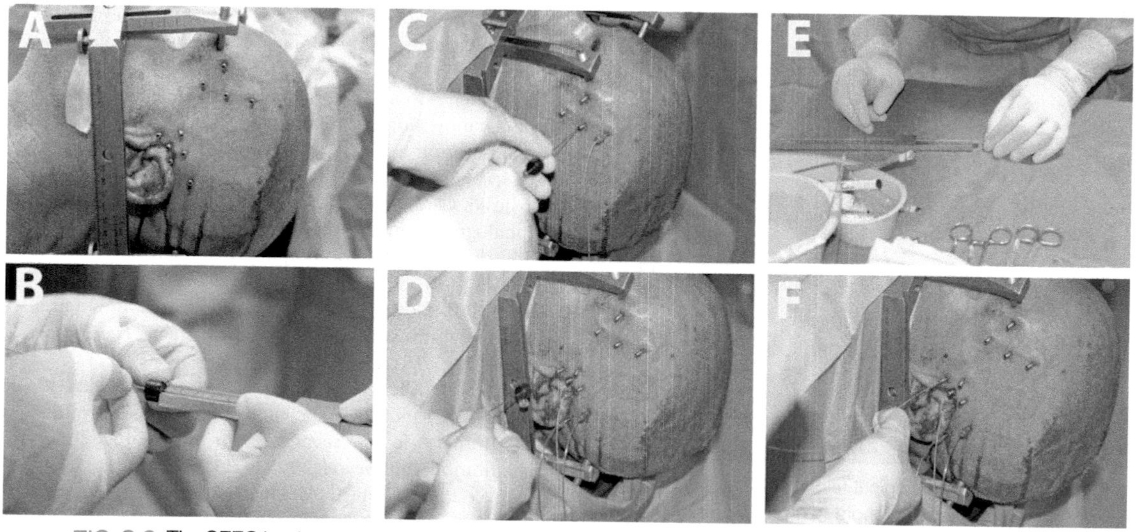

FIG. 3.6 The SEEG implantation technique. (A) An intraoperative lateral aspect during a right frontal-temporal SEEG exploration, after the implantation of the guiding bolts in orthogonal and semi-orthogonal orientations. (B) Measurements of the external stylet, matching the length of the specific trajectory. (C and D) depicting the insertion of the external stylet, moments before the implantation of the SEEG depth electrode. (E) Final measurements of the SEEG depth electrode. (F) Final aspect of the electrode implantation, through the guiding bolt.

from SEEG electrode placement. In a more extensive work, Cardinale et al.[20] most recently presented their experience with 6496 electrodes stereotactically implanted in 482 epilepsy patients with refractory epilepsy. These authors identified two patients (0.4%, or 0.03% per electrode) with permanent neurological deficits in their series; 14 patients (2.9%, or 0.2% per electrode) with hemorrhagic complication; two patients (0.4%, or 0.03% per electrode) with infection; and one mortality (0.2%) resulting from massive brain edema and concomitant hyponatremia following electrode implantation. Finally, in a more recent retrospective analysis of 549 consecutive SEEG implantations, McGovern et al. described an incidence of 19% of any type of hemorrhage findings on postimplant CT. Of these, 93 (16.9%) were asymptomatic and 12 (2.2%) were symptomatic, with three implantations (0.6%) resulting in either a permanent deficit (2, 0.4%) or death (1, 0.2%). Male sex, increased number of electrodes, and increasing age were associated with increased risk of postimplant hemorrhage (Fig. 3.7).

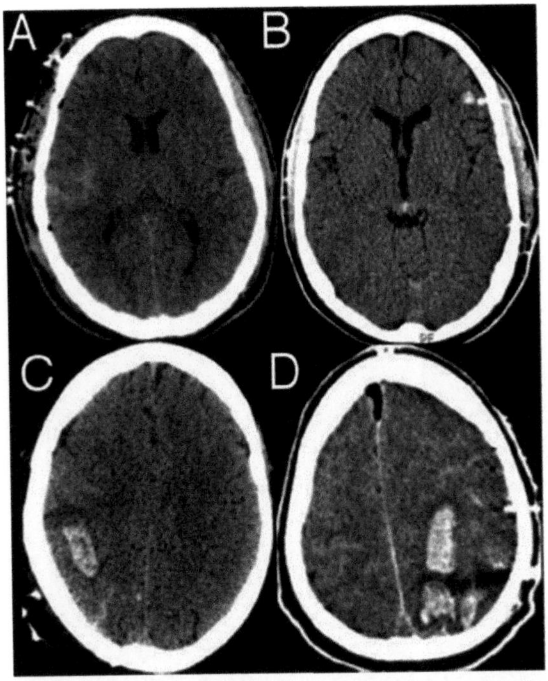


FIG. 3.7 Examples of radiological findings (CT scans) after SEEG explorations. (A) Subarachnoid hemorrhagic in the right sylvian cistern. (B) Small asymptomatic intraparenchymal hemorrhage located in the left frontal lobe. (C) Symptomatic intraparenchymal hemorrhage located in the right perirolandic areas. (D) Large intraparenchymal hemorrhage, with the presence of midline shift.

## CONCLUSIONS

The SEEG method provides the possibility to study the epileptogenic neuronal network in its dynamic and tridimensional aspect, with an optimal time and space correlation with the clinical semiology of the patient's seizures. Within the method, the SEEG stereotactic technique has proven its efficacy and safety over more than half century. More recently modern image and stereotactic device has incremented the technique, providing further stereotactic capabilities, efficiency, and precision.

## REFERENCES

1. Bancaud J. Surgery of epilepsy based on stereotactic investigations—the plan of the SEEG investigation. *Acta Neurochir Suppl*. 1980;30:25–34.
2. Bancaud J, Angelergues R, Bernouilli C, et al. Functional stereotaxic exploration (SEEG) of epilepsy. *Electroencephalogr Clin Neurophysiol*. 1970;28(1):85–86.
3. Bancaud J, Angelergues R, Bernouilli C, et al. Functional stereotaxic exploration (stereo-electroencephalography) in epilepsies. *Rev Neurol (Paris)*. 1969;120(6):448.
4. Bancaud J, Talairach J. Methodology of stereo EEG exploration and surgical intervention in epilepsy. *Rev Oto-Neuro-Ophtalmol (Paris)*. 1973;45(4):315–328.
5. Chauvel P, Rheims S, McGonigal A, Kahane P. French guidelines on stereoelectroencephalography (SEEG): editorial comment. *Neurophysiol Clin*. 2018;48(1):1–3.
6. Gonzalez-Martinez J, Lachhwani D. Stereoelectroencephalography in children with cortical dysplasia: technique and results. *Childs Nerv Syst*. 2014;30(11):1853–1857.
7. Talairach J, Bancaud J, Bonis A, Szikla G, Tournoux P. Functional stereotaxic exploration of epilepsy. *Confin Neurol*. 1962;22:328–331.
8. Cardinale F, Cossu M, Castana L, et al. Stereoelectroencephalography: surgical methodology, safety, and stereotactic application accuracy in 500 procedures. *Neurosurgery*. 2013;72(3):353–366.
9. Cossu M, Cardinale F, Colombo N, et al. Stereoelectroencephalography in the presurgical evaluation of children with drug-resistant focal epilepsy. *J Neurosurg*. 2005; 103(4 Suppl):333–343.
10. Chauvel P, Gonzalez-Martinez J, Bulacio J. Presurgical intracranial investigations in epilepsy surgery. *Handb Clin Neurol*. 2019;161:45–71.
11. Chauvel P, Kliemann F, Vignal JP, Chodkiewicz JP, Talairach J, Bancaud J. The clinical signs and symptoms of frontal lobe seizures. Phenomenology and classification. *Adv Neurol*. 1995;66:115–125.
12. Chauvel P, McGonigal A. Emergence of semiology in epileptic seizures. *Epilepsy Behav*. 2014;38:94–103.
13. Talairach J. Stereotaxic radiologic explorations. *Rev Neurol (Paris)*. 1954;90(5):556–584.
14. Talairach J, Bancaud J, Bonis A, et al. Surgical therapy for frontal epilepsies. *Adv Neurol*. 1992;57:707–732.

15. Talairach J, David M, Fischgold H, Metzger J. Radiography, encephalography, and angiography in lipoma of the corpus callosum. *Rev Neurol (Paris)*. 1951;85(6):511–517.
16. Gonzalez-Martinez J. Convergence of stereotactic surgery and epilepsy: the stereoelectroencephalography method. *Neurosurgery*. 2015;62(Suppl 1):117–122.
17. Gonzalez-Martinez J, Bulacio J, Alexopoulos A, Jehi L, Bingaman W, Najm I. Stereoelectroencephalography in the "difficult to localize" refractory focal epilepsy: early experience from a North American epilepsy center. *Epilepsia*. 2013;54(2):323–330.
18. Gonzalez-Martinez J, Bulacio J, Thompson S, et al. Technique, results, and complications related to robot-assisted stereoelectroencephalography. *Neurosurgery*. 2016;78(2):169–180.
19. Gonzalez-Martinez J, Mullin J, Vadera S, et al. Stereotactic placement of depth electrodes in medically intractable epilepsy. *J Neurosurg*. 2014;120(3):639–644.
20. Cardinale F, Lo Russo G. Stereo-electroencephalography safety and effectiveness: some more reasons in favor of epilepsy surgery. *Epilepsia*. 2013;54(8):1505–1506.
21. Munari C, Hoffmann D, Francione S, et al. Stereo-electroencephalography methodology: advantages and limits. *Acta Neurol Scand Suppl*. 1994;152:56–67.
22. Guenot M, Isnard J, Ryvlin P, et al. Neurophysiological monitoring for epilepsy surgery: the Talairach SEEG method. StereoElectroEncephaloGraphy. Indications, results, complications and therapeutic applications in a series of 100 consecutive cases. *Stereotact Funct Neurosurg*. 2001;77(1–4):29–32.
23. Tanriverdi T, Ajlan A, Poulin N, Olivier A. Morbidity in epilepsy surgery: an experience based on 2449 epilepsy surgery procedures from a single institution. *J Neurosurg*. 2009;110(6):1111–1123.

# Neural Scales in SEEG: Biophysical Principles and Technological Advances

TEJA MANNEPALI, PHD • JAY R. GAVVALA, MD, MSCI • JOHN C. MOSHER, PHD

## INTRODUCTION

To highlight the challenges and interpretations of SEEG modeling, we begin the discussion of this chapter with Fig. 4.1 of a unilateral implantation. The left figure, Fig. 4.1A, is a standard coronal view of a single SEEG electrode with multiple contacts. The other two images are of the same electrode and several others with respect to a 3D rendering of the cortical surface. The cortical surface is tessellated with nearly 540,000 small triangles, comprising nearly 270,000 vertices. As we will discuss, each triangular vertex can be modeled as the surface point of an elemental cortical column that descends directly below the point for about 2 mm. Since the adult human cortical surface is approximately 240,000 square mm,[1] each vertex nominally represents about a square mm of the pial surface. The challenges we discuss in this chapter center on the scales of the neural models that comprise these cortical columns, and, correspondingly, on the scales of the recordings possible with conventional SEEG electrodes. We also briefly examine the next generation of SEEG electrodes in prototype and design that may enhance our ability to differentiate multiple sources of neural activity.

## NEURONAL ACTIVITY: FROM MICROSCALE TO MACROSCALE

### The Single Cortical Column

To illustrate the scales discussed in this chapter, we begin with a detailed cortical column created in our labs for research and proposal purposes, shown in Fig. 4.2. The cylindrical column model is 2 mm long and 0.2 mm in diameter, comprising over 12,000 cells spanning about 40 different cell types. For our purposes here, the types of cells are not important. The column spans the classic model of six layers of the cortex, with representative densities given in the figure. The top six cell types are displayed in the central figure, with each cell indicated by a point.

Each of these individual neurons creates "micro-current sources.[3]" These micro-current sources are synaptic and action potentials at neuronal membranes.[4] The post-synaptic potentials could be excitatory (EPSPs), with inflow of Na + ions at the apical dendrites, or inhibitory (IPSPs) with an inflow of Cl-ions at the soma. Excitatory synapses predominate on dendrites while inhibitory synapses predominate on soma and basal dendrites. The potential difference between the synaptic area and the rest of the cell causes intracellular and extracellular currents. The synapse outside the cell now will equivalently be an "active sink" of negative polarity. The soma and basal dendrites can be assumed as a distributed "passive source" resulting in an extracellular potential of positive polarity. A similar mechanism follows for the IPSPs.[5]

Using a detailed NEURON[6] model of activation for these cellular sources, the final panel of Fig. 4.2 shows a raster plot of cellular activation for all of the cells. In Fig. 4.3, we calculated the voltage signal that might be recorded at distances of 1−2 mm from this column, over the one second course of the activations shown by the raster plot in Fig. 4.2. As the right-most panel in Fig. 4.3 shows, the measured voltage falls off rapidly in this logarithmic scale, for even just 2 mm from this cell population. Indeed, at even these short distances of a few mm, the exquisite details of the cortical model rapidly become the approximate simple model shown in Fig. 4.4. The simplified cortical column now emphasizes the dominant sources and sinks within the column, with corresponding positive and negative charges. These in turn are more simply modeled as a single charge separation within the column, with current "pumped" from the negative charge to the positive charge, as indicated by the current dipole arrow, giving

The Fundamentals of Stereoelectroencephalography. https://doi.org/10.1016/B978-0-443-10877-8.00011-5

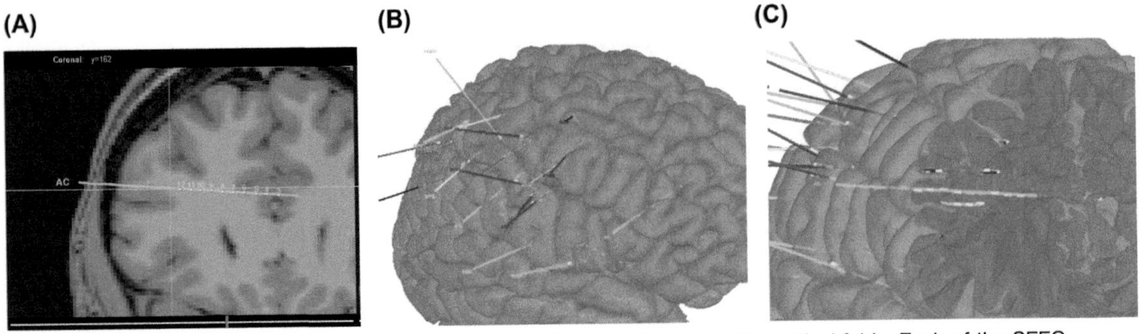


FIG. 4.1 SEEG electrode placement and 3D visualization with respect to cortical folds. Each of the SEEG contacts shown in *yellow* are cylinders 2 mm long by 0.8 mm diameter, shown to scale with the cortex. Renderings were created in Brainstorm.[2] (Courtesy Mosher Lab at UTHealth Houston.)

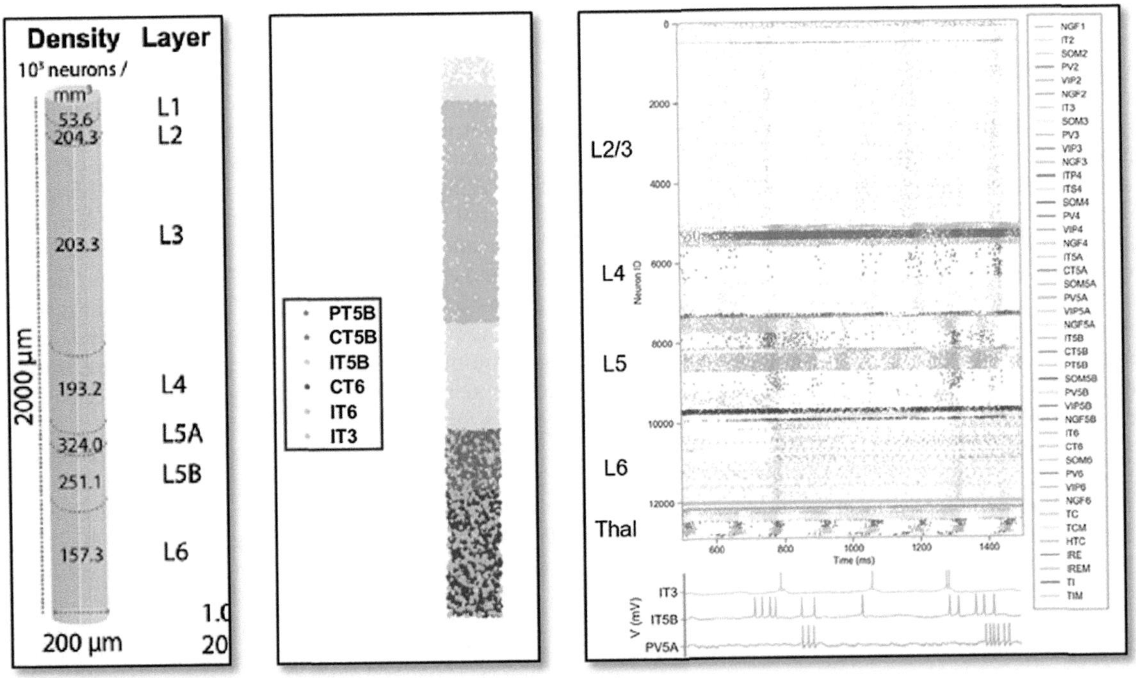


FIG. 4.2 A single cylindrical model of the cortex, 2 mm high by 0.2 mm diameter. The *left* figure indicates the cell densities per cubic mm for the cortical layers of this column. The *central* picture color codes the top six neuronal populations of the model of the column, comprising over 12,000 cells spanning nearly 40 cell types. The *right* picture shows a NEURON simulation of activation sequences for the thousands of cells in this single column, viewed as a raster plot of activations. (Courtesy Salvador Dura-Bernal SUNY Downstate Health Sciences University and Seymour Lab UTHealth Houston. Center picture courtesy Mosher Lab UTHealth Houston.)

us the simple model of "primary current" within the cortical column.

## The Neural Scales

Because of this rapid fall-off of potentials as a function of relatively small distances, we may break our cortical column model down into four recording scales, as summarized by Nunez[3]:

1. *Micro-scale recordings*: The micro recordings of the surface or transmembrane potentials correspond to the actions of the individual cells, such as we have modeled above. In this chapter, we generally assume

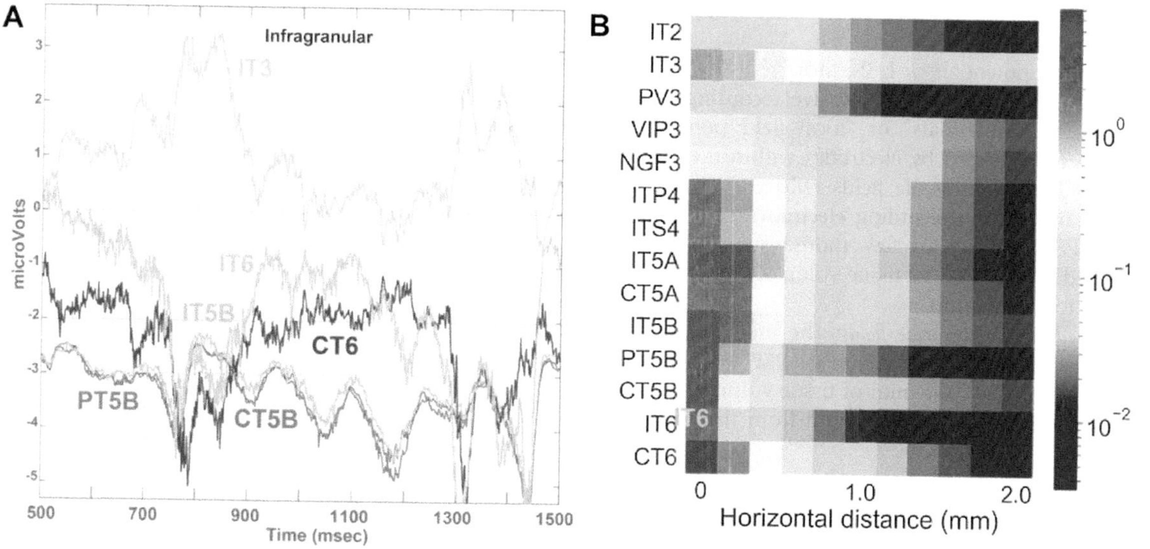


FIG. 4.3 Activation patterns of the dominant cell types, measured within a few mm of the cortical column, as shown in panel A. Note the logarithmic scale of voltages in panel B, which shows the power of cell types as a function of distance to the column. (Courtesy Salvadore Dura-Bernal of SUNY Downstate Health Sciences Center.)

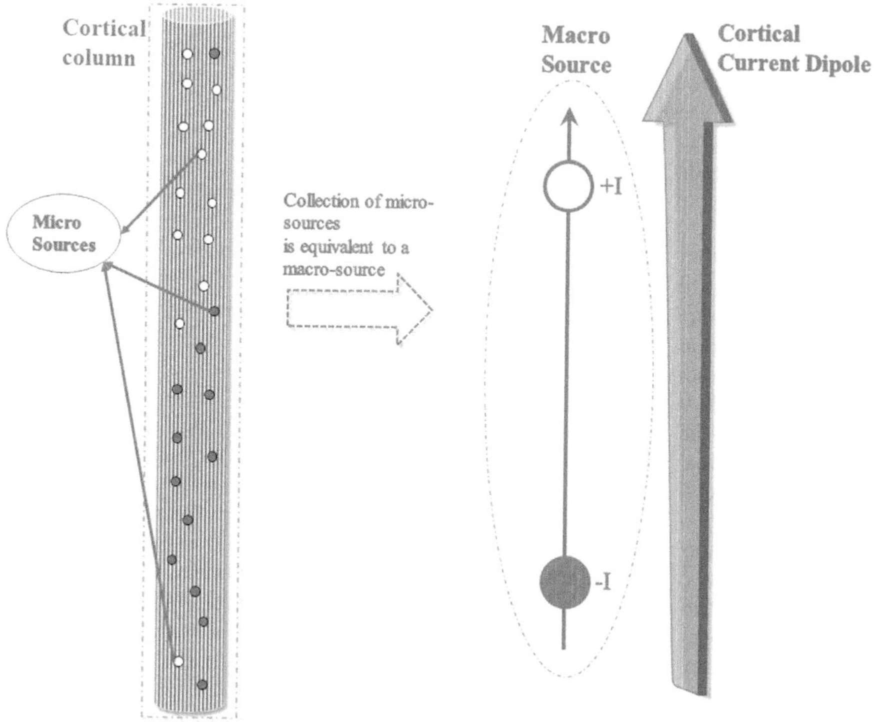


FIG. 4.4 The fine details of the column are rapidly lost at any minor distance, and the complex cell becomes instead a net separation of sources and sinks in the column. At distances approaching a cm, even this distinction in detail is lost and the cortical column simply becomes a current dipole, indicated by an arrow, in which current is "pumped" from negative to positive within the column. (Courtesy Mosher Lab.)

that this level of recording is not available in human recording.

2. Local field potentials or LFPs: More realistically for SEEG and related human invasive recordings, the "small-scale potentials" or "local field potentials (LFP)" are recorded by electrodes within the brain tissue. These small-scale fields reflect PSPs within 0.1–1 mm of the recording electrodes. This summed PSPs activity of few thousand neurons is referred to as LFPs. The tissue volumes are typically 0.001 to 1 cubic mm.
3. *Intermediate (meso) scale fields*: The meso-scale potentials reflect summed neuronal PSPs activity of typically 1 to 20 cubic mm of tissue volume, representing distances about 2–5 mm from the cortical column.
4. *Macro-scale fields*: At distances greater than about 5–8 mm from the column, we are essentially in the macro field. Nunez denotes this macro distance as roughly four times the height of the source, and our columnar sources are nominally 2 mm high.

For the non-invasive measurements made by scalp EEG and MEG, only the macro field model is useful due to the combination of CSF, skull, and scalp thickness. Indeed, even subdural electrocorticography (ECoG) mostly employs a macro model, except perhaps for sources directly in contact with a sensor at the pial surface of a gyrus. The SEEG electrode is therefore unusual in its ability to come close enough to a wide range of sources at many depths, such that we may consider additional LFP or meso scale models, in addition to the macro scale.

## Dipoles, Quadrupoles, and Patches

By electromagnetic superposition, the total measured potential or magnetic field is simply the summation of the fields from all the individual sources. Because each source has a direction, then some sources will be parallel and directly sum together, while other sources will be in opposition and cancel each other. While the micro-scale represents the individual cells in a column, for SEEG purposes the more useful elemental model sums these tens of thousands of cells into a single cortical column, as was shown above in Fig. 4.4. The classic cortical model aligns these cortical columns as perpendicular to the cortical surface, representing the columnar organization of the pyramidal cells in the gray matter. We caution this columnar organization is only an approximate model of the neocortex, since as noted by Nunez,[3] many regions of cortex may not be as simply columnar in organization; nonetheless, we find the columnar model useful at many scales.

In Fig. 4.5, we show an exemplar region of interest (ROI), the pars opercularis (left) of the Desikan-Killiany segmentation. The MRI is the widely available "Colin27" template model,[7] and the pial surface has been segmented and labeled by Freesurfer,[8] with rendering in the Brainstorm[2] program. The ROI spans about 3000 square mm of cortex and is tessellated here with about 3000 vertices. Thus each triangular vertex nominally represents one square mm of surface of the cortex, and the cortical column extends down into the gray matter in the direction of the vertex normal, a direction readily calculated by any surface rendering software. We therefore find the cortical column model to be a readily achievable model in practice, simply modeling each triangle vertex as a cortical column.

At this scale of the cortical column, we may simply model the column as a current dipole, represented by a source and a sink, with the "primary current" being forcibly driven from the source (negative) to the sink (positive).[9] We next address the question of how much current might we anticipate for a square mm of cortex, i.e., one of the vertices in Fig. 4.5. From Okada,[10] their experimental results suggest an upper limit of about 1 nA-m per square mm for many animals, with the human subjects measured close to 0.2 nA-m. We emphasize that this "Okada Constant" simply sets the plausible upper range of current, but this limit is nonetheless quite useful when we consider later "extended" regions of activity on the cortical surface. Given the nominal electrical length of the column to be about 2 mm, the model therefore suggests an upper limit of 0.5 microamps flowing up and down the column.

Rather than just a single cortical column, however, models of evoked responses and interictal spikes suggest several square cm of cortex are involved in the generation and observation of neural activity. For example, in Fig. 4.6, we show a subregion of the pars opercularis of Fig. 4.5, spanning about 500 square mm of cortex. In this "patch," we now observe that individual cortical columns are nominally radially oriented to the sphere of the head, or tangentially oriented, and/or on opposing sides of the sulcal wall. If we assume that all cortical columns are uniformly active, then by electromagnetic superposition, we have a complicated combination of elemental sources that may constructively or destructively add to each other.

For this subregion, we can simplify the details of the nominally 500 columnar sources into the net single equivalent current dipole (ECD), which represents the net constructive sum of all of the dipolar currents, which can be viewed as the net current flowing through the region, represented by the large green arrow

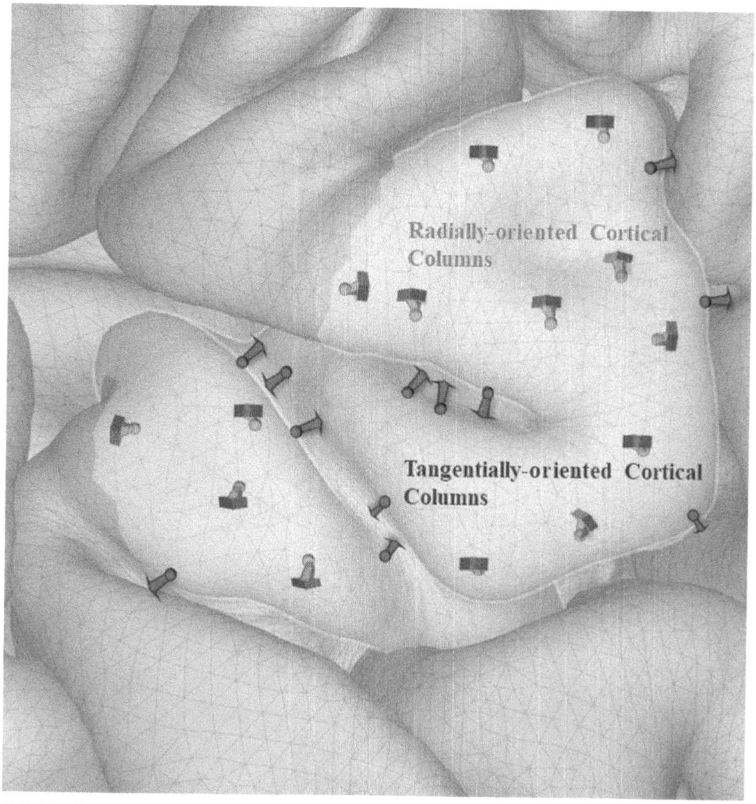


FIG. 4.5 Highlighted region of interest here is the pars opercularis of the Desikan-Killiany segmentation. Freesurfer was used with the widely available Colin27 MRI dataset to segment and label this region of interest, rendered here in Brainstorm. The "Okada Constant" sets an upper limit of about 1 nA-m per square mm, here nominally represented by each triangular vertex in this image. (Brainstorm rendering courtesy Mosher Lab at UTHealth Houston.)

traversing the patch. Not all currents constructively add, such as the opposing currents shown in the sulcal wall. When these opposing currents are viewed from a distance, the currents cancel each other in a simple sum, but their horizontal separation nonetheless can create a "circulation" of current in the immediate vicinity. We can model this "vorticity" as an equivalent current quadrupole (ECQ), representing the net of these opposing sources. While the ECD represents the current flowing through the patch, the ECQ which represents the current that is "rotating" figuratively around in this patch. Neither the ECD nor ECQ "exists" in the physical sense, but rather represents a model of the net effect of currents in the cortical columns of this patch.

These first two models of currents within the patch, the ECD and ECQ, are part of a "multipolar expansion" that continues with octupoles and higher.[11] These multipoles are mathematical representations of how currents flow into and out of this region. The emphasis, however, is on the scale at which we are measuring this patch, i.e., the distance from our electrode to this patch. Each of these multipolar components is measurable at rapidly decreasing distances from the patch, as a function of increasing order. The dipolar component has a field strength that decays with the distance squared to the electrode. By comparison, the quadrupole decays as the distance cubed, and the octupolar as the distance to the fourth power. Just as we showed in Fig. 4.4 how the complex microcellular model rapidly decays into a cortical column dipole at relatively short distances, so does the physiological patch of activity rapidly decay into just a single ECD. Thus, while the Okada Constant suggests an upper limit of 1 nA-m per vertex (cortical column) in our subregion of interest, the ECD for this same subregion is often modeled as tens of nA-m in evoked responses and hundreds of nA-m in interictal spikes. At the macro model level, such as in EEG and

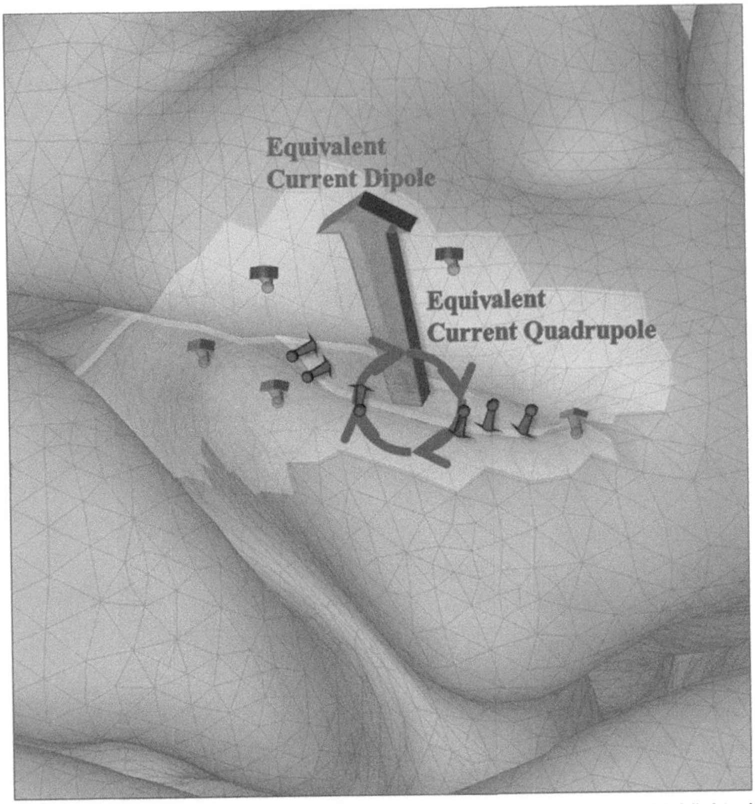


FIG. 4.6 Subregion of interest of the pars opercularis from Fig. 4.5. The region highlighted spans about 500 square mm, roughly the region that is activated in an interictal spike. We note that the cortical columns in this "patch" are nominally radial, tangential, and opposing, greatly complicating the full model. The equivalent current dipole (ECD) model represents the net additive sum of all currents similarly oriented, represented by the large current arrow. The *blue arrows* are oppositely opposed, so they cancel in the sum representing the ECD, but their separation in the sulcal fold nonetheless causes a circulation of current. The equivalent current quadrupole (ECQ) represents this net tendency for these currents to "spin" around the patch, represented here by the *blue circle*. (Brainstorm rendering courtesy Mosher Lab at UTHealth Houston.)

MEG, we often ignore the higher order multipolar models, as discussed and justified by Jerbi,[11] and thus the ECD is the emphasized model of choice in much of epilepsy work.

In summary, at distances of even just a few mm, a cortical column can be reasonably modeled as an elemental cortical dipole, and we may ignore the fine details of individual neurons. The Okada Constant sets an upper bound of 1 nA-m per square mm of cortex for this column, and indeed, empirical evidence suggests much lower current densities. Analogously, at a larger scale, the superposition of hundreds of these cortical columns in a region of interest (ROI) further collapses the model into an ECD representing the net current passing through the ROI. We next examine the role of the SEEG electrodes in measuring these currents at various scales.

## LEAD FIELD ANALYSIS

The previous section emphasized the scales of the neural source, from micro to macro models, where the scale of the source changes based on the distance from the source. In this section, we now examine an analogous scaling from the perspective of the measurement sites, i.e., the contacts on the SEEG electrodes, then detail the meso- and LFP recordings that are possible from SEEG contacts.

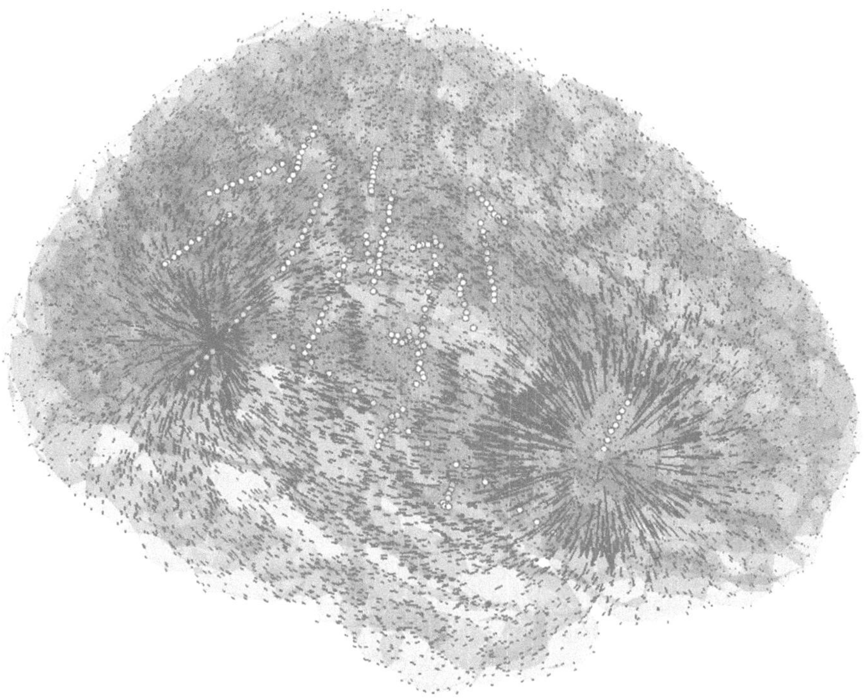

FIG. 4.7 Macro lead fields between two widely separated contacts, on a relatively coarse grid. The view is from oblique orientation above the sagittal plane, as approximately shown in Fig. 4.1, and the small spheres are the SEEG contacts. The lead fields flow from the *green* contact in the anterior portion of the brain (the "anode") to the contact in the posterior regions of the brain (the "cathode"). The fields have been sampled on the cortical surface between the two contacts. (Brainstorm rendering courtesy Mosher Lab at UTHealth Houston.)

## Macro-scale Lead Fields: Referential Montage

In Fig. 4.7, we show samples of the "lead field[12]" between two contacts on two widely separated SEEG electrodes, located in the posterior and anterior regions of the brain. The lead fields are defined as the lines of current that would occur if a current were driven from one contact to the other. In other words, the figure shows samples of the current that would appear in a deep brain stimulation (DBS), if such stimulation were attempted across two such widely separated contacts. At each point on this grid, we see the orientation and relative strength of the lead field. These field lines are relatively intuitive, with very strong lead fields in the immediate vicinity of each contact, here flowing outward from the "anode" in the anterior region of the brain, then mostly aligning and flowing relatively uniformly across the gap of the brain between the two contacts, before arriving at the "cathode" in the posterior region of the brain.

These lead fields are generated readily by "forward" or "head model" software, such as found in research electrophysiology software such as Brainstorm,[2] MNE,[13] Fieldtrip,[14] and DAiSS (SPM12).[15] The forward model includes the effects of head geometry, conductivities, and sensor configurations, relating how each current dipole in the brain relates to each measurement point in the sensor array. Different types of head model calculations include spheres, overlapping spheres, boundary elements, and finite elements,[16,17] and variations of these models and others are found in the forward modeling routines of these research software.

By the Theorem of Reciprocity, the forward models are identically the lead field models. The lead field matrix is arranged such that each row of the matrix represents a different sensor (EEG, MEG, SEEG, etc.), and each set of three columns of the matrix represents a different unconstrained dipole location sampled on a cortical grid, volume grid, or some combination. Thus the columns of the matrix are the forward field of a current dipole, sampled at many sensor locations, and the rows of this same matrix are the lead fields of the sensors, sampled at the dipole locations. The two viewpoints are interchangeable, and all of the research software listed above can generate these matrices.

We can use these lead fields to understand how neural activity at any point in the brain would be recorded by these two contacts. At a given grid point, we calculate the net ECD moment of the neural activity, as discussed in the last section, with emphasis on both its amplitude and orientation. We then take the "inner product" of this ECD with the lead field at this point, which is to say we consider the cosine of the angle between the ECD and the lead field. If the ECD is perpendicular to the lead field, then this contact pair records zero voltage, i.e., the contact pair is "blind" to the ECD. Conversely, we achieve the maximum recorded voltage if the ECD is parallel to the lead field. The voltage recorded is the product of the ECD amplitude and the lead field amplitude (the units of the lead field models, i.e., head models such as in Brainstorm, have already been calibrated to give the overall correct units of voltage). For any arbitrary angle between the lead field and the ECD, then the recorded voltage at the contacts is this maximum voltage times the cosine of the angle.

We can therefore make several observations at this point with this "macro" (large scale) recording between two contacts as shown in Fig. 4.7. For a given ECD amplitude, then the pair of contacts obviously records the highest voltage in the immediate vicinity of either contact, as evidenced by the relatively large lead field vectors in the figure. Thus, an ECD in the vicinity of a contact can be recorded, for almost any orientation of the ECD, as we note the lead field lines also spread in nearly all directions in the immediate vicinity, i.e., the field lines are "diverse." In the distant region between contacts, however, the contact pair records a relatively much smaller voltage, and the maximum voltage recorded is possible only if the ECD is aligned with the mostly uniform flow of lead field vectors. Many ECD orientations and more complicated activity patterns on regions of interest may not be adequately recorded by this contact pair, due to the combination of small amplitude lead fields and misaligned orientations with the ECDs.

The solution to this problem is two-fold. First, we employ more sensors in the vicinity of the desired ROIs, i.e., we get closer to the ECDs, which is an obvious solution. The lead field vectors will be larger and therefore more sensitive to the ECDs. The second solution may not be as obvious: We increase the "diversity" of the lead fields passing through the desired ROIs, which is to say we place additional contact pairs such that the field lines passing between them flow in dramatically different angles from the other contact pairs. Hence, we need more SEEG contacts to "surround" the ROI, so that their lead field lines can intersect the ROI in many different angles.

## Bipolar Montage

In Fig. 4.7, the contact pair is widely separated, as might be used in a "referential" montage, where the reference is chosen in an otherwise "uninvolved" region of the brain, selected at the user's discretion (to include possibly scalp electrodes, not shown here). As we noted, the voltage measured at this pair could come from any point in this wide lead field pattern, yet sources halfway between the two contacts could be entirely missed if they are not aligned with the fields. We therefore have possibly "detected" an ECD, but we cannot adequately "locate" where this ECD is, for a measured voltage signal in the contact pair.

To combat this uncertainty, a widely used alternative in SEEG recording is the "bipolar" montage, in which the contact pairs are directly adjacent to each other on an SEEG electrode. In Fig. 4.8, we show the lead fields between two such contacts, with two notable features over that of the referential montage in Fig. 4.7. First, the diversity and strength of the lead fields in the immediate vicinity of the pair is greatly increased, and second, the rapid decrease in lead field strength and diversity at even minor distances from the pair.

An obvious key benefit is that more complicated sources in the vicinity of the bipolar pair can be recorded, although we do note that the lead field lines are still somewhat dipolar in appearance, and therefore the predominant component of a patch of cortex will nonetheless be its ECD that aligns with this lead field. Another obvious feature is that the voltage measured by this contact pair must have necessarily occurred in the vicinity of this pair, yielding insight into the location of the source. We contrast this obvious statement with the referential montage, which may record a voltage, but with uncertainty as to where in the lead field pattern this activity occurred. Therefore, this bipolar feature is obviously double-edged: We must know accurately where to implant the electrode if we are to measure and locate the source.

Nonetheless, SEEG electrode arrays are often implanted in suspected regions of the brain, locations that are drawn from prior hypotheses, and therefore neural sources may indeed be adjacent to the contacts. The bipolar montage can yield a greater wealth of information from these sources that are in the immediate vicinity. As we detailed in the prior section, the local field potentials can be measured within a few mm of the

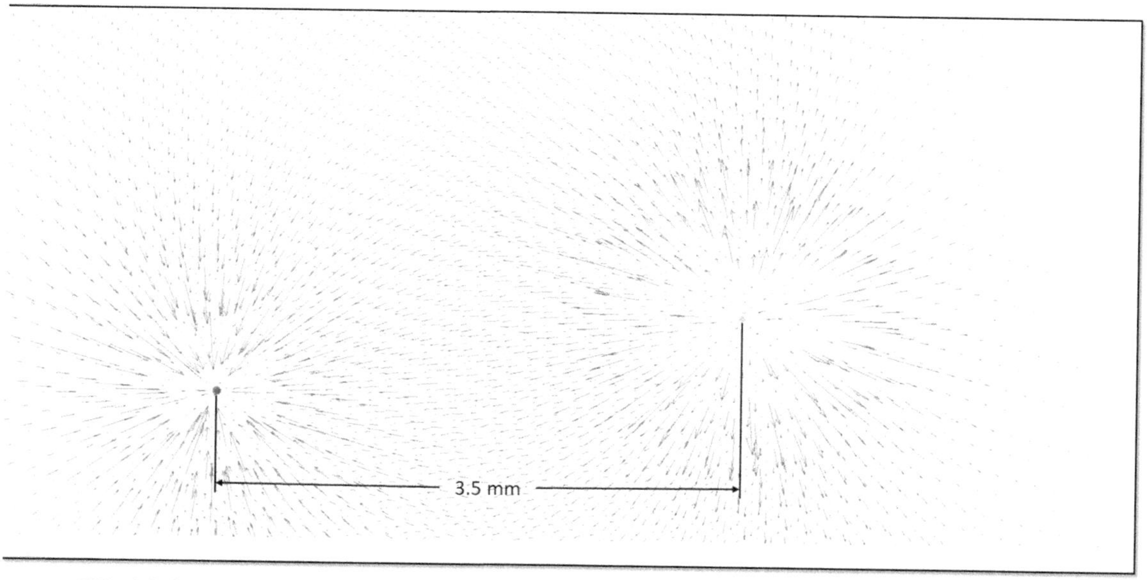


FIG. 4.8 Lead fields in bipolar mode, between two cylindrical SEEG contacts, sampled on a 0.25 mm grid in three dimensions. The centers of the two contacts are 3.5 mm apart, and the physical size of the contact and the device itself have not been taken into account, with only the point approximation for each contact used. We observe the compact and centered field lines that rapidly diminish at even relatively short distances from the pair. (Brainstorm figure, courtesy Mosher Lab.)

contacts, and some of the higher-order (non-ECD) components of the cortical region are also captured.

## Diverse Montages of the SEEG

As noted above, the SEEG bipolar montage can only record in its immediate vicinity, and thus surgical implantations often use more than a dozen devices, as shown in Fig. 4.1, to increase the odds of capturing the source. Each additional SEEG electrode comprises 8 to 16 contacts, which increases the diversity of lead fields that can traverse the regions of interest. Each electrode implantation, however, is not without risk, and therefore new devices are being developed that increase the diversity of measurements without incrementally increasing the risk above that of a device implantation. In Fig. 4.9, we present theoretical work by our groups in designing just such arrays.

The source and time series in Fig. 4.9 are the same as in Fig. 4.2, where the source now is the 2 mm long object next to a theoretical SEEG device, with novel arrays of contacts. The surface of the 0.8 mm diameter device is 1 mm from the surface of the 0.2 mm diameter source. On the sides of the device, we have arranged contact points in each of four quadrants around the device, and we have repeated these points every 0.25 mm along the axis of the device. We examined the voltage that would be recorded by a 2 mm long SEEG contact (blue points) versus a "mini" SEEG contact that is 0.5 mm long (black points). The theoretical voltage recorded by each is simply the weighted sum of these closely spaced analysis points. Because the mini-SEEG is shorter, yet nonetheless circumferential, it simply records a smaller voltage than a regular length SEEG, as shown by the black versus blue traces in the simulated response curve. In this simulation, the regular SEEG contact is of equal length to the simulated 2 mm cortical column, and exactly and optimally aligned vertically with the source. Because the mini-SEEG contacts are smaller, however, more of them can be placed above and below each other, leading to greater sensitivity along the axis of the device as to where the source is located vertically. We do not explore further this advantage of mini-SEEG arrays here, but we focus instead on a second type of "directional" array in development.

In the envisioned array, contacts are isolated on the sides of the device, rather than as isolated cylinders along the axis of the device, indicated as green and red components in Fig. 4.9. This "directional and scalable" (DiSc) array[18] has the feature that not only are contacts that are closest to the source (green points) have the strongest voltages, but conversely contacts on

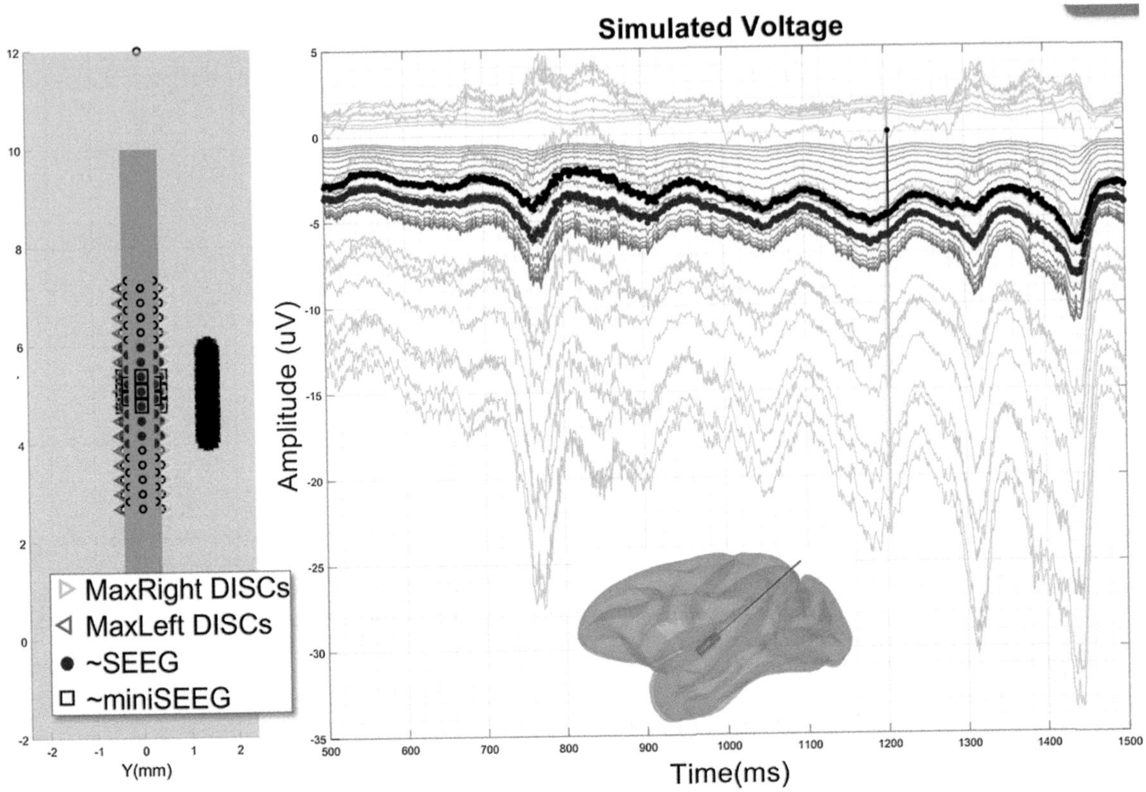


FIG. 4.9 Directional and scalable (DiSsC) depth array. (Courtesy Seymour, Mosher, and Leahy labs.)

the far side of the device (red points) have the weakest. As compared to the cylinder, we therefore achieve a directionality to the source. As we move vertically along the device, we also observe rapid changes in the amplitude, giving us sensitivity to the vertical location of the source, and, indeed, possible sensitivity to the layers of the column.

These DiSc devices are presently in prototype development with grant support to test their feasibility. In Fig. 4.10 we show the lead fields calculated in the immediate vicinity of a DiSc electrode, between two prototype contacts on opposite sides of the device and separated by about a small distance along the axis of the device. As distinct from Figs. 4.7 and 8.8, in this figure we have taken into account the physical size of the contact and the insulating properties of the device itself in order to calculate and display the lead field lines. We observe that these contacts show a strong preferential direction away from the side of the device, before quickly diminishing at relatively small distances from the device. Hence Figs. 4.9 and 4.10 show that the DiSc is sensitive both circumferentially and vertically to sources in the immediate vicinity of each contact.

Fig. 4.11 presents a macaque cortical model developed in the NetPyNe multiscale modeling toolbox.[19,20] We computed the lead fields not only along the device, i.e., in a bipolar configuration, but also between two adjacent and perpendicular alignments in a theoretical macaque brain, targeting the auditory cortex. The perpendicular orientations give "diversity" to the patterns of lead fields traversing the brain region between them. The iso-contours show the "dumbbell" pattern of sensitivity between the two devices, allowing us to "target" specific regions of the auditory cortex of the macaque.

Since the DiSc device itself remains the same dimensions as the existing SEEG devices, the risk of implantation of these novel devices in the human brain is not incrementally increased. We therefore anticipate rapid approval and adoption of these novel directional arrays once feasibility of production and acquisition are demonstrated.

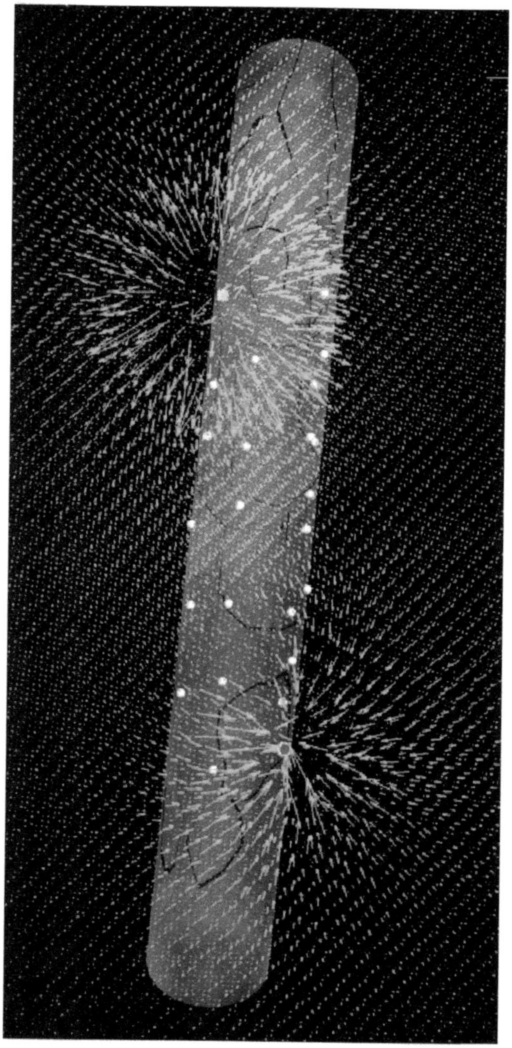

FIG. 4.10 DiSc contacts on opposite sides of the device, which is 0.8 mm in diameter, and the contacts are also separated vertically, with the lead fields sampled on a very fine grid between two such point. (Courtesy Leahy and Mosher Labs.)

## DISCUSSION

We have demonstrated a duality in scales between the generation of complex neural patterns and the arrays of diverse sensors to measure them. The scales of neural activity – LFPs, meso-scale, and macro-scale models – are dependent on the observable distance to the neural cluster. We find it convenient to model the gray matter as nominally 2 mm tall cortical columns. Although such columnar organization oversimplifies the trans-cortical connections, it does emphasize the six layers of neural activity found within the column, comprising thousands of cells and many dozens of cell types.

At even short observation distances, quasi-static electromagnetic superposition of the activity in this column results in the suppression of most of the fine distinctions. The column can be simply modeled as a charge pair, which in turn is equivalently modeled as a cortical current dipole, with current being pumped from negative to positive charges. We can therefore model the pial surface as a set of cortical columns descending below the surface, for an effective electrical length of 2 mm. MRI segmentation and labeling software render detailed triangular tessellations of the pial surface, where we can assign a cortical column to each vertex of the triangles, with a corresponding orientation normal to the local surface. We can then effectively model each region of interest (ROI) as a collection of gyral (radial) and sulcal (tangential) cortical column sources.

Just as the relatively small distance from the cortical column yielded the simple cortical dipole model, so does a relatively small distance from a ROI yield a simplification of the patch. ECD is the net summation of all of the dipolar current within a patch, and ECQ is the net tendency for the currents in this patch to cause the currents to circulate or spin. Therefore, LFPs are the potentials measured in the immediate vicinity of cortical columns, and ECDs and ECQs are the models used for meso- and macro distances from these sources.

The second part of our discussion is how to record this neural activity.

Magnetoencephalography (MEG) is the measurement of the extracranial magnetic fields generated by this activity, and electroencephalography (EEG) is the corresponding scalp potentials. Although not discussed, MEG and EEG have complementary lead field patterns that interrogate the superficial regions of interest with great diversity. We focused in this chapter on the invasive measurement of SEEG, which bypasses modeling concerns of the skull and brings measurement points much closer to the deeper regions of interest. The duality of the discussion is that SEEG contact pairs can create patterns of lead fields that are strongest and most diverse in the vicinity of the contacts but become weak and more uniform at distances from the contacts. Referential and bipolar montages help discriminate detection and location of many types of sources.

A new generation of SEEG devices under development greatly increases the number and diversity of contacts on the device, for the same form factor and therefore same relative risk of implantation. Not

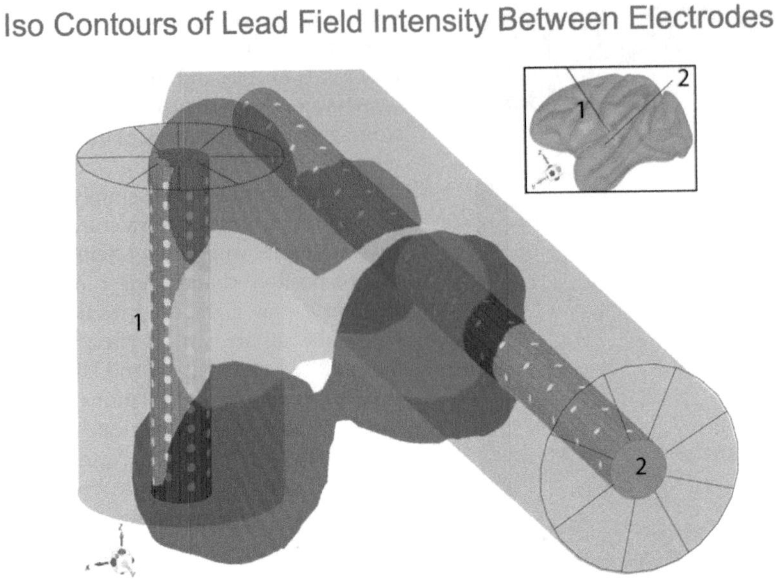


FIG. 4.11 Lead field analysis between two DiSc devices in a macaque brain. (Courtesy Seymour lab.)

discussed, but under active research by us, are advanced source localization algorithms that exploit this diversity of numerous contacts to better detect and localize neural activity found between the "forest" of SEEG contacts, but not necessarily directly adjacent in a single contact.

## ACKNOWLEDGMENTS

We thank John Seymour of UTHealth Houston Department of Neurosurgery, Salvadore Dural-Bernal of SUNY Downstate Health Sciences Center, and Takfarinas Medani of the University of Southern California Signal & Image Processing Institute for the use of their figures and discussions with them about the practicalities of micro cellular models and SEEG finite element modeling. Research reported in this publication was supported in part by the National Institute of Neurological Disorders and Stroke under R01NS128924 and by the National Institute of Biomedical Imaging and Bioengineering under R01EB026299, both of the National Institutes of Health. The content is solely the responsibility of the authors and does not necessarily represent the official views of the National Institutes of Health.

## REFERENCES

1. Toro R, Perron M, Pike B, et al. Brain size and folding of the human cerebral cortex. *Cerebr Cortex*. 2008;18(10): 2352–2357. https://doi.org/10.1093/cercor/bhm261.
2. Tadel F, Baillet S, Mosher JC, Pantazis D, Leahy RM. Brainstorm: a user-friendly application for MEG/EEG analysis. *Comput Intell Neurosci*. 2011;2011. https://doi.org/10.1155/2011/879716.
3. Nunez PL, Nunez MD, Srinivasan R. Multi-scale neural sources of EEG: genuine, equivalent, and representative. A tutorial review. *Brain Topogr*. 2019;32(2):193–214. https://doi.org/10.1007/s10548-019-00701-3.
4. Nunez PL, Wingeier BM, Silberstein RB. Spatial-temporal structures of human alpha rhythms: theory, microcurrent sources, multiscale measurements, and global binding of local networks. *Hum Brain Mapp*. 2001;13(3):125–164. https://doi.org/10.1002/hbm.1030.
5. Moini J, Piran P. Cerebral cortex. In: *Functional and Clinical Neuroanatomy*. Elsevier; 2020:177–240. https://doi.org/10.1016/b978-0-12-817424-1.00006-9.
6. Carnevale NT, Hines ML. *The NEURON Book*. Cambridge University Press; 2006. https://doi.org/10.1017/CBO9780511541612.
7. Holmes CJ, Hoge R, Collins L, Woods R, Toga AW, Evans AC. Enhancement of MR images using registration for signal averaging. *J Comput Assist Tomogr*. 1998;22(2): 324–333.
8. Dale AM, Fischl B, Sereno MI. *Cortical Surface-Based Analysis I. Segmentation and Surface Reconstruction*; 1999. http://www.idealibrary.com.
9. Williamson SJ, North Atlantic Treaty Organization, Scientific Affairs Division. *Biomagnetism : An Interdisciplinary Approach*. Plenum Press; 1983.
10. Murakami S, Okada Y. Invariance in current dipole moment density across brain structures and species: physiological constraint for neuroimaging. *Neuroimage*. 2015;

111:49–58. https://doi.org/10.1016/j.neuroimage.2015.02.003.
11. Jerbi K, Mosher JC, Baillet S, Leahy RM. On MEG forward modelling using multipolar expansions. *Phys Med Biol.* 2002;47(4):523–555. https://doi.org/10.1088/0031-9155/47/4/301.
12. Malmivuo J, Suihko V, Eskola H. Sensitivity distributions of EEG and MEG measurements. *IEEE Trans Biomed Eng.* 1997; 44(3):196–208. https://doi.org/10.1109/10.554766.
13. Gramfort A, Luessi M, Larson E, et al. MEG and EEG data analysis with MNE-python. *Front Neurosci.* 2013;(7 DEC). https://doi.org/10.3389/fnins.2013.00267.
14. Oostenveld R, Fries P, Maris E, Schoffelen JM. FieldTrip: open source software for advanced analysis of MEG, EEG, and invasive electrophysiological data. *Comput Intell Neurosci.* 2011;2011. https://doi.org/10.1155/2011/156869.
15. Litvak V, Mattout J, Kiebel S, et al. EEG and MEG data analysis in SPM8. *Comput Intell Neurosci.* 2011;2011. https://doi.org/10.1155/2011/852961.
16. Mosher JC, Leahy RM, Lewis PS, Alamos L. *Matrix Kernels for the Forward Problem in EEG and MEG.* 1997.
17. Medani T, Garcia-Prieto J, Tadel F, et al. Brainstorm-DUNEuro: an integrated and user-friendly Finite Element Method for modeling electromagnetic brain activity. *Neuroimage.* 2023;267. https://doi.org/10.1016/j.neuroimage.2022.119851.
18. Abrego AM, Khan W, Wright CE, et al. Title: sensing local field potentials with a directional and scalable depth array: the DISC electrode array. *J Neural Eng.* 2023;20. https://doi.org/10.1101/2021.09.20.460996.
19. Dura-Bernal S, Suter BA, Gleeson P, et al. NetPyNE, a tool for data-driven multiscale modeling of brain circuits. *Elife.* 2019;8(e44494). https://doi.org/10.7554/eLife.44494.001.
20. Dura-Bernal S, Griffith EY, Barczak A, et al. Data-driven multiscale model of macaque auditory thalamocortical circuits reproduces in vivo dynamics. *Cell Rep.* 2023;42(11). https://doi.org/10.1016/j.celrep.2023.113378.

CHAPTER 5

# The SEEG Signal—Understanding Human Intracranial Electrophysiology

MELISSA M. ASMAR, MD, MSC • NIGEL P. PEDERSEN, MBBS, FAES, FANA

## INTRODUCTION

This chapter provides an overview of the principles of human intracerebral electrophysiology in the context of the stereo-electroencephalographic (SEEG) method. SEEG is an approach to determining a patient's seizure network(s) and should be considered distinct from the mere addition or use of intracerebral "depth" electrodes. While the approach to the SEEG method involves knowledge of an analysis of seizure semiology—the temporal progression of clinical symptoms and signs in association with a seizure—this chapter will help understand the basis and interpretation of electrophysiological signals.

In outline, we include a brief history of intracerebral electrophysiologic recordings in the context of the SEEG method. We then review the pragmatics of obtaining a recording, the general principles behind the biological basis of consequent local field or "mesoscale" electrophysiologic signals, an approach to reviewing data, and some core elements of clinical interpretation. We follow this by emerging approaches to analysis, especially signal processing. We also emphasize that careful analysis of the SEEG signal can only be as good as hypotheses and implantation planning—topics covered in other chapters.

## HISTORICAL FOUNDATIONS

Technical advances have driven the history of neuroscience, as well as the evolution of intracerebral electrophysiology. Building on the work of Hitzig and Ferrier,[1,2] Richard Caton was the first to describe intrinsic electrical activity from regions of the cerebral cortex in the 1870s, achieved through subdural electrode placement in cats, rabbits, and monkeys.[3] About 20 years later, Hans Berger suffered a near-death experience, seemingly simultaneously predicted by his sister and father. This unusual inspiration led to his career-long interest in psychophysics and the study of electric fields of the brain as a potential means to understand the action of neural phenomena at a distance. Hans Berger obtained a string galvanometer with a smoked drum, enabling him to study small voltage fluctuations. With foil electrodes applied to the front and back of his young son's head, he could record an approximately 10 Hz oscillation that appeared when his son closed his eyes.[4] This first rhythm was denoted "alpha" followed by the appreciation of "beta" activity with mental math. This was not met with much interest until it was validated by Adrian, who expanded the repertoire of rhythms to include faster "gamma" activity of the intracranially recorded olfactory area in hedgehogs during sniffing behavior.[5] "Delta" activity was soon added in association with sleep,[6] completing the core pantheon of EEG rhythms. Berger expanded his approach to include intracerebral recordings after 1924, as published in his series of papers on electroencephalography.[4] After validating electric field voltage recordings in humans, this method was turned to clinical disorders with an underlying oscillatory basis. Given the speculation of Hughlings Jackson, the idea that seizures were a disorder of abnormal rhythmic cerebral activity,[7] attention was particularly turned toward epilepsy. Much of what we consider with montages and the rhythms characterizing inter- and ictal abnormalities in epilepsy was pioneered by Erna and Fred Gibbs (a spousal scientific partnership) in the 1930s, resulting in the classic and first EEG atlas of epilepsy.[8] This was made possible by collaboration with another spousal team, Ellen and Albert Grass. The Grasses were able to create a three-channel electronic amplifying encephalograph in only 3 months, which, with further development and evolution, resulted in the Grass Instrument company, a major manufacturer of EEG and stimulation equipment up until the beginning of the 21 century.[9]

The Fundamentals of Stereoelectroencephalography. https://doi.org/10.1016/B978-0-443-10877-8.00012-7

Intraoperative stimulation studies were developed by Ottfried Foerster in the 1920s and later accompanied by acute intracranial recordings, influencing Wilder Penfield—a mentee of Foester—and Penfield's collaboration with Herbert Jasper from 1937.[10,11] An oft-forgotten chapter in the history of intracranial electrophysiology is the achievement, by a collaboration of Penfield, Jasper, and Donald Hebb, of the first prolonged extraoperative epidural recording in 1938.[12] This is the first case of extraoperative monitoring to identify the seizure onset zone, along with subsequent surgical resection that monitored language function during resection.

The work of Penfield and Jasper, in the context of a strong history of neurologic thinking and localization in France, was a major inspiration to Jean Bancaud.[13] The collaboration of Bancaud, a neurologist, and Jean Talairach, originally a psychiatrist prior to becoming a neurosurgeon, ultimately resulted in the SEEG method. This method was made possible by Talairach's creation of the stereotactic method, Talairach space, and its functional correlations.[14] These developments enabled localization of semiology to study a patient's epilepsy in an individualized manner with the implantation of depth electrodes. Their work, characterized in several papers and then a key monograph,[15] described much of the SEEG method and approaches to interpreting intracerebral electrophysiology. At the heart of this method was the correlation of gross regional anatomy, the functional localization of semiology, and its electrophysiologic correspondences—the *anatomo-electroclinical correlation.* This fundamental approach has remained, bolstered by technical innovations in amplifiers, surgical techniques, neuroimaging, and signal processing. The reliance of this approach on both clinical experience and the wellspring of systems neuroscience has resulted in an evolution of the practice that continues to this day. While the ultimate "signal" we seek in SEEG is the anatomo-electroclinical correlation, this chapter focuses on the electrophysiological component of this triad.

## THE PRAGMATICS OF SEEG ELECTROPHYSIOLOGY

### Instrumentation and Considerations When Recording

The SEEG signal is obtained by recording small voltage differences between two points in the forebrain, most often within the cerebral cortex (which includes specializations such as the amygdala and hippocampal formation), and less often subcortical structures such as the thalamus and hypothalamus. Subcortical recordings remain uncommon, with emerging clinical use of this information,[16] such as in hypothalamic hamartoma.[17] Recordings of deep cortical malformations resulting from impaired cellular migration are common, such as in periventricular nodular heterotopia.

While early EEG and SEEG recordings were made with analog pen-chart recorders, modern recordings are acquired digitally. The organization of hardware for typical modern digital recording is shown in Fig. 5.1. As we will see, digital recording has several advantages related to storing raw data that can then be manipulated both online and offline with respect to montage, filters, and other signal processing.

### Electrodes

SEEG electrodes are typically made of platinum-iridium (Pt–Ir, 95% Pt, 5% Ir) contacts with plastic spacers between them. Pt–Ir contacts are chosen for their electrochemical properties, and stability is partly due to the iridium oxide layer on the surface of these electrodes. Iridium oxide is more electrochemically stable and therefore resistant to metal deposition during the application of charge (as in radiofrequency ablation and electrical stimulation).

### References, Ground, and Recording Contacts

Although reference and ground can be common, they have distinct purposes. The ground electrode on the patient helps to prevent voltage offset between the patient and recording equipment. Because an electrode cannot measure absolute voltage, the EEG amplifier measures the difference between each recording contact and the chosen reference electrode. In stereo EEG, separate contacts on a subgaleal electrode at the vertex are often used for ground and reference due to their consistent signal quality and relatively low susceptibility to artifacts. This most commonly used reference is active, however, picking up vertex activity, especially prominent in sleep. Another approach is to use an extracranial ground that is sometimes switched to a relatively quiet white matter reference shortly after connecting the patient, but white matter references are not inactive and also include intracerebral field potentials. Ground and reference electrodes should have a low impedance and be composed of the same material as the recording contacts to prevent electrochemical current production. The reference often has a similar impedance to the recording contacts. The location of the system reference should not then be changed during subsequent recording, and an alternate computed reference can also be used (see below). Many centers use the system

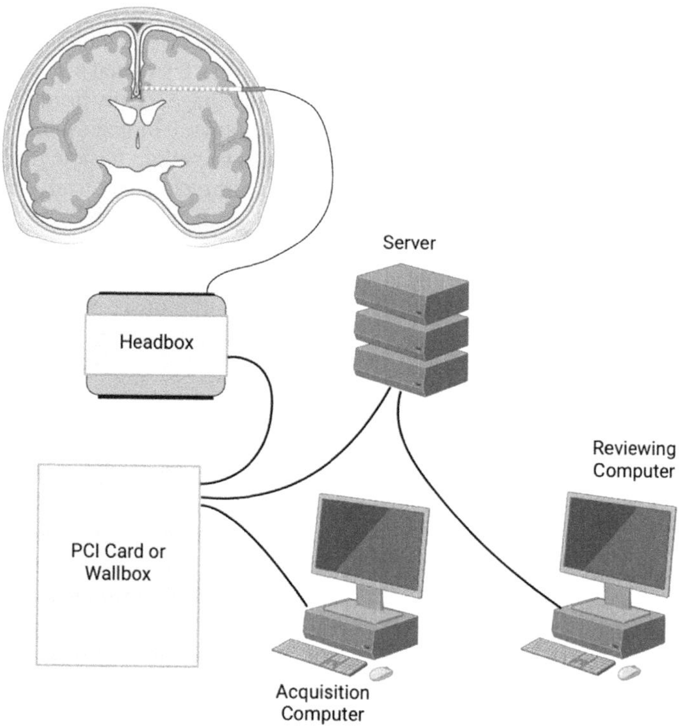


FIG. 5.1 **Modern Recording Setup.** The head box typically includes most components of the acquisition hardware, with hardware high pass filter, amplifier, anti-aliasing filter, sampler, and multiplexer. The multiplexed signal is then sent to a wall unit or PCI card for de-multiplexing or sending the signal via a serial or Ethernet connection.

reference for a referential montage, which is often adequate.

## Sampling

It is important to consider sampling rate when recording the SEEG signal. The sampling rate is the frequency at which samples are taken from each recording contact from the analog signal. While it has been suggested that the manual review of raw SEEG data can tolerate sampling rates around 100 Hz,[18] this is not recommended for the reasons discussed below. Identifying low-voltage fast activity in SEEG, which often has frequencies above 80 Hz, and embedded higher frequency activity, is critical. To identify low-voltage fast activity, compared to other contacts (typically requiring signal processing as described below), it is critical to sample in a way that captures activity up to at least 200 Hz. Sampling at a minimum of ~500 S/second is therefore recommended. If there is any current or future interest in high-frequency oscillations or pathological ripples in the SEEG signal, it is necessary to record frequencies of up to 500 Hz.[19,20] Therefore, it is recommended to sample at 2 kS/second where possible. The large data files generated are often smaller than accompanying compressed video but can make sharing and storing data more onerous.

## Noise

Noise arises from many sources and is generally divided into two categories: biological and non-biological. Non-biological noise and artifacts commonly result from electromagnetic interference in the recording environment. Principal among sources is line-noise frequency artifact due to the electromagnetic fields accompanying power lines, switching power supplies, fluorescent lights, and alternating-current power equipment in the immediate environment. Sometimes, interference from cell phone networks and wireless devices is present. These sources of noise can be minimized: if wires are bundled together (so that they encounter the same ambient noise), and a driven ground is used,[21] there can be a very clean signal despite the electromagnetically noisy environment of a hospital room. All recording equipment should also be on the same electrical circuit (or have common ground), and "wall wart" switching power supplies may need to be moved away from the patient and recording equipment. Most importantly, ensure that all recording, reference, and ground contacts have a low impedance. When contact impedance is high, the apparent voltage measured is increased (consider the equation *voltage* = *current* × *impedance*) and may report high amplitude electromagnetic noise (typically line noise, which is 60 Hz in the Americas and some parts of Asia, mostly 50 Hz elsewhere), rather than biological signal. While a notch filter can be used, it should be avoided where possible given the potential for filter ringing, and removal of some biological signal at this and immediately adjacent frequencies.

## Montages

EEG has 1/f amplitude characteristics,[22,23] meaning that lower frequencies have higher voltages than faster oscillations. Relatedly, slow potentials generally affect a larger tissue region than high frequencies.[24] Exclusion of low frequencies by comparison of near electrode contacts helps to visually emphasize fast activity, which is usually important in defining seizure onset. Contrarily, using distant electrode contacts helps visualize slow activity and ictal baseline shifts.

There are three common types of referential montage in SEEG. Firstly, there is a *system reference montage*. These are the signals as recorded against a system reference. This is distinct from a *computed referential montage*, where each derivation is re-calculated against a chosen, often white matter, contact. Unless there is a failure of the system physical reference, one should never move the recording system reference to another site after initial selection—this creates a discontinuity in the dataset. Instead, the computed reference should be created digitally, typically in the reviewing software. An *average reference montage*, computed after removing noisy or artifact-containing contacts, is typically only used in research.

In addition to the referential montage mentioned above, interpreting the SEEG signal requires a *bipolar montage*. The bipolar montage is computed by subtracting each subsequent contact on the electrode shaft, starting from the contact at the end of the depth electrode. A *laplacian montage* may also be useful in interpreting the SEEG signal, though the loss of the end contacts is a limitation.[25] Screening of SEEG data is generally performed with a bipolar montage, as the derivations of this montage generally help discriminate the generators of faster activity and interictal discharges. It is also possible to overlook background suppression and fast activity on a referential montage, given the potential that higher voltage activity from an active reference electrode may obscure biological low-voltage fast activity.

It is also important to note that referential montage provides complementary and necessary information. Very slow potentials such as an ictal baseline shift,[26] typically occur in a larger tissue area, and therefore may be obscured on a bipolar montage that compares signals at a millimeter scale. A referential montage may also help define the more precise location of a phenomenon noted on bipolar review.

## Artifacts

The reader is assumed to be familiar with scalp EEG recording and interpretation. In comparison to scalp or extracranial EEG recordings, intracranial artifacts are much less prevalent. Contacts adjacent to the muscles of mastication will encounter a higher frequency, mostly aperiodic electromyographic signal. Rhythmic muscle artifacts encountered from the neck muscles in scalp EEG may rarely be seen. Pulsatile artifacts from CSF flow or adjacent blood vessels are also rarely present. Common-mode biological artifacts and non-biological noise are typically more prevalent when using an extracranial system reference that is also used for a referential montage.

## Filters

Filters should principally be used to exclude recording artifacts. A secondary use of filters is to examine specific frequency components of the signal—this use of filters should only be performed with all necessary caveats in mind. The various types of filters are extensively reviewed elsewhere.[27,28]

There are three commonly used filters in EEG recording: A high-pass filter (allows higher frequency activity to pass, colloquially called a low-frequency filter), a low-pass filter (that allows low frequencies to pass, sometimes called a high-frequency filter), and a band-stop or notch filter that attenuates the signal at a specific frequency. There are several important things to keep in mind when using filters. Firstly, while the cut frequently represents a "corner" in the fall-off of signal power, this is not a clean cut-off but a roll-off. Secondly, filters can "ring" when a sudden deflection in the signal occurs, resulting in artifactual higher frequency oscillations (Gibb's phenomenon or filter ringing).[29] This is typically a problem with high-frequency filters such as the line-noise 60 Hz notch filter or other low-pass and band-pass filters. These principles are important to consider when the clinician is looking for superimposed fast activity. This may be mitigated by examining the signal with filters off or by using more advanced approaches (see Signal Processing below). Thirdly, and typically of less consequence for clinical interpretation, filters can slightly shift the time base. This becomes important when using different filter settings for channels that are compared in the same recording. Lastly, given the high noise attenuation by the "driven ground" used in modern clinical EEG systems, the need for a line-noise notch filter should alert the reader and team to technical problems and should not be used routinely.

An anti-aliasing filter is often configured automatically. The Nyquist frequency is the highest frequency that can be sampled at a given sampling rate. If the sampling rate is 2 kS/second, the Nyquist frequency is 1 kHz. Frequencies above the Nyquist frequency will "alias" at a lower frequency. In order to prevent this, an anti-aliasing filter is applied that is half or less of the sampling rate. If there were a signal at the Nyquist frequency, this could only be recorded as a sample that occurs twice each cycle and would therefore appear as a triangular waveform. It is typically desirable to have a higher resolution for a sampled waveform, so the anti-aliasing filter is often below the Nyquist frequency.[28]

## CELLULAR, SEEG, AND SCALP EEG RECORDINGS

### Types of Intracranial Recording—Cellular and Field Potential

Extracellular intracranial (and intra-parenchymal) electrophysiological recordings in the nervous system are broadly divided into cellular versus field potential recordings. The size of electrode contacts is directly related to the size of the field recorded. Small electrodes can record both cellular activity and highly localized field potentials. When recording voltage fluctuations from a region or field around an electrode, we either remove or do not obtain individual cellular potentials, we speak of a *field potential* (sometimes local field potential or LFP). Field potential recording measures voltage changes in nervous tissue due to the activity of large numbers of neuronal cell bodies and, more importantly, their dendrites.

Given the size of SEEG electrode contacts, the net activity of millions of neurons are recorded. Such field potential recordings in large "macrocontact" SEEG electrodes arise from the neuropil of gray matter, with individual units' activity too focal to obtain. This also means that dendritic potentials, accounting for a large component of extracellular space in gray matter, are the source of recordings. Obtaining field potentials is also assisted by the arrangement and morphology of neurons, particularly pyramidal cells, whose cellular long axis is aligned with other pyramidal cells, forming aligned dipoles. Common activity in the dendritic compartments of these neurons enables the recording of higher voltage field potentials. It is important to recognize that when we examine the SEEG signal, we are looking at the activity of dendrites in a large population of pyramidal cells, and these may be sinks or sources of intracerebral currents. This has critical implications for our interpretation of the SEEG signal, since we are recording synchronized population activity in dendrites that may not reflect underlying action potentials in these neurons. If this always held, we would be measuring the inputs to a sampled area, not local neuronal firing. Under normal physiological conditions, high-frequency components of the SEEG signal, particularly high gamma (possibly 50, definitely 80 Hz and above) correspond well to underlying unit activity.[30,31] In the context of seizures and low-voltage fast activity, gamma activity likely arises principally from local inhibitory neurons and their effects on pyramidal dendrites, but still reflects local neuronal firing.[32]

### Scalp EEG Versus the SEEG Signal

While point electric fields decay as an inverse square of the distance, the combined and synchronized action of many dendritic arbors over a larger area of the cortex results in less rapid decay that can even be measured on the scalp. Given the orientation of the dipoles in the cerebral cortex in relation to scalp EEG electrodes, the signal is dominated by dendritic activity in pyramidal cells in the crest of the gyrus.[33] Thus, unlike SEEG, the scalp EEG consists only of summated dendritic potentials of pyramidal cells. As an example of summation, high voltage spindles are relatively simultaneous in frontocentral areas of the adult brain but not completely synchronized in SEEG. Still, on the scalp, they are summated and appear synchronous. Generally, it is held that several centimeters of gyral crest activity are summated in scalp EEG.[34] Thus scalp EEG potentials are recorded when sufficiently synchronous at a particular frequency in a contiguous area of cortical gyri. High gamma activity is typically not measurable in adult scalp EEG (owing to it not being synchronized over a large area and having low voltage). Instead, flattening of the record on scalp EEG likely reflects the involvement of a large cortical area in higher frequency activity, manifesting as suppression.

In contrast, the "listening zone" for SEEG contacts is only up to a few millimeters,[35] providing an accurate review of what is happening locally and is therefore complementary and non-identical to scalp EEG. Furthermore, the ability to record high-frequency activity on SEEG allows one to suspect that there are underlying local action potentials, likely of local inhibitory neurons,[32,36] measured by their effect on pyramidal cell dendrites, and therefore not just representing inputs from other components of a circuit.

Another key distinction between scalp EEG and SEEG is that the scalp EEG electrodes, as with subdural recording, are always above and orthogonal to the apical dendrites of gyral crest pyramidal cells, as described above. This means that the orientation and location of EEG contacts are not variable in relation to the generators of scalp EEG potentials. This means that much of the normal background in scalp EEG has a typical voltage and polarity, encouraging the use of a standard calibration (7 μV/mm). In contrast, SEEG electrode contacts may have almost any orientation and location in relation to generators. Polarity flips as the depth electrode advances through generators, and there is no standard calibration for all electrodes. However, a starting point is often 100–150 μV/mm, often less, and modified further depending on the structure sampled.

## The SEEG Signal Varies Between Regions of the Cerebral Cortex

There are three further implications for the practice of SEEG. Firstly, cellular morphology and architecture determine how much we can obtain high-voltage potentials. Some regions of the cerebral cortex show less cellular alignment or columnar organization producing lower voltage signals and different morphology for epileptiform and ictal discharges. The best example is the amygdala, which has a heterogeneous organization in its various nuclei.[37] From a practical standpoint, this means that a higher gain is needed to see discharges and low-voltage activity.[38] Therefore, the amygdala's high amplitude spikes and sharp waves are especially salient given that it requires marked synchrony to provide these field potentials. It should also encourage the reader to consider that high-voltage potentials recorded in the amygdala may originate from the adjacent and medial cerebral cortex or the head of the hippocampus. Conversely, the high cell density and arrangement of pyramidal neurons in *cornu ammonis* of the hippocampus result in high voltage potentials—the gain for these channels can be reduced.

Secondly, electrode orientation matters and will change the orientation of the recording contacts to cortical dipoles. Therefore orthogonal implantation of gray matter tends to provide better recordings given alignment with pyramidal cell dipoles and the bipolar montage that is typical for reading SEEG. Overall, these observations prevent standard voltage calibration in SEEG; not all channels should necessarily have the same gain setting.

Lastly, the frequency of recorded rhythms varies by the network or region sampled, as is discussed below (Section The normal intracranial EEG background).

## Near and Far Fields in SEEG

We have briefly mentioned far-field effects, which are important to consider when reading SEEG electrophysiological studies. The alternative is a near-field potential that arises locally. While direct cortical recordings have been conceptualized as near-fields, in contrast to MEG and EEG far-fields,[39] it seems likely that some far-field phenomena can be recorded on SEEG contacts, particularly in a referential montage. There are two situations in which far fields should be considered: the first is obvious and relates to using a distant reference electrode. The signal can be contaminated with an active reference. This is due to the montage and is not due to far field contamination at the recording contact. More importantly, however, is that large portions of synchronous adjacent cortex show a reduced spatial decay of the electric field. This means that the listening zone of an SEEG contact may be greater for large, synchronized, and more planar generators. Clinical interpretation of SEEG may not need to take this into account, and there is no ready way to do so at present. Theoretically, the large generators associated with seizures may lead to electric fields having less spatial decay than some normal brain activity. This also applies to spatial large ictal baseline shifts. The term "volume conduction" should be avoided and should not be confused with far fields—volume conduction instead refers to tissue conduction (e.g., recording electrocardiogram signal in the feet and hands).

## Mesoscale Potentials or Field Potentials?

An alternative set of descriptors can help draw parallels to work in other domains. Arising from studies of brain connections, *connectomics*, the terms micro-, meso-, and macro-scale are used.[40] Respectively, these terms refer to cellular connections, connections of local processing units (sometimes cortical columns vs. functional units), and large-scale connections between brain areas. This could correspond to microelectrode recording of brain cells (see below), versus local field potentials, versus the activity of large cortical regions, as in EEG. If we make a parallel schema from electrophysiology, SEEG is within the domain of mesoscale potentials, but the difficulty of this being somewhat ill-defined persists, with the size of the local field varying depending on electrode type. Generally, it might be reasonable to use a broad term for the SEEG signal—field potentials—and appreciate distinctions from scalp EEG. In fact, the term SEEG is inaccurate: Intracerebral field potentials are distinct from EEG for the above reasons.

## CLINICAL INTERPRETATION OF THE SEEG SIGNAL

In this section, we will provide an overview of the clinical interpretation of the SEEG signal. Before we embark, we must clearly understand common terms used in SEEG, and differentiate these terms from those that arose in the context of subdural recording. This section helps clarify the use of terms for SEEG and avoids the confusion that often arises when using subdural terminology in SEEG. We will then discuss normal findings, abnormal findings, interictal epileptiform abnormalities, the ictal preparation, ictal transition, and electrographic correlates of seizures.

### Terminology

*Epileptogenic Network*—There are three definitions of epileptogenic tissue: (1.) The earliest definition is operational, not theoretical, and refers the network involved in the principal organization of the seizure.[41,42] (2.) Later, from Lüders and colleagues, the tissue that needs to be removed to cure the epilepsy, and is a theoretical region (styled as "epileptogenic zone").[43] (3.) And, while it makes the most sense based on the word's etymology, the most recent and least common usage is: The tissue that gives rise to the patient's epilepsy.[44] An example of this latter definition might be Bruton's "dual" or "double" pathology,[45] where one discharging lesion kindles the hippocampus over time (e.g., a tumor or cavernoma). It is important to understand how the term is used in the book or article being read, and the term should be clearly defined whenever it is used. The first definition is most used in the context of the SEEG and, along with the lesional and irritative zones or networks should be clearly documented at the end of an SEEG exploration. As will be further described below, in SEEG these are not theoretical concepts but are based on the SEEG signal and should be described topographically and in relation to networks when possible.

*Ictal Transition* versus *Ictal (Seizure) Onset*—It is often difficult to identify exactly where a seizure starts. For example, increasingly prominent bursts of fast activity may appear riding upon discharges which evolve before low-voltage fast activity appears. These discharges are commonly similar to interictal discharges. The question about whether a seizure has occurred is more important than the time of precise onset. It typically makes more sense to identify a period of ictal transition—the time over which findings that may be similar to interictal abnormalities evolve into a seizure, and where these appear causally related to the following seizure.[46] Generally, in SEEG, it is more helpful to think about the ictal transition and commonly preceding ictal preparation. Seizure onset can be appropriate when the ictal transition is sharp and clear.

*Ictal Preparation ("pre-ictal" phase)* is the period preceding or overlapping with the ictal transition, which is typically similar to interictal epileptiform abnormalities but is reproducibly and convincingly causally related to the ictal transition. For example, repetitive spiking might always be seen before the ictal transition in a particular electrode.

*Anatomo-Electroclinical Correlation*—this concept is at the heart of SEEG methodology and refers to the interpretation method of SEEG.[15,47,48] One must correlate the anatomical substrates of the seizure with the electrophysiological pattern and clinical manifestations throughout each part of the seizure. The missing yet critical piece of information from this triumvirate of anatomy, EEG and clinical semiology is the pathophysiology. Electrophysiology patterns and clinical manifestations are determined by the precise large-scale, local and microscopic circuits involved in the seizure. The involvement of these circuits is in turn determined by the underlying pathology and connectivity. In many SEEG patients, the pathology is unclear. Even when the etiology is known, the way that this gives rise to seizures and affects cortical microcircuits is often unclear. Similarly, the connectivity of the human forebrain is incompletely understood, as is how pathology modifies this connectivity. Modern clinical and fundamental research in epilepsy should address these questions to allow clearer anatomopathological electroclinical correlations in the future. This incomplete knowledge leaves some unaccounted variability in seizure onsets, as will become clear below where we discuss the electrographic patterns of seizures.

*Subdural* Versus *SEEG Concepts of the Symptomatogenic Zone, Irritative Zone, Lesional Zone, Ictal Onset Zone*—these concepts have also been defined in a more theoretical way in the context of subdural recording, as developed and popularized by Rosenow and Luders.[49] While each has a clear definition, the concepts of symptomatogenic and ictal onset zones do not fit as well with the SEEG method and approach.[50] One of the main reasons in each case is that symptoms/signs, seizure triggering, and seizure onset are all conceived as network phenomena in SEEG, rather than being foci. In Rosenow and Luder's schema, the *symptomatogenic zone* is conceived of as a localized area that gives rise to the symptom(s) characteristic of the patient's seizure. This has some limitations: In SEEG, the clinical correlation unfolds over time, so the area of the symptom generation migrates. Secondly, in SEEG, the presumption is that network activity (i.e., across a group of connected structures) is modified, not a single focus. Additionally, the seizure may be asymptomatic at onset. Finally, clinical and subjective manifestations differ in correlation with ictal electrophysiology according to not only spatial (anatomic) but also temporal features of epileptic discharge (see below).[50] A common example of all three concerns: while the symptoms of a somatosensory aura may be localized to a somatosensory "symptomatic zone", it can be that the high-frequency activity in the motor cortex does not result in a movement but drives the somatosensory cortex to produce a somatosensory symptom.

The *irritative zone* term is used on both SEEG and in subdural recording and is defined as the area that demonstrates interictal abnormalities. This may be linked to the regions that produce the seizure or give rise to the process of epileptogenesis itself. Further complicating matters, while the term "irritable cortex" is circular (on scalp EEG the cortex can be said to be irritable because of interictal discharges, and that it has interictal discharges because it is irritable without any further useful conceptual information being supplied), it is often used to refer to any cortex where interictal discharges are noted. In SEEG, this is operationalized by documentation of the regions or networks in which interictal discharges occur.[42] The primary irritative zone defines the spikes located in the epileptogenic network, and the secondary are those outside—these can only be defined once seizures are recorded.[51]

The *Lesional Zone* is electrophysiologically determined in SEEG, particularly by the presence of continuous or sub-continuous slowing,[42] not to be confused with a radiologic lesion. This term was first defined in SEEG in the setting of tumors. In contrast, Rosenow and Lüders defined the "epileptogenic lesion" as hypothesized or actual tissue pathology and best identified by radiologic findings.[49] This would include areas or networks that show pathologic slowing or interictal discharges. This can, again, often be a network rather than a discrete zone. It is important to note that the lesional zone often is distinct from, or extends beyond, an area of imaging abnormality.

Finally, the *Ictal Onset Zone* can often be more than one discrete area of cortex and refers to where one can see the point at which clear evolution of the seizure commences. The terms *ictal onset* as a point in time, and either *early ictal network* or *ictal onset network* may be preferred. In SEEG it is important to describe the electrophysiology (with topography and clinical accompaniments) of seizure onset, rather than describing this as an anatomical zone alone.

## The Normal Intracranial EEG Background

The normal intracranial EEG background was first described in the era of Jasper and Penfield from intraoperative recordings from the pial surface.[52] The anterior-posterior gradient evident on scalp EEG recording was redemonstrated in these studies: they described a preponderance of beta activity anterior to the central sulcus, with posterior alpha activity that increased in voltage as electrode recording approached the occipital cortex. Though these studies were performed solely by visual analysis, more recent intracranial data, which allows for frequency analysis and improved anatomical resolution, has generally substantiated the anterior-posterior gradient of frequency and amplitude.

While there is at least one comprehensive atlas of subdural EEG electrophysiological findings,[53] there is not yet a comprehensive atlas of intracranial findings on SEEG. There is ongoing work in this area and there are descriptions of background frequencies by brain region. Frauscher and colleagues collected data from patients undergoing intracranial EEG across three surgical centers,[54] most of which had depth electrodes. In wakefulness, the posterior dominant rhythm correlated with a robust alpha peak in the occipital lobe; a less prominent alpha peak was seen in the parietal lobe, which also exhibited an additional beta band. Higher beta and gamma bands were more anteriorly found in the frontal lobe (Fig. 5.2). Wang and colleagues found an additional tendency toward higher frequencies in the medial cortices.[55]

Perhaps of particular importance in epilepsy patients, intracranial data has allowed for isolation of the medial temporal structures from lateral neocortex. Jasper and Penfield described 14–16 Hz activity overriding polymorphic slow waves from electrodes placed intraoperatively on the basal temporal surface.[52] A modest $<3$ Hz delta peak seen by Frauscher and colleagues was in agreement with these slow-wave findings when analyzing the temporal lobe in its entirety, though they found the most significant peak to be

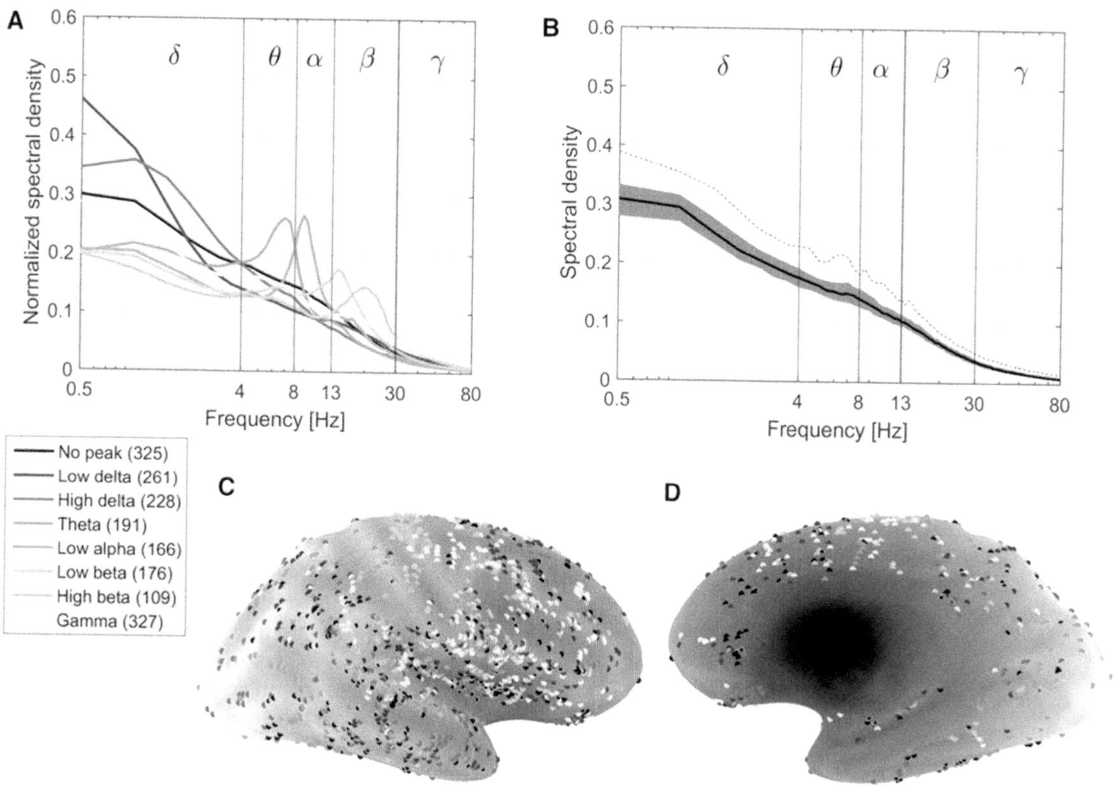


FIG. 5.2 **Unsupervised Classification of Channels and No-peak Set.** (A) Median normalized spectral density of the eight different groups obtained by the classification. Channels with delta or gamma activity usually do not show sustained rhythms (no peaks) but simply an increase in the low or high-frequency activity. (B) The spectral density of the no-peak set is derived from the group of channels with no peak in their spectrum. (C and D) Distribution of the groups in the inflated cortex (lateral and mesial views). Even though the frequency resolution of this unsupervised classification is poor, the figure gives a rough global idea of the distribution of rhythms in the brain. It shows a posterior-to-anterior gradient of increasing frequencies. (Reproduced with permission from Frauscher et al. (permission pending).[56])

rather in the low alpha range.[54] However, when analyzed in isolation, the hippocampus and amygdala lacked this higher frequency peak: both exhibited significant delta, with an additional low theta band seen only in the amygdala recordings.

Despite a general redemonstration of the anterior-posterior gradient as above, SEEG recordings have less consistent polarity and amplitude than subdural and scalp data, as described above. This is understood when considering the increased variability of distance and orientation between a source and its recording allowed by the implantation of depth electrodes versus scalp and subdural placement. Normal EEG features are more difficult to recognize and, at times, may be incorrectly identified as pathological. For this reason, understanding the precise anatomical location of all contacts is critical.

A hallmark of normal N2 sleep, sleep spindles are seen independently in regions throughout the brain on intracranial studies, though, as could be expected, are most prevalent in the parietal and frontal lobes. Simultaneous scalp and intracranial electrode activity reveal significant asynchrony of intracranial spindle activity, in contrast to synchronous spindles seen concurrently in scalp EEG channels. In contrast to typical scalp EEG findings, intracranial recording of sleep spindle frequency is inconsistent between regions, with a tendency toward faster frequencies in the centroparietal region and hippocampus versus the occipital and basal temporal regions.[56]

Mak-McCully and colleagues found that K complexes also had variable distribution and could occur more focally than expected based on scalp data.[57] They were generated throughout the cortex, with a weak tendency toward an anterior-posterior direction of propagation. POSTS and vertex waves are other normal NREM sleep features; the former has been recorded only in the occipital lobe, and the latter is more broadly seen bilaterally in electrodes close to the midline central region. The waking correlate of POSTS—lambda waves—are also limited to the occipital lobe. Mu rhythm has been described across the entirety of the sensorimotor cortex and can be present at the temporoparietal junction.

## Interictal Abnormalities

It is important to note both non-epileptiform and epileptiform background abnormalities in SEEG, and report on both. A necessary prerequisite is, therefore, to understand expected background rhythms as described above. Given less clear and specific cutoff for normal background activity, it is often useful to compare to adjacent anatomically similar recordings or, perhaps more accurately, to compare to contralateral normal tissue correlate where possible.

### *Non-epileptiform background abnormalities*

Lesional tissue, whether evident on MRI or not, is nearly always sampled in SEEG study of an epilepsy. The hallmark of this tissue is continuous or near continuous focal slowing; in fact, this slowing is often used to define a "lesional zone," as opposed to an irritative or epileptogenic zone, with this concept first being used on the context of tumor surgery in the pre-MRI era.[42] This continuous slowing, often higher amplitude compared to adjacent electrodes due to the inverse relation of amplitude to frequency, is easier to appreciate than absence of normal background rhythms, another hallmark of the lesional zone. Normal sleep features, particularly spindles, are often absent or poorly formed. Lesional tissue may fail to organize a posterior dominant and mu rhythm in occipital and motor regions, respectively. Warren and colleagues showed that in patients with epilepsy, there was decreased synchrony of local field potentials between seizure generating brain and other brain regions, suggesting some functional uncoupling of the epileptogenic or lesional zones.[58]

### *Epileptiform abnormalities*

As in all aspects of stereo-EEG, interictal epileptiform abnormalities must be considered as part of a network, rather than discrete and independent points of data. One should avoid listing consecutive electrode sites containing these abnormalities, and instead describe the breadth and propagation of the network. Details including morphology, frequency and prevalence may provide more information than the presence or absence of a discharge alone.

Malinowska and colleagues described large interictal networks, confirmed on magnetoencephalography (MEG), which acted in synchrony. Upon closer inspection, a lead–in was evident in these cases, defined either as temporally preceding or frequently occurring independently of more remote sites.[59] This abnormal interictal network may or may not persist with the transition to ictus; the relationship between the irritative and epileptogenic zone is complex. Makhalova, Bartolomei, and colleagues quantified a spike index and epileptogenicity index (SI and EI) separately. They showed that while they more frequently overlapped, in a significant proportion of patients, EI and SI regions were dissociated.[60]

## Electrophysiology of Seizures

### *The ictal transition*

The transition from interictal to ictal background has been described in multiple ways. Early data supported differentiation into two groups: those with preictal spiking preceding onset of fast discharge, and those without. Bartolomei and coworkers described increased synchronicity of temporal lobe regions during this transition state in patients with temporal lobe epilepsy.[61] More recently, time frequency analysis has allowed for description of an "ictal fingerprint."[62] While this method employs a machine learning based classifier, it relies on three components that can be seen visually—preictal spiking, onset of fast activity, and suppression of the background rhythms—and fourth that can be appreciated with further signal processing: bands of fast activity that are non-harmonic (see below).

### *Common seizure onset patterns*

Several studies have examined distinct species of seizure onset electrophysiological patterns. A key study of 252 SEEG patients described eight patterns organized into three larger categories: low-voltage fast activity (LVFA), rhythmic slow spikes, and sinusoidal sharp activity (see Fig. 5.3).[63] Patterns were predictive of surgical outcomes: patients who lacked LVFA at seizure onset were less likely to achieve seizure freedom. Further, LVFA preceded by a burst of polyspikes at ictal onset predicted the highest chance of seizure freedom, in accord with the "ictal fingerprint."

### *Correlation of onset patterns with underlying pathology*

Multiple groups have found a tendency toward specific ictal onset patterns predicted by anatomical lesion

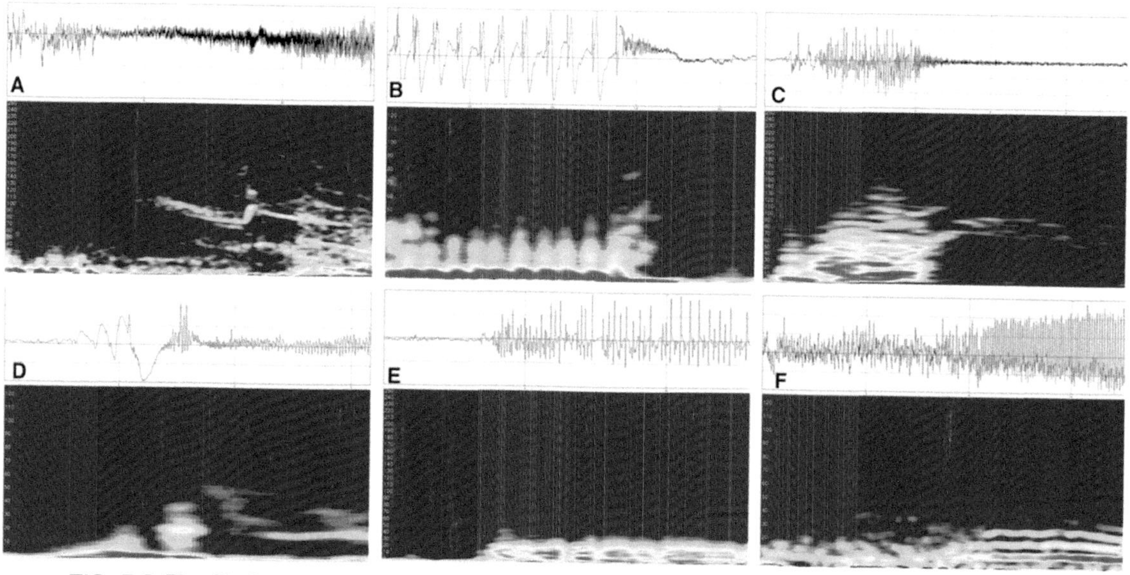


FIG. 5.3 **The Six Patterns of Seizure Onset According to the Time-Frequency Representation From SEEG Trace.** (A) Low-voltage fast activity (LVFA), (B) preictal spiking with rhythmic spikes of low frequency followed by LVFA. (C) burst of polyspikes of high frequency and amplitude followed by LVFA. (D) Slow wave or baseline shift followed by LVFA. (E) rhythmic spikes or spike-waves, at low frequency and with high amplitude. (F) theta/alpha sharp activity with progressive increasing amplitude. (Reproduced with permission from Lagarde et al. (permission pending).)

pathology of the epileptogenic zone. Lagarde and colleagues found that, of the eight seizure onset patterns they described, only focal cortical dysplasias had ictal onset with polyspikes preceding low-voltage fast activity.[64] Although Perucca evaluated the prevalence of individual onset pattern components separately (i.e., the presence of LVFA and the presence of polyspikes rather than polyspikes preceding LVFA), their data did not support that polyspikes were unique to FCDs, though they were significantly correlated.[65] Interestingly, they did find that a delta brush onset pattern was specific to two patients with FCDS. Giacomo described a statistically significant association of repetitive fast spike bursts with FCD types IIa and IIb.[66] Figs. 5.4 and 5.5, Table 5.1 summarize the onset patterns described by these three groups.

## Anatomo-electroclinical Correlations

SEEG allows for the direct documentation of seizure electrophysiology as it spreads across electrodes and contacts—thus characterizing the timing and spatial extent of a seizure within a sparsely sampled brain. There are hundreds of years—if including pathologic correlations—and thousands of papers examining the localization, to network or region, of brain functions. Seizures perturb these functional networks; ictal disturbances of the normal physiological networks are responsible for the production of seizure semiology. Thus there is an enormous and growing evidential basis for analyzing seizure semiology—the collection of symptoms and signs associated with a seizure and how these unfold in time. An area of ongoing study is the correlation between electrophysiological patterns and way in which function of a cortical region or network is altered. For example, repetitive spiking in the primary motor cortex has been shown to correlate with clonic jerks. Even in primary cortex, however, semiology has been shown to have frequency-dependent expression. Maillard reported a patient with positive and negative motor signs within the same ictal onset zone; when the predominant discharge band was in the alpha-beta range, tonic contraction occurred. When discharge exceeded approximately 45 Hz, there was instead a transient paralysis in the same muscle group.[68]

Given the relative complexity of the normal language network in comparison to primary cortical areas, it follows that disturbance of this network is also more complex. Generally, ictal language disorders are described in two categories: speech arrest and vocalization, though there are multiple subtypes within these categories. In a review by Chauvel and McGonigal,

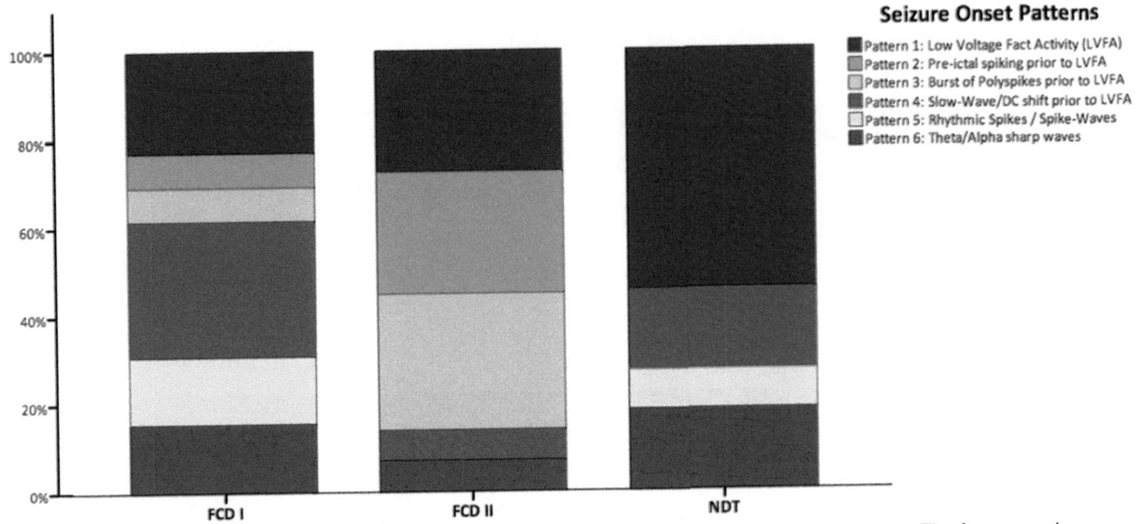


FIG. 5.4 **Frequency of the Seizure-onset Patterns According to the Histologic Types.** The frequency is expressed in percentage of the total number of patients for each histologic type. Patterns without fast activity (5–6) are almost always absent in patients with FCD type II.[65] (Reproduced with permission from Lagarde et al. (Permission pending).)

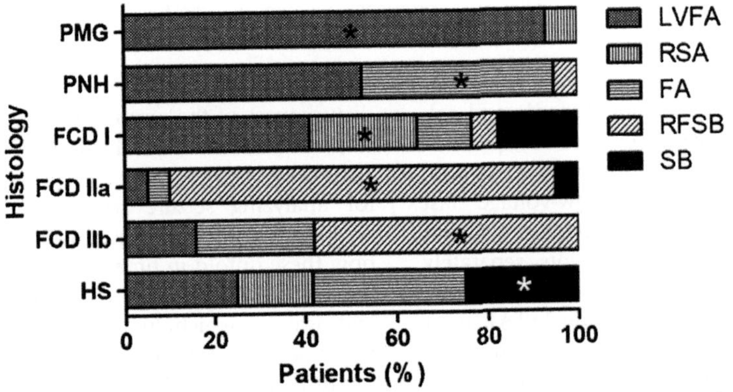


FIG. 5.5 **SEEG-SOZ Pattern Grouping with Respect to Their Histopathology.** *FA:* Fast activity; *FCD:* Focal cortical dysplasia; *HS:* Hippocampal sclerosis; *LVFA:* Low-voltage fast Activity; *PMG:* Polymicrogyria; *PNH:* Periventricular nodular heterotopia; *RFSB:* Repetitive fast spike bursts; *RSA:* Rhythmic sharp activity; *SB:* Slow burst of high amplitude polyspikes or spikes and wave complex. *The *P* value was obtained using the Fisher exact test. We considered statistically significant the *P* values obtained with the Fisher exact test and Bonferroni correction for multiple comparisons with a factor of 30 (6 histopathologies by five ictal patterns), corresponding to a significative adjusted alpha of $P < .00167$. (Reproduced with permission from Giacomo et al. (Permission pending).[67])

they summarized existing studies describing jargon aphasia in seizures emerging from the basal temporal language area, and verbal automatisms in non-dominant temporal epilepsies. Ictal aphasia was rarer and did not consistently correlate with a specific ictal onset zone but may have a particular network to electrophysiological pattern correlate.[67]

Synchrony between components of a network is also important for the emergence of semiology. For example, deja vu appears to be more common when stimulation of medial temporal lobe structures is associated with increased electrophysiological coherence among these structures; stimulation that did not result in increased synchrony were less likely to produce this

**TABLE 5.1**
**Distribution of Intracranial EEG Seizure-onset Patterns Across Different Epileptogenic Lesions**

| | EPILEPTOGENIC LESIONS, NUMBER OF SEIZURES (%) | | | | | |
|---|---|---|---|---|---|---|
| | **Mesial Temporal Atrophy/ Sclerosis** | **Focal Cortical Dysplasia** | **Periventricular Nodular Heterotopia** | **Tuberous Sclerosis Complex** | **Polymicrogyria** | **Cortical Atrophy** |
| Low-voltage fast activity | 4 (19) | 7 (58) | 4 (80) | 1 (33) | 3 (75) | 4 (50) |
| Low-frequency high-amplitude periodic spikes | 11 (52) | – | – | – | – | – |
| Sharp activity at <13 Hz | 4 (19) | – | 1 (20) | 1 (33) | 1 (25) | 1 (12.5) |
| Spike-and-wave activity | 3 (14) | 1 (8) | – | – | – | 1 (12.5) |
| Burst of polyspikes | – | 2 (17) | – | – | – | 1 (12.5) |
| Burst suppression | – | – | – | 1 (33) | – | 1 (12.5) |
| Delta brush | – | 2 (17) | – | – | – | – |

Values in cells indicate the number of seizures arising from a certain lesion that displays a specific pattern at onset (% of all seizures arising from that lesion).
Reproduced with permission from Perucca et al. (Permission pending).[68]

semiology.[69] Overall, enormous evidence from systems neuroscience that supports semiological analysis continues to emerge. However, the relationship between electrophysiological patterns, underlying pathology, and alterations in function is a lively area of ongoing research and must be considered when analyzing semiology.[50]

## ADVANCED TOPICS

### Signal Processing—Time-Frequency Analysis

The SEEG recording provides time-series data—a series of voltage readings over time. This data can be graphed as a time series, as in the typical review of clinical data, after the application of necessary (high pass and anti-aliasing) and potentially further filtering. In addition to this, we can look at data in the frequency domain, or as a time-frequency plot. An example of a review of the frequency domain would be to take a block of time series data, and then decompose this into its constituent frequencies using some transformation of the data. A typical example might be a Fourier transform, where the data is decomposed into a series of sine waves with a particular phase and amplitude. The amplitude of these sine waves can then be plotted by frequency, with frequency on one access and power on the vertical axis. We will examine different approaches and limitations to the Fourier transform and alternative methods below. Alternatively, this frequency domain information can be plotted over time by representing amplitude with a color or grayscale. In most instances, except for specialized applications, phase information from these transforms is discarded.

The key approaches to the spectral (frequency domain) analysis of SEEG are the Fourier series-related methods and wavelet transforms. A Fourier series is a set of harmonically related sine or cosine functions that, when added together, produce another function. The harmonic relationship refers to the numeric frequency interval between functions. It is not possible to completely model some arbitrary functions with a Fourier series. For example, one single square pulse could be approximated by a series of functions with specific amplitudes. Still, for a perfect square wave pulse an infinite Fourier series would only approach the modeled function. When the reverse approach is taken, the discrete Fourier transform, a given input function can be decomposed into a Fourier series. If one has an invariant oscillatory signal that has somewhat sinusoidal morphology, a reasonable Fourier series can be produced. When we consider EEG or SEEG signals, there are three difficulties. Firstly, some rhythms are not sinusoidal—for example, the typically comb-shaped posterior dominant rhythm. While there might be one oscillation with comb-shaped morphology at a given frequency, say 10 Hz, the attempt to express this as a Fourier series of sine waves will result in higher frequency harmonics in the time-frequency plot. The second limitation is that the Fourier series is best suited for a *stationary* input—one that does not vary over time. The human EEG and SEEG signal vary substantially at a subsecond level, with periods of more clear oscillation and periods that are aperiodic or have mixed frequencies. This difficulty can be partially surmounted by *windowing*, where the input function for the Fourier transform is broken up into short time-segments. When selecting a window length, the sampling rate must be considered so that there are enough cycles of the underlying oscillations to compute a Fourier series. Additionally, the number of functions in the Fourier series is determined by the number of samples in the window: When more points are provided, the frequency resolution is increased. The trade-off is that temporal resolution is decreased because of longer windows. Thirdly, when there are discontinuities, such as an epileptiform discharge, a broad increase in power across the Fourier series is noted.

A further refinement of the Fourier method is the use of various windows. Above, we implied the use of a rectangular window that would take all consecutive samples of a given period of time, and, so doing, introduce windowing artifacts.[27] When the input function for each of these windows is varying, two modifications can be made. Firstly, one can use overlapping windows that are partially averaged, and has the empiric effect of improved temporal resolution. In addition, and partly overcoming windowing artifact, one can use a window function that places more weight on the center of the window and less on the edges of the window. This is obtained by multiplying the input function over the time of interest with the window function. Another even more advanced approach is the multitaper method that computes a range of functions that are multiplied with the signal—tapers—and can thereby provide some statistical information about the confidence intervals for the spectral estimate.[70] Finally, the number of cycles of an oscillation in the input function will be higher for high frequencies and fewer, eventually less than one, for lower frequencies. Some of these limitations can be overcome by the use of wavelet transforms.

Wavelet analysis is better suited to signals with fluctuating frequency content—non-stationary signals—such as EEG. In particular, a one-dimensional (given a series of single values or voltage in EEG) and continuous (repeatedly applied to consecutive time blocks) wavelet is used for signal analysis in EEG. This can be plotted similarly to a spectrogram, with time on the x-axis and frequency on the y-axis, with amplitude conveyed by shading. In the case of wavelet transforms, this is called a *scalogram*. A "mother" wavelet is used and is a spindle-like oscillation with a particular number of cycles and frequency. Consequently, a wavelet at low frequencies is longer in duration than one at higher frequencies. Larger scales are longer in duration, and shorter scales of the wavelet function include higher frequencies. Conceptually, the value generated represents an estimate to which scales fit the input function. This method is suited to non-stationary neural signals and treats lower and higher frequencies in the same way but does not provide a stable estimate and estimates improve with multiple similar aligned events or trials. Given the very short duration of smaller scales, the wavelet transform has better time resolution for high-frequency activity and can better represent the precise timing of varied frequency components of the signal. In addition, artifactual harmonics produced by non-sinusoidal oscillations are not present. These advantages are especially useful when examining seizure onset. These and other methods have been reviewed, including comparison to a more recent methods.[71]

## Examining High-Frequency Components of the SEEG Signal

It is important to consider higher frequency components of the SEEG signal. While it has been argued that sampling or resampling intracranial EEG at a low frequency such as 100 Hz does not substantially impact conventional clinical interpretation,[18] some features of intracranial EEG require higher sampling rates, as described above. Raw conventional review of data does not readily enable the appreciation of high-frequency components, leading to the above conclusion. Given the approximately 1/f properties of the intracranial signal,[22,23] high frequency components can be of low amplitude and hard to appreciate during clinical review. When using high pass filters to examine these higher frequencies, interictal discharges cause Gibbs phenomenon or filter ringing that can be misinterpreted as ripples or high-frequency oscillations.[29] Recognition of low-voltage fast activity and high frequency oscillations (HFOs) are important in determining areas of seizure onset, and, in the case of HFOs, broader epileptogenicity.

When considering fast components of the interictal intracranial signal, frequencies in the 80–500 Hz range are relevant, requiring sampling at 2 kS/second or above. Such high-frequency oscillations (HFO) were noted during clinical SEEG, subdural recordings and a pre-clinical model at seizure onset,[72–74] particularly at 250–500 Hz (fast or pathologic ripples), forming a spectrum with physiologic ripples at 80–250 Hz. Further characterization of interictal HFO in human macroelectrodes recordings launched many studies of HFO in human epilepsy.[75–77] This topic has been extensively reviewed,[20,78] subject to meta-analysis,[79] and with a recent consensus statement on the recording and detection of ripples.[19] This continues as an active area of research. Overall, studies show that fast ripples have some diagnostic value in determining the region of cortex that can be excised to provide a good surgical outcome. However, predictivity may not be practically increased in comparison to spikes alone.[80] One common limitation is that HFO can only be recorded where electrodes are placed, as with the seizure onset: If the pre-implantation hypotheses are incorrect and given that sampling is sparse, HFOs may be found but may not indicate the full extent of the epileptogenic network. Recently, it has been shown that the combination of fast ripples with, or the use of ictal signal characteristics predicts better outcomes that the use of interictal fast ripples/HFO alone.[60] Key information is added by examining the propagation of seizures over time, with the possibility of anatomo-electroclinical correlation and determination of the early ictal network. The difficulty of detecting and analyzing a plethora of HFO events has limited the practicality of wide adoption of this method in analyzing intracranial EEG.

While there are a variety of seizure onset patterns, a key type of seizure onset includes low-voltage fast activity, as described above. Spectral analysis of seizure onsets, using the "ictal fingerprint,"[62,81] and "epileptogenicity index" methods,[60,82] can help identify key epileptogenic tissue. The former depends on machine learning classification of ictal onset wavelet transforms, with the limitation that it focuses on low-voltage fast onset only. The index method is relative, identifying the area of fastest activity, with respect to time from onset, again in the setting of low-voltage fast onset seizures. These methods are more practical for clinical use because they depend on examining the early ictal period alone. Some commercial EEG software provides spectrograms or scalograms that can be helpful but do not fully implement these approaches. An important question for SEEG practitioners is whether the standard of care should be to employ these methods, or at a minimum, to examine the time-frequency plots of channels involved in seizure onset. If this is the case, we believe sampling at a rate sufficient to capture high frequency gamma activity is necessary, at least 500 S/second.

In the case of all analytic methods, the most critical question is whether electrodes have been placed to truly sample the epileptogenic networks and normal margins for resection planning. Examination of the intracranial literature reveals frequent cases with imperfect sampling, highlighting the importance of careful semiology analysis in relation to continually evolving knowledge of cortical functional organization and connectivity, as well as integration of this information with data from other imperfect methods such as neuropsychological testing, MRI, scalp EEG, PET, SPECT, and MEG. It is important to note that the analysis of the SEEG signal can be unhelpful or even misleading in the case of poor implantation planning and hypotheses.

## Unit Recording and Special Electrodes

The recording of single neurons or the activity of several neurons—respectively *unit* or *multi-unit* activity—has become more common in SEEG. As far as we are aware, these methods are not yet used for clinical decision-making. Three main methods are available to achieve this: Microwires, microcontacts, and tetrodes. Firstly, Behnke-Fried microwire electrodes typically include nine ~38-micron microwires that extend beyond the terminal end of the electrode.[83,84] Spike sorting can typically be performed despite the uncertain relationship between microwire tips.[85,86] The major clinical concern with these electrodes is the absence of a terminal clinical macrocontact. While this likely does not prevent sampling of the field potential of seizure onset in adjacent contacts, the presence of microwires in the terminal gray matter of the trajectory and the absence of a clinical contact means that stimulation—typically a standard of care in SEEG—is not possible in medial cortices. These electrodes are often used in the temporal lobe, resulting in some gray matter (often the entorhinal cortex or parahippocampal gyrus) that cannot be stimulated for network exploration or habitual seizure reproduction. Implanting the microwires in still less medial structures (e.g., hippocampus vs. entorhinal cortex) means that the terminal macrocontact may not be in the "listening zone" of the most medial cortices. As an example, this can be problematic given the heterogeneity of medial temporal lobe epilepsy,[87,88] where it is important to include or exclude the medial cortices in the early ictal network. This has become increasing important with the use of less invasive methods of surgical treatment such as radiofrequency and laser ablation. We also know that memory outcomes are improved with sparing of medial cortices from primate studies and human epilepsy surgery experience.[89–91] In addition, the difference in electrode diameter and contact surface area compared with other implanted electrodes results in a different safety limit for stimulation as well as threshold for stimulation effect at a particular charge density—the neurologist performing stimulation should take this into account.

Tetrodes have been the most widely used approach for studying single units in non-human research settings. Four microwires are glued or twisted and annealed together, with wire diameters in pre-clinical studies of ~14 microns.[92] The fixed geometry of the electrodes enables the recording of a single cell on each wire. Spike sorting is based broadly on the morphology and amplitude of the four wires and enables reliable sorting of single units. This has recently become available in otherwise typical SEEG electrodes.[93] Tungsten is used for its electrophysiological properties and rigidity. These tetrodes are deployed after implantation from a depth electrode that therefore has a terminal contact as well as the same diameter (0.8 mm) as other depth electrodes, overcoming safety limit disparities, and enabling stimulation of medial terminal gray matter.

Other electrode types are becoming increasingly popular and useful preclinically, including silicon substrate electrodes with large numbers of contacts (e.g., silicon probes and Neuropixel).[94] Still, these cannot serve conventional clinical purposes, for LFP recording or stimulation, and can only be used in limited settings given some risk of bleeding and breakage of a device that does not meet any current clinical need. SEEG electrodes with smaller contacts and shorter inter-contact spacers, or with microcontacts between macrocontacts, have also been used.

### Stimulation and Stimulus Artifacts

As mentioned above, electrical stimulation is a core part of intracranial exploration in SEEG. While the approach to stimulation is beyond the scope of this chapter, it is worth briefly reviewing the interpretation of consequent electrophysiological signals. Firstly, the main types of clinical stimulation in SEEG are low-frequency, often 1 Hz, and higher-frequency stimulation, often 50 Hz.[47,95] Both are used to examine function, as well as to elicit discharges and seizures. In both cases, stimulus pulses produce a stimulation artifact and can potentially saturate the amplifier. After-discharges—epileptiform discharges or runs following stimulation—may be noted. Of note, these are typically interpreted in SEEG as a failure to mount a seizure from the stimulated region, rather than used to directly guide surgery.[96] Cortico-cortical evoked potentials can also be studied in the context of averaged—typically at least 20 trials—low frequency (so called single pulse) stimulation. The evoked potentials occur about 20 ms after stimulus onset,[97,98] and thus likely represent oligosynaptic responses. It is not possible to infer direct connectivity using this approach, and the clinical use of these to determine relevant functional connectivity and seizure propagation is in development. Stimulation methods in SEEG are described in other chapters in this book.

### The Future of SEEG

Much remains to be discovered. SEEG draws upon the systems neuroscience of functional networks—a field that continues to evolve. The analysis of semiology is also therefore evolving, as is our understanding of seizure initiation and propagation, particularly at a cellular level. Electroclinical correlations are still being described and will certainly change as new signal processing methods and electrode technologies are developed. While the approach to SEEG remains similar to its conception in the 1960s, technological improvements and further observations ensure continued evolution of the method with accumulation of knowledge.

## CONCLUSIONS

The SEEG intracranial field potential signal is a core component of the triad of anatomo-electroclinical correlation, and the approach to this method continues to develop alongside our knowledge of clinical semiology and the anatomy of the human forebrain. We propose that stereoelectroencephalography is presently the best way to evaluate a clear anatomical network hypothesis generated from careful consideration of high-quality phase I and related data. Given sparse sampling and the small local fields that are recorded with SEEG, this distinct and complementary method to scalp EEG, needs to be interpreted in the context of its underlying biology and is only as useful as the hypotheses informing implantation. There are numerous areas of active research, and the SEEG method is far from solidified. Advancement is ongoing for electrode design, signal processing, and the understanding of cortical functional organization, all with the goal to better define the anatomo-electroclinical correlation. Semiological manifestations are of particular clinical interest: There is a complex interplay between the normal physiological network, its interruption by interictal abnormalities, and the transition from interictal signal to unstable, rapidly change, and propagating seizure. Making this even more complex is the way in which these ongoing physiological shifts affect behavior and subjective experience in patients with individualized sparse implantations. The wellspring of SEEG is full and rich for informing our understanding of the functional organization of the human brain.

## REFERENCES


1. Fritsch G, Hitzig E. Electric excitability of the cerebrum (Uber die elektrische Erregbarkeit des Grosshirns). *Epilepsy Behav.* 2009;15(2):123–130. https://doi.org/10.1016/j.yebeh.2009.03.001.
2. Ferrier D. *The Localisation of Cerebral Disease*. Smith, Elder; 1878.
3. Caton R. The electric currents of the brain. *Br Med J.* 1875; 2(765):278.
4. Berger H. *On the Electroencephalogram of Man: Fourteen Original Reports on the Human Electroencephalogram*. Elsevier; 1969.
5. Adrian ED. Olfactory reactions in the brain of the hedgehog. *J Physiol.* 1942;100(4):459–473.
6. Kuhlo W, Lehmann D. Experience during the onset of sleep and its neuropohysiological correlates. *Arch fur Psychiatr Nervenkrankh.* 1964;205(6):687–716. https://doi.org/10.1007/bf00344881.
7. York GK, Steinberg DA. Hughlings jackson's neurological ideas. *Brain.* 2011;134:3106–3113.
8. Gibbs FA, Gibbs EL. *Atlas of Electroencephalography*. Lew A. Cummings; 1941.
9. Zottoli SJ. The origins of the grass foundation. *Biol Bull.* 2001;201(2):218–226. https://doi.org/10.2307/1543336.
10. Tan TC, Black PMcL. *The Contributions of Otfrid Foerster (1873–1941) to Neurology and Neurosurgery*; 2001. https://journals.lww.com/neurosurgery/Fulltext/2001/11000/The_Contributions_of_Otfrid_Foerster__1873_1941_.38.aspx. Accessed February 6, 2024.
11. Vannemreddy P, Stone JL, Vannemreddy S, Slavin KV. Psychomotor seizures, Penfield, Gibbs, Bailey and the development of anterior temporal lobectomy: a historical vignette. *Ann Indian Acad Neurol.* 2010;13(2):103–107. https://doi.org/10.4103/0972-2327.64630.
12. Almeida AN, Martinez V, Feindel W. The first case of invasive EEG monitoring for the surgical treatment of epilepsy: historical significance and context. *Epilepsia.* 2005;46(7): 1082–1085. https://doi.org/10.1111/j.1528-1167.2005.66404.x.
13. Kahane P, Arzimanoglou A, Benabid AL, Chauvel P. Epilepsy surgery in France. In: Lüders H, ed. *Textbook of Epilepsy Surgery*. CRC Press; 2008:86–93. https://doi.org/10.3109/9780203091708-11.
14. Talairach J, Tournoux P. *Co-Planar Stereotaxic Atlas of the Human Brain: 3-D Proportional System: An Approach to Cerebral Imaging*. Thieme; 1988.
15. Bancaud J, Talairach J. *La Stereo-Electroencephalographie Dans l'Epilepsie*. 1st ed. Masson; 1965.
16. Gadot R, Korst G, Shofty B, Gavvala JR, Sheth SA. Thalamic stereoelectroencephalography in epilepsy surgery: a scoping literature review. *J Neurosurg.* 2022;137(5): 1210–1225. https://doi.org/10.3171/2022.1.jns212613.
17. Kahane P, Ryvlin P, Hoffmann D, Minotti L, Benabid AL. From hypothalamic hamartoma to cortex: what can be learnt from depth recordings and stimulation? *Epileptic Disord.* 2003;5(4):205–217.
18. Davis KA, Devries SP, Krieger A, et al. The effect of increased intracranial EEG sampling rates in clinical practice. *Clin Neurophysiol.* 2018;129(2):360–367. https://doi.org/10.1016/j.clinph.2017.10.039.
19. Liu AA, Henin S, Abbaspoor S, et al. A consensus statement on detection of hippocampal sharp wave ripples and differentiation from other fast oscillations. *Nat Commun.* 2022;13(1):6000. https://doi.org/10.1038/s41467-022-33536-x.
20. Frauscher B, Ellenrieder N von, Zelmann R, et al. High-frequency oscillations in the normal human brain. *Ann Neurol.* 2018;84(3):374–385. https://doi.org/10.1002/ana.25304.
21. Winter BB, Webster JG. Reduction of interference due to common mode voltage in biopotential amplifiers. *IEEE Trans Biomed Eng.* 1983;BME-30(1):58–62. https://doi.org/10.1109/tbme.1983.325167.
22. Jasper HH. Cortical excitatory state and variability in human brain rhythms. *Science.* 1936;83(2150):259–260. https://doi.org/10.1126/science.83.2150.259.
23. Pritchard WS. The brain in fractal time: 1/F-like power spectrum scaling of the human electroencephalogram. *Int J Neurosci.* 1992;66(1–2):119–129. https://doi.org/10.3109/00207459208999796.
24. Freeman W. *Mass Action in the Nervous System*. Academic Press; 1975.
25. Dickey AS, Alwaki A, Kheder A, Willie JT, Drane DL, Pedersen NP. The referential montage inadequately localizes corticocortical evoked potentials in stereoelectro encephalography. *J Clin Neurophysiol.* 2022;39(5): 412–418. https://doi.org/10.1097/wnp.0000000000000792.
26. Lee S, Issa NP, Rose S, et al. DC shifts, high frequency oscillations, ripples and fast ripples in relation to the seizure onset zone. *Seizure.* 2020;77:52–58. https://doi.org/10.1016/j.seizure.2019.05.001.
27. Drongelen W van. *Signal Processing for Neuroscientists*. 2nd ed. Academic Press; 2018.
28. Burgess RC. Chapter 4 Filtering of neurophysiologic signals. *Handb Clin Neurol.* 2019;160:51–65. https://doi.org/10.1016/b978-0-444-64032-1.00004-7.
29. Oppenheim AV, Willsky AS, Nawab H. *Signals and Systems*. 2nd ed. Prentice Hall; 1996.

30. Ray S, Crone NE, Niebur E, Franaszczuk PJ, Hsiao SS. Neural correlates of high-gamma oscillations (60-200 Hz) in macaque local field potentials and their potential implications in electrocorticography. *J Neurosci.* 2008;28(45): 11526–11536. https://doi.org/10.1523/jneurosci.2848-08.2008.
31. Ray S, Maunsell JHR. Different origins of gamma rhythm and high-gamma activity in macaque visual cortex. *PLoS Biol.* 2011;9(4):e1000610. https://doi.org/10.1371/journal.pbio.1000610.
32. Schevon CA, Tobochnik S, Eissa T, et al. Multiscale recordings reveal the dynamic spatial structure of human seizures. *Neurobiol Dis.* 2019;127:303–311. https://doi.org/10.1016/j.nbd.2019.03.015.
33. Gloor P. Neuronal generators and the problem of localization in electroencephalography: application of volume conductor theory to electroencephalography. *J Clin Neurophysiol.* 1985;2(4):327–354. https://doi.org/10.1097/00004691-198510000-00002.
34. Cooper R, Winter AL, Crow HJ, Walter WG. Comparison of subcortical, cortical and scalp activity using chronically indwelling electrodes in man. *Electroencephalogr Clin Neurophysiol.* 1965;18(3):217–228. https://doi.org/10.1016/0013-4694(65)90088-x.
35. McCarty MJ, Woolnough O, Mosher JC, Seymour J, Tandon N. The listening zone of human electrocorticographic field potential recordings. *eNeuro.* 2022;9(2). https://doi.org/10.1523/eneuro.0492-21.2022.
36. Elahian B, Lado NE, Mankin E, et al. Low-voltage fast seizures in humans begin with increased interneuron firing. *Ann Neurol.* 2017;84(4):588–600. https://doi.org/10.1002/ana.25325.
37. Yilmazer-Hanke DM. Amygdala. In: Mai JK, Paxinos G, eds. *The Human Central Nervous System.* 3rd ed. Elsevier; 2012:401–424.
38. Khoo HM, Hall JA, Dubeau F, et al. Technical aspects of SEEG and its interpretation in the delineation of the epileptogenic zone. *Neurol Medico Chir.* 2020;60(12): 565–580. https://doi.org/10.2176/nmc.st.2020-0176.
39. Fuchs M, Wagner M, Kastner J. From ECoG near fields to EEG and MEG far fields. *Int Congr Ser.* 2007;1300: 125–128. https://doi.org/10.1016/j.ics.2006.12.077.
40. Sporns O, Tononi G, Kötter R. The human connectome: a structural description of the human brain. *PLoS Comput Biol.* 2005;1(4):e42. https://doi.org/10.1371/journal.pcbi.0010042.
41. Bartolomei F, Lagarde S, Wendling F, et al. Defining epileptogenic networks: contribution of SEEG and signal analysis. *Epilepsia.* 2017;58(7):1131–1147. https://doi.org/10.1111/epi.13791.
42. Talairach J, Bancaud J. Lesion, "irritative" zone and epileptogenic focus. *Stereotact Funct Neurosurg.* 1966;27(1–3): 91–94. https://doi.org/10.1159/000103937.
43. Lüders H, Engel J, Munari C. General principles. In: Engel J, ed. *Surgical Treatment of the Epilepsies.* 2nd ed. Raven Press; 1993:137–153.
44. Engel J. *Seizures and Epilepsy.* 2nd ed. Oxford University Press; 2012.
45. Bruton CJ. *The Neuropathology of Temporal Lobe Epilepsy.* Oxford University Press; 1988.
46. Wendling F, Hernandez A, Bellanger JJ, Chauvel P, Bartolomei F. Interictal to ictal transition in human temporal lobe epilepsy: insights from a computational model of intracerebral EEG. *J Clin Neurophysiol.* 2005;22(5): 343–356.
47. Isnard J, Taussig D, Bartolomei F, et al. French guidelines on stereoelectroencephalography (SEEG). *Neurophysiol Clin.* 2018;48(1):5–13. https://doi.org/10.1016/j.neucli.2017.11.005.
48. Chauvel P, Rheims S, McGonigal A, Kahane P. French guidelines on stereoelectroencephalography (SEEG): editorial comment. *Neurophysiol Clin.* 2018;48(1):1–3. https://doi.org/10.1016/j.neucli.2017.12.001.
49. Rosenow F, Lüders H. Presurgical evaluation of epilepsy. *Brain.* 2001;124(9):1683–1700. https://doi.org/10.1093/brain/124.9.1683.
50. McGonigal A, Bartolomei F, Chauvel P. On seizure semiology. *Epilepsia.* 2021;62(9):2019–2035. https://doi.org/10.1111/epi.16994.
51. Chauvel P, Gonzalez-Martinez J, Bulacio J. Presurgical intracranial investigations in epilepsy surgery. *Handb Clin Neurol.* 2019;161:45–71. https://doi.org/10.1016/b978-0-444-64142-7.00040-0.
52. Jasper H, Penfield W. Electrocorticograms in man: effect of voluntary movement upon the electrical activity of the precentral gyrus. *Arch für Psychiatr Nervenkrankh.* 1949; 183(1–2):163–174. https://doi.org/10.1007/bf01062488.
53. Sperling MR. Intracranial electroencephalography. In: Sperling MR, Clancy RR, eds. *Atlas of Electroencephalography.* Vol. 3. Elsevier; 1993.
54. Frauscher B, Ellenrieder N von, Zelmann R, et al. Atlas of the normal intracranial electroencephalogram: neurophysiological awake activity in different cortical areas. *Brain.* 2018;141(4):1130–1144. https://doi.org/10.1093/brain/awy035.
55. Wang HE, Scholly J, Triebkorn P, et al. VEP atlas: an anatomic and functional human brain atlas dedicated to epilepsy patients. *J Neurosci Methods.* 2021;348:108983. https://doi.org/10.1016/j.jneumeth.2020.108983.
56. Frauscher B, Ellenrieder N von, Ferrari-Marinho T, avoli M, Dubeau F, Gotman J. Facilitation of epileptic activity during sleep is mediated by high amplitude slow waves. *Brain.* 2015;138(Pt 6):1629–1641. https://doi.org/10.1093/brain/awv073.
57. Mak-McCully RA, Deiss SR, Rosen BQ, et al. Synchronization of isolated downstates (K-complexes) may be caused by cortically-induced disruption of thalamic spindling. *PLoS Comput Biol.* 2014;10(9):e1003855. https://doi.org/10.1371/journal.pcbi.1003855.
58. Warren CP, Hu S, Stead M, Brinkmann BH, Bower MR, Worrell GA. Synchrony in normal and focal epileptic brain: the seizure onset zone is functionally disconnected. *J Neurophysiol.* 2010;104(6):3530–3539. https://doi.org/10.1152/jn.00368.2010.
59. Malinowska U, Badier J, Gavaret M, Bartolomei F, Chauvel P, Bénar C. Interictal networks in

magnetoencephalography. *Hum Brain Mapp*. 2014;35(6):2789–2805. https://doi.org/10.1002/hbm.22367.
60. Makhalova J, Madec T, Villalon SM, et al. The role of quantitative markers in surgical prognostication after stereoelectroencephalography. *Ann Clin Transl Neurol*. 2023;10(11):2114–2126. https://doi.org/10.1002/acn3.51900.
61. Bartolomei F. Coherent neural activity and brain synchronization during seizure-induced loss of consciousness. *Arch Ital Biol*. 2012;150(2–3):164–171. https://doi.org/10.4449/aib.v150i2.1252.
62. Grinenko O, Li J, Mosher JC, et al. A fingerprint of the epileptogenic zone in human epilepsies. *Brain*. 2018;141(1):117–131. https://doi.org/10.1093/brain/awx306.
63. Lagarde S, Bonini F, McGonigal A, et al. Seizure-onset patterns in focal cortical dysplasia and neurodevelopmental tumors: relationship with surgical prognosis and neuropathologic subtypes. *Epilepsia*. 2016;57(9):1426–1435. https://doi.org/10.1111/epi.13464.
64. Lagarde S, Buzori S, Trébuchon A, et al. The repertoire of seizure onset patterns in human focal epilepsies: determinants and prognostic values. *Epilepsia*. 2019;60(1):85–95. https://doi.org/10.1111/epi.14604.
65. Perucca P, Dubeau F, Gotman J. Intracranial electroencephalographic seizure-onset patterns: effect of underlying pathology. *Brain*. 2014;137(Pt 1):183–196. https://doi.org/10.1093/brain/awt299.
66. Giacomo RD, Uribe-San-Martin R, Mai R, et al. Stereo-EEG ictal/interictal patterns and underlying pathologies. *Seizure*. 2019;72:54–60. https://doi.org/10.1016/j.seizure.2019.10.001.
67. Chauvel P, McGonigal A. Emergence of semiology in epileptic seizures. *Epilepsy Behav*. 2014;38:94–103. https://doi.org/10.1016/j.yebeh.2013.12.003.
68. Maillard L, Gavaret M, Régis J, Wendling F, Bartolomei F. Fast epileptic discharges associated with ictal negative motor phenomena. *Clin Neurophysiol*. 2014;125(12):2344–2348. https://doi.org/10.1016/j.clinph.2014.03.023.
69. Bartolomei F, Barbeau EJ, Nguyen T, et al. Rhinal-hippocampal interactions during déjà vu. *Clin Neurophysiol*. 2012;123(3):489–495. https://doi.org/10.1016/j.clinph.2011.08.012.
70. Babadi B, Brown EN. A review of multitaper spectral analysis. *IEEE Trans Biomed Eng*. 2014;61(5):1555–1564. https://doi.org/10.1109/tbme.2014.2311996.
71. Ks SC, Mishra A, Shirhatti V, Ray S. Comparison of matching pursuit algorithm with other signal processing techniques for computation of the time-frequency power spectrum of brain signals. *J Neurosci*. 2016;36(12):3399–3408. https://doi.org/10.1523/jneurosci.3633-15.2016.
72. Allen PJ, Fish DR, Smith SJM. Very high-frequency rhythmic activity during SEEG suppression in frontal lobe epilepsy. *Electroencephalogr Clin Neurophysiol*. 1992;82(2):155–159. https://doi.org/10.1016/0013-4694(92)90160-j.
73. Fisher RS, Webber WR, Lesser RP, Arroyo S, Uematsu S. High-frequency EEG activity at the start of seizures. *J Clin Neurophysiol*. 1992;9(3):441–448. https://doi.org/10.1097/00004691-199207010-00012.
74. Bragin A, Engel J, Wilson CL, Vizentin E, Mathern GW. Electrophysiologic analysis of a chronic seizure model after unilateral hippocampal KA injection. *Epilepsia*. 1999;40(9):1210–1221. https://doi.org/10.1111/j.1528-1157.1999.tb00849.x.
75. Jacobs J, Zelmann R, Jirsch J, Chander R, Dubeau CCF, Gotman J. High frequency oscillations (80–500 Hz) in the preictal period in patients with focal seizures. *Epilepsia*. 2009;50(7):1780–1792. https://doi.org/10.1111/j.1528-1167.2009.02067.x.
76. Jirsch JD, Urrestarazu E, LeVan P, Olivier A, Dubeau F, Gotman J. High-frequency oscillations during human focal seizures. *Brain*. 2006;129(6):1593–1608. https://doi.org/10.1093/brain/awl085.
77. Urrestarazu E, Jirsch JD, LeVan P, et al. High-frequency intracerebral EEG activity (100–500 Hz) following interictal spikes. *Epilepsia*. 2006;47(9):1465–1476. https://doi.org/10.1111/j.1528-1167.2006.00618.x.
78. Chen Z, Maturana MI, Burkitt AN, Cook MJ, Grayden DB. High-frequency oscillations in epilepsy: what have we learned and what needs to be addressed. *Neurology*. 2021;96(9):439–448. https://doi.org/10.1212/wnl.0000000000011465.
79. Wang Y, Xu J, Liu T, et al. Diagnostic value of high-frequency oscillations for the epileptogenic zone: a systematic review and meta-analysis. *Seizure*. 2022;99:82–90. https://doi.org/10.1016/j.seizure.2022.05.003.
80. Roehri N, Pizzo F, Lagarde S, et al. High-frequency oscillations are not better biomarkers of epileptogenic tissues than spikes. *Ann Neurol*. 2018;83(1):84–97. https://doi.org/10.1002/ana.25124.
81. Li J, Grinenko O, Mosher JC, Gonzalez-Martinez J, Leahy RM, Chauvel P. Learning to define an electrical biomarker of the epileptogenic zone. *Hum Brain Mapp*. 2020;41(2):429–441. https://doi.org/10.1002/hbm.24813.
82. Bartolomei F, Chauvel P, Wendling F. Epileptogenicity of brain structures in human temporal lobe epilepsy: a quantified study from intracerebral EEG. *Brain*. 2008;131(Pt 7):1818–1830. https://doi.org/10.1093/brain/awn111.
83. Fried I, MacDonald KA, Wilson CL. Single neuron activity in human Hippocampus and amygdala during recognition of faces and objects. *Neuron*. 1997;18(5):753–765. https://doi.org/10.1016/s0896-6273(00)80315-3.
84. Fried I, Wilson CL, Maidment NT, et al. Cerebral microdialysis combined with single-neuron and electroencephalographic recording in neurosurgical patients: technical note. *J Neurosurg*. 1999;91(4):697–705. https://doi.org/10.3171/jns.1999.91.4.0697.
85. Tankus A, Yeshurun Y, Fried I. An automatic measure for classifying clusters of suspected spikes into single cells versus multiunits. *J Neural Eng*. 2009;6(5):056001. https://doi.org/10.1088/1741-2560/6/5/056001.
86. Rutishauser U, Schuman EM, Mamelak AN. Online detection and sorting of extracellularly recorded action potentials in human medial temporal lobe recordings, in vivo.

*J Neurosci Methods.* 2006;154(1–2):204–224. https://doi.org/10.1016/j.jneumeth.2005.12.033.
87. Maillard L, Vignal JP, Gavaret M, et al. Semiologic and electrophysiologic correlations in temporal lobe seizure subtypes. *Epilepsia.* 2004;45(12):1590–1599. https://doi.org/10.1111/j.0013-9580.2004.09704.x.
88. Bartolomei F, Khalil M, Wendling F, et al. Entorhinal cortex involvement in human mesial temporal lobe epilepsy: an electrophysiologic and volumetric study. *Epilepsia.* 2005;46(5):677–687. https://doi.org/10.1111/j.1528-1167.2005.43804.x.
89. Zola-Morgan S, Squire LR, Ramus SJ. Severity of memory impairment in monkeys as a function of locus and extent of damage within the medial temporal lobe memory system. *Hippocampus.* 1994;4(4):483–495. https://doi.org/10.1002/hipo.450040410.
90. Liu A, Thesen T, Barr W, et al. Parahippocampal and entorhinal resection extent predicts verbal memory decline in an epilepsy surgery cohort. *J Cognit Neurosci.* 2017;29(5):869–880. https://doi.org/10.1162/jocn_a_01089.
91. Drane DL, Willie JT, Pedersen NP, et al. Superior verbal memory outcome after stereotactic laser amygdalohi ppocampotomy. *Front Neurol.* 2021;12:779495. https://doi.org/10.3389/fneur.2021.779495.
92. Gray CM, Maldonado PE, Wilson M, McNaughton B. Tetrodes markedly improve the reliability and yield of multiple single-unit isolation from multi-unit recordings in cat striate cortex. *J Neurosci Methods.* 1995;63(1–2):43–54. https://doi.org/10.1016/0165-0270(95)00085-2.
93. Despouy E, Curot J, Reddy L, et al. Recording local field potential and neuronal activity with tetrodes in epileptic patients. *J Neurosci Methods.* 2020;341:108759. https://doi.org/10.1016/j.jneumeth.2020.108759.
94. Jun JJ, Steinmetz NA, Siegle JH, et al. Fully integrated silicon probes for high-density recording of neural activity. *Nature.* 2017;551(7679):232–236. https://doi.org/10.1038/nature24636.
95. Trébuchon A, Chauvel P. Electrical stimulation for seizure induction and functional mapping in stereoelectroencephalography. *J Clin Neurophysiol.* 2016;33(6):511–521. https://doi.org/10.1097/wnp.0000000000000313.
96. Trebuchon A, Racila R, Cardinale F, et al. Electrical stimulation for seizure induction during SEEG exploration: a useful predictor of postoperative seizure recurrence? *J Neurol Neurosurg Psychiatry.* 2021;92(1):22–26. https://doi.org/10.1136/jnnp-2019-322469.
97. Prime D, Rowlands D, O'Keefe S, Dionisio S. Considerations in performing and analyzing the responses of cortico-cortical evoked potentials in stereo-EEG. *Epilepsia.* 2018;59(1):16–26. https://doi.org/10.1111/epi.13939.
98. Matsumoto R, Kunieda T, Nair D. Single pulse electrical stimulation to probe functional and pathological connectivity in epilepsy. *Seizure.* 2017;44:27–36. https://doi.org/10.1016/j.seizure.2016.11.003.

CHAPTER 6

# What Is Seizure Onset? Interictal, Preictal/Ictal Patterns, and the Epileptogenic Zone

THANDAR AUNG, MD, MS • PATRICK CHAUVEL, MD

## INTRODUCTION

The epileptogenic zone (EZ) concept arises from the stereoelectroencephalography (SEEG) method introduced by Talairach and Bancaud.[1,2] The term "EZ" was proposed by Bancaud and defined as "the regions of the brain involved in the primary organization of the ictal discharge", which refers to the cortical areas, not necessarily anatomically contiguous, bound together through an excessive synchronization at seizure onset and "early spread".[2] Thus, the concept of "network" in EZ has been introduced since 1965,[2] recognizing both spatial and temporal aspects of seizure dynamics. The EZ definition mentioned above is practical yet challenging as the term "primary organization" seems arbitrary, leading to difficulty in accurately delineating the EZ's boundaries. With the spread of the SEEG methodology to North America, where the subdural grid (SDG) intracranial (IcEEG) recording dominated, an additional definition of the EZ was introduced. The EZ was defined as "the area of cortex indispensable for generating seizures" and "total resection or disconnection is necessary and sufficient for seizure freedom", implying that the concept of EZ is a theoretical one.[3,4] Thus, the seizure onset zone (SOZ) was introduced as the "area of cortex from which clinical seizures are generated" as a "practical" counterpart of the EZ.[3] This new definition doesn't eliminate the challenge of accurately delineating the EZ's boundaries in SEEG. In fact, the interchangeable usage of the terms "EZ" and "SOZ" makes the fellow reader more muddled as the SOZ in SDG doesn't mean the same as the SOZ in the SEEG, as SDG and SEEG are two different methodologies.[5] This chapter aims to demonstrate the important interplay between the lesional zone (or network), based on the background activity in SEEG, the irritative zone (or network), based on the interictal epileptiform discharges (IEDs), and the EZ (or network) based on seizure onset structures. Please be mindful that the main concept of SEEG methodology is based on anatomo-clinico-electrical correlations. Due to the scope of our chapter, we will not delve deeper into this concept. In this chapter, we aim to illustrate that defining the SOZ as a specific temporal time point proves impractical within the framework of the SEEG methodology and to describe the importance of the spatiotemporal dynamics transition of the interictal phase to the ictal phase as the key to localizing the EZ in the SEEG methodology, together with the main concept being anatomo-clinico-electrical correlations.

## INTERICTAL SEEG ACTIVITIES

Before the era of SEEG and EZ concept, Penfield and Jasper used the concept of the epileptogenic lesion based on interictal spikes localization using intraoperative electrocorticogram (ECoG) together with intraoperative electrical cortical stimulation, in which ECoG's interictal epileptiform discharges (IEDs) extended far beyond the structural lesion in patients with tumors.[6] Jasper et al. reported a landmark paper on a strong correlation between the complete removal of IEDs guided by the ECoG and seizure freedom in patients with lesional epilepsy, but not in all the cases, illustrating that IEDs alone were insufficient to define an epileptic focus and IEDs could be seen to be more extensive than the epileptogenic lesions.[7,8] Thus, Jasper et al. concluded that not all the IEDs had the same significance in acute intraoperative ECoG recording. With further studies, the importance of the background activity was stressed in relation to the spikes. It was documented that the IEDs seen in abnormal cortical regions, defined based on abnormal background

The Fundamentals of Stereoelectroencephalography. https://doi.org/10.1016/B978-0-443-10877-8.00005-X

activity in ECoG, needed to be surgically treated, but not those IEDs seen at the variable distances from lesional borders, which were defined as transmitted or propagated IEDs.[8–10]

The concept is further advanced with the SEEG methodology, which allows subacute prolonged extra-operative recording of interictal and seizure activities. In the late 1950s, Bancaud and Talairach, equipped with the capacity to record seizures, documented for the first time recording of seizures using stereoelectroencephalography (SEEG). Bancaud introduced the concepts of the irritative zone (IZ) and lesional zone (LZ), emphasizing that abnormal interictal activities and lesions were not consistently colocalized with the epileptogenic zone (EZ) as a rule.[2,11,12] IZ is defined as cortical regions with increased cortical excitability indicated by the presence of spontaneous spikes or spike-wave activity.[11] LZ is defined as cortical regions of underlying cerebral dysfunction with or without structural anomaly characterized by the presence of continuous or sub-continuous slowing.[12] Subsequent studies have consistently substantiated that the IZ could be entirely colocalized, partially localized, or even independent of the EZ. Subsequently, IZ can further be divided into either primary IZ (confined within the EZ) or secondary IZ (extending beyond the EZ).[2,11,12] Notably, a meticulous analysis of IZ is crucial in SEEG analysis to estimate the dynamic changes of an IZ network or multiple IZ networks, thereby enhancing the accuracy in delineating and mapping the EZ.[5,13,14]

Before identifying IZ and LZ, it is important to recognize baseline physiological SEEG activity to define abnormality.[14] Distinct physiological rhythms are observed across distinct cortical regions of the brain. A multicenter ICEEG atlas (https://mni-open-ieegatlas.research.mcgill.ca) is available to reference neurophysiological awake activity in various cortical areas.[15] The significant differences in the spectral density distributions between different frequencies are noted across the different brain regions[15] (Fig. 6.1). Hence, it is crucial to emphasize the significance of electrode reconstruction. If the designated electrodes are positioned incorrectly, there is a risk of misinterpretation as pathological slowing originating from white matter SEEG activity.[5,16] As illustrated in Fig. 6.2, C′ mesial contacts (1–4) were initially targeted to the posterior hippocampus, but the SEEG activities in C′ one to four showed low amplitude delta and alpha activity similar to the C′ 4–10 mid-electrode contacts, which were not expected to be in the posterior hippocampus. Was it an abnormal lesional activity? In fact, the electrode anatomical reconstruction confirmed that electrode C′s mesial contacts were in the white matter outside the hippocampus (Fig. 6.2C). Thus, before concluding about the abnormality in SEEG analysis, one must understand the three-dimensional anatomical regions where the electrodes are in the individual brain. After the confirmation of electrode location, one needs to rule out the effect of anesthesia or sedation as the physiological SEEG signal can be mistaken as slowing if analysis and confirmation is made with a first few days. Thus, it is better to analyze and study at least 24–72 h following SEEG placement before considering the background activity as being abnormal.[5,15–19]

Regarding LZ, the relationship between the MRI lesional cortex and SEEG-defined lesional cortex needs to be well-defined, as the lesional zone defined by SEEG from neurophysiological data can be far more extensive than the structural lesion noted in the MRI. After confirming the abnormal background, one needs to rule out the physiological EEG activity as the physiological SEEG signal can be mistaken as a spiking activity.[5,15–19] Thus, extra caution is required in order to avoid overcalling the normal physiological activity or missing the abnormal spike activity. Also, one should keep in mind that physiological and pathological activities can co-exist in the same region.[5,15–19] Thus, the following step-by-step analysis is recommended before defining the lesional or irritative zone (Table 6.1). In elucidating the aforementioned practical observation, we present a case exemplified in Fig. 6.3. The SEEG exploration was conducted in a patient diagnosed with bilateral occipital epilepsy. Anticipated within this context were normal physiological activities, specifically lambda waves, given the placement of SEEG electrodes in the occipital cortices. During the side-to-side eye movement, lambda activities were noted to be co-occurring over the right and left occipital electrode contacts (right occipital (L) and left occipital (L′) mesial and lateral contacts) (Fig. 6.3A and C). Although the L and L′ were symmetrically placed, the activation of lambda activity was more pronounced over the left lateral occipital cortex (L′ and V′ electrodes) compared to the right occipital cortex (L and V electrodes) (Fig. 6.3C). Following the reduction of ASM, the emergence of polyspikes and sharp waves in the lateral occipital cortices (L and L′ lateral contacts) was observed (Fig. 6.3D and E). This underscores the imperative of a thorough analysis of SEEG data and emphasizes the need for vigilant scrutiny of dynamic changes in SEEG IED activities, particularly in response to modifications in factors such as alterations in ASM.

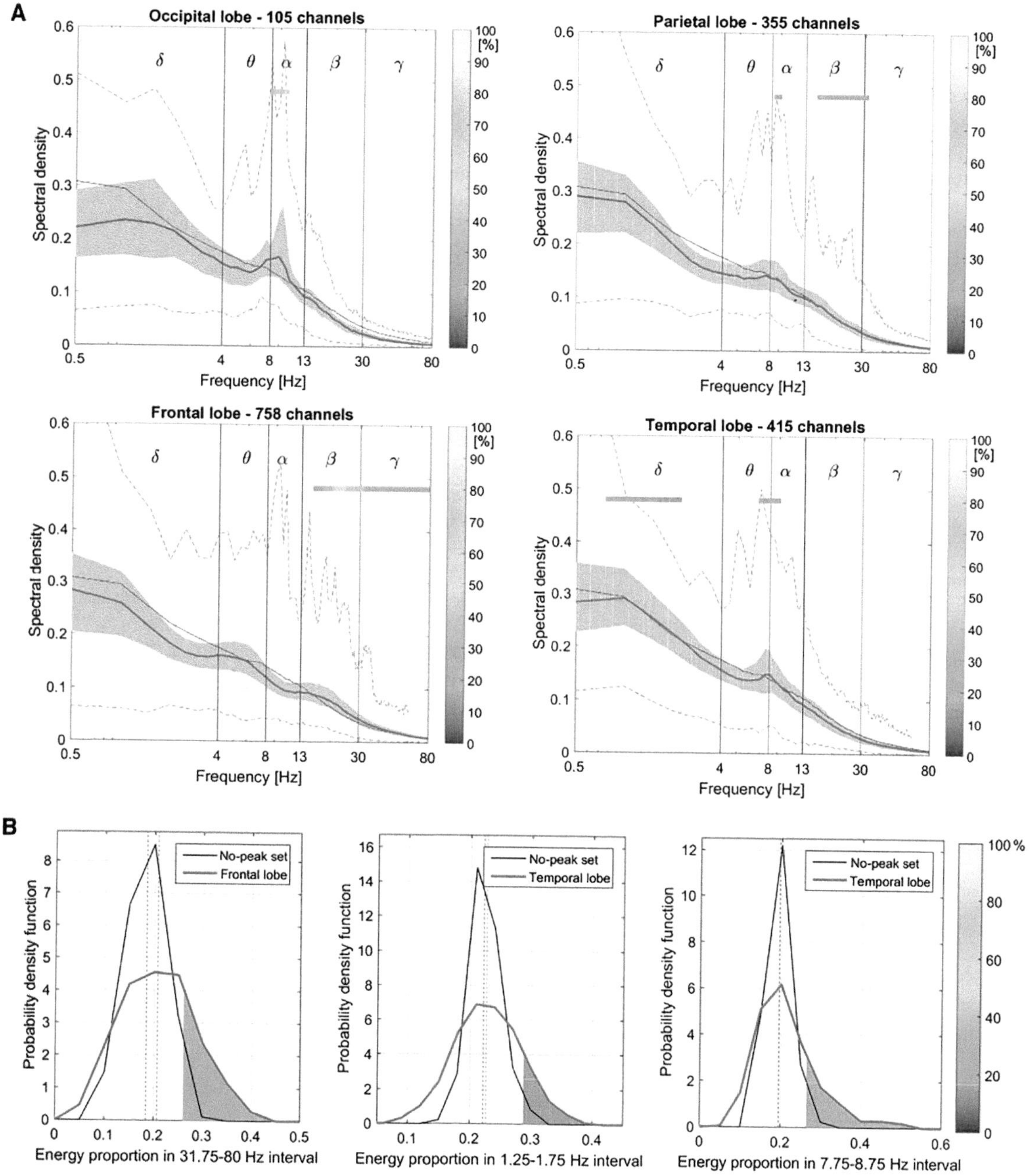


FIG.6.1 Lobar differences in EEG frequences. (A) Spectra of the different brain lobes in semi-logarithmic graph. The red line corresponds to the median spectral density of all the channels in the region. The 25 and 75 percentiles are indicated by the *pink shaded region*. The *broken red lines* show the upper and lower bounds of the spectral distribution at every frequency. The *thin black line* shows the median spectrum of the no-peak set used to determine the presence of peaks. *Vertical black lines* separate the common clinical frequency bands indicated by Greek letters. The colored horizontal segments in the *upper part* of each graph indicate the presence of peaks. If the segment is present, it indicates that the distribution of the channel spectral densities is significantly higher than the distribution of the no-peak set. The color of the *line* indicates the percentage of channels that have a significant deviation compared to the no-peak set at each frequency. (B) Illustration of differences not clearly visible in A. Each panel shows in *black* the distribution of the energy in the no-peak set

Thus, in summary, after the abnormal SEEG activities were confirmed, as illustrated in Fig. 6.3, one needs to identify interictal epileptiform discharges (IEDs) morphology and frequency, their prevalence or abundancy, their evolution over temporal distribution (i.e., occurrence earlier in the recording right after the SEEG implantation, occurrence during sleep stage changes, occurrence after medications changes, occurrence before or after seizures) and the evolution over spatial distribution (i.e., occurrence between different regions and in relation to each other) in order to map the IZ (or network (s)).[5,15,16,20]

Regarding morphology, a spectrum of interictal epileptiform discharges (IEDs) presenting diverse patterns is evident (Fig. 6.4). These patterns encompass (1) spikes, characterized by a large-amplitude rapid component lasting 50–100 ms, typically followed by a slow wave spanning 200–500 ms; (2) sharp waves, featuring a rapid component lasting between 100 and 300 ms; (3) bursts of spikes; (4) fast oscillations; and (5) repetitive, paroxysmal slow waves.[21–23] Various IEDs are known to be mediated by distinct neurobiological mechanisms, playing divergent roles in ictogenesis.[21,24] While the occurrence of different IED types in the same patients or regions is not uncommon, these distinct patterns hold clear diagnostic value. For instance, continuous high-frequency spikes and polyspikes strongly suggest Taylor-type II focal cortical dysplasia.[25] Therefore, the manifestation of IEDs can vary based on cortical regions, structural dysfunction, and electrode placement relative to the sources of epileptiform discharges. Amidst the diverse IEDs, the prevalence of fast activities, particularly high-frequency oscillation activities (HFOs 80–400 Hz), associated with the IEDs is of paramount significance. Such activities have been demonstrated to correlate with interictal biomarkers in specific types of focal epilepsy.[13,26] Additionally, Guth and colleagues demonstrated that IEDs with HFOs are prominent in the epileptogenic zone and exhibit a tendency to increase during the transition to seizure activity.[27] Moving beyond morphology and frequency, the signal amplitude in SEEG is contingent on the source orientation relative to the recording electrode. As such, amplitude lacks absolute significance; for example, amygdala spikes generally exhibit smaller amplitudes compared to hippocampal spikes (see also chapter in this book on The SEEG Signal). Moreover, the amplitude of spikes can vary based on regions of structural dysfunction, such as encephalomalacia.

Analyzing both temporal and spatial synchronization of interictal activities is vital to studying and differentiating primary from secondary IZ.[28] Topographical analysis of co-occurrence of interictal activities can help understand the IZ network.[29] In patients with mesial temporal lobe epilepsy, studies have confirmed that interictal spikes are reproducible subsets of co-activated mesial temporal structures. However, lateral temporal regions in most patients are involved only secondarily or with clonic discharges, representing interictal propagation.[23] A similar finding is also reported in neocortical epilepsies, with the interictal network overlapping with the ictal network.[30,31] In addition, it has been shown that IEDs networks' analysis can identify its most active generators, and its resection can lead to better postsurgical outcome.[32] Notably, the identification of multiple or extensive interictal networks can be indicative of the presence of multiple EZs.[33]

Thus, in conclusion, large varieties of IED patterns can be seen in a single patient or region, generated by distinct neurobiological mechanisms and pathologies, and have differing roles in ictogenesis.[34,35] Thus, it is imperative to analyze interictal activity autonomously, distinct from preictal and ictal activity, while recognizing their interdependence and inseparability. The precise interpretation of background activities and IEDs in SEEG recordings enables the discernment of the dynamic transition to ictal onset.

for the given frequency interval, and the *red line* shows the distribution in different brain regions (frontal lobe and temporal lobe). The *broken vertical lines* indicate the median value, and the colored area under the curve indicates the percentage of channels that has significantly higher power than the no-peak set in the corresponding frequency interval. The figure illustrates situations in which the test can find differences, not always obvious looking only at the median (in A). *Left*: Different position (mean, median) in the gamma band of the frontal lobe. *Middle*: Equal median but different dispersion (SD) in the delta band of the temporal lobe. *Right*: Equal median but asymmetric distribution (skewness) in the alpha band of the temporal lobe. (With permission from Frauscher B, Von Ellenrieder N et al. Atlas of the normal intracranial electroencephalogram: Neurophysiological awake activity in different cortical areas. Brain. 2018; 141(4):1130–1144. https://doi.org/10.1093/brain/awy035)

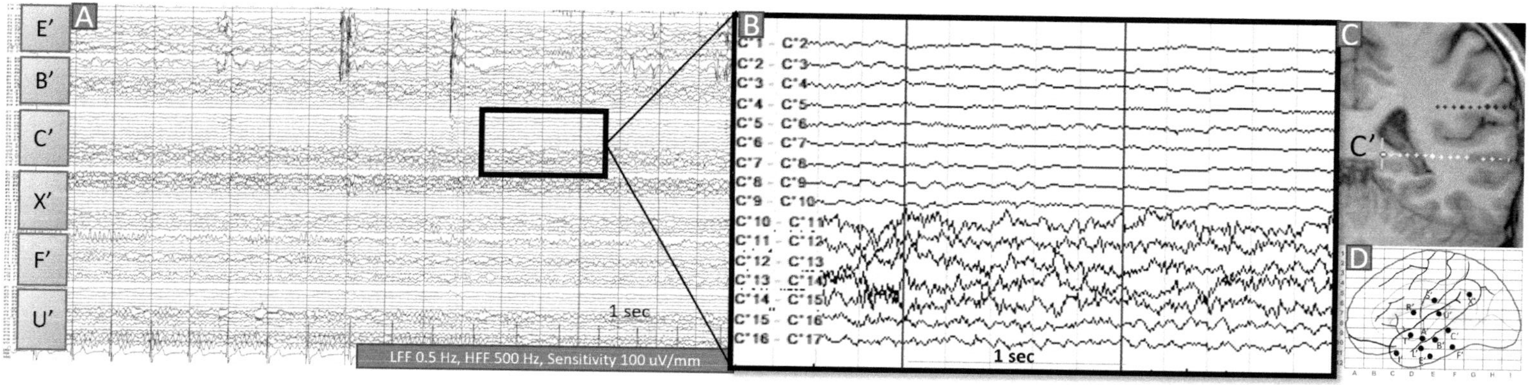


FIG. 6.2 Illustrating the importance of electrode co-registration and knowledge of electrode location. Panels A and B:The C′ mesial electrodes (one to four contacts), which were intended for targeting the posterior hippocampus. However, SEEG activities in the C′ one to four contacts exhibited low-amplitude alpha/theta activity, similar to the remaining electrodes in the C′ mid-electrode contacts. This unexpected finding contradicted typical posterior hippocampus activities. Panel C showing the anatomical reconstruction of the electrodes, confirming that the mesial contacts of electrode C were located in the white matter outside the hippocampus. This emphasizes the significance of electrode reconstruction before drawing conclusions about abnormal activity in SEEG analysis. Panel D illustrates the electrode implantation map of the patients, exploring the temporo-perisylvian regions.

**TABLE 6.1**
**Step-by-step Approach to Analyze and Differentiate SEEG Background Physiological or Pathological Activities.**

| The following steps are recommended to analyze baseline SEEG physiology or pathological activities. | |
|---|---|
| 1. | Understanding and expectation of normal activity based on the cortical regions that are being explored by the SEEG electrodes |
| 2. | Individual effects on the anesthesia are different, and thus, baseline activity needs to be studied at least 24–72 h following SEEG electrode placement. |
| 3. | The changes in the background activities between stage changes, such as awake and sleep, should be analyzed. |
| 4. | Routine baseline activation procedures are recommended if exploring functional cortex (photic stimulation, hyperventilation, eye closure, eye saccades (side to side or up and down movement, unilateral motor movements as well as sleep and awake) |
| 5. | The changes in the background SEEG activities with antiepileptic (ASM) medication as well as sleep deprivation |

## PREICTAL AND ICTAL EEG ACTIVITIES IN RELATION TO EZ

The preictal period is defined as a state immediately before the "onset" of an epileptic seizure, but at this point, there is no way to clearly estimate the exact duration of a preictal phase before the transition to the seizure, i.e., it may vary from seconds to days.[36,37] Studies on seizure prediction have often brought some confusion about the concept of a preictal period. Although the duration may not be definite, it has been shown that preictal neuronal activities are different from the interictal (resting state) neuronal activities in focal epilepsy.[36] Levesque et al. reported differences in the mechanisms of IEDs depending on interictal and preictal stages.[38] More and more data are pointing out whether the focal IEDs with paroxysmal depolarization shift during the interictal stages may be viewed as an attempt to inhibit ictal transition rather than promote the ictal transition.[39,40] A distinction between preictal and ictal periods has been documented in temporal lobe epilepsy.[41] As illustrated in Fig. 6.5, when compared to the background interictal phase, an increase in synchrony between the hippocampus and entorhinal cortex is observed during the preictal spiking phase, followed by a desynchronization when the higher frequency activity arises. A similar phenomenon is observed in neocortical epilepsy, as illustrated in Fig. 6.6, showing a comparison of synchronous preictal spikes/fast activity sequence in a mesial temporal and a neocortical seizure. Fig. 6.6A demonstrates the emergence of synchronous spikes in the mesial temporal network, encompassing the amygdala, hippocampus, and entorhinal regions, followed by a transition to fast activity. A similar pattern of preictal synchronization is evident in the anterior perisylvian network, involving the insula, orbitofrontal, and anterior cingulate areas, ultimately transitioning to fast activity (Fig. 6.6B). Hence, it is imperative to questions the definition of the seizure onset zone (SOZ) as a precise time point, and the emphasis should be placed on analyzing the temporal dynamics of frequency changes throughout the transition from preictal to ictal phases.

Presently, no single noninvasive presurgical or intraoperative ECoG investigation is currently operative to define the EZ and its extent. The conceptualization of the EZ is intrinsically linked with SEEG methodology. The initial purpose of this concept was to make a methodical distinction between lesion, interictal activity, and seizure topography. The pioneers/founders observed that a very focal localized onset was a rare observation, due to the early "synchrony" within the epileptogenic network, leading them to adopt the term "primary organization", meaning a consistent assembly of areas bound together.[2] Most of the time, seizure onset involves multiple areas/regions with distinct morphology and frequency patterns. Regarding the frequency pattern, fast activity at the primary organization has been acknowledged as a hallmark of the EZ in focal epilepsies since the beginning of SEEG.[2]The relative latencies of onset for these areas may vary from one seizure to another. "Primary organization," encompassing ictal onset and early spread, represents the fixed and reproducible structure of this paroxysmal assembly. Notably, its discharge can be triggered in its entirety by stimulation.[2]

Primary organization can differ from patient to patient, even with the same type of epilepsy. In individuals with mesial temporal lobe epilepsy, synchronized discharges can be confined to the mesial temporal structures, with fast activity exclusively present in these regions (Fig. 6.7). Alternatively, synchronized preictal discharges may extend beyond the mesial temporal lobe structures, encompassing the temporal pole and insular cortex, while the transition to fast activity

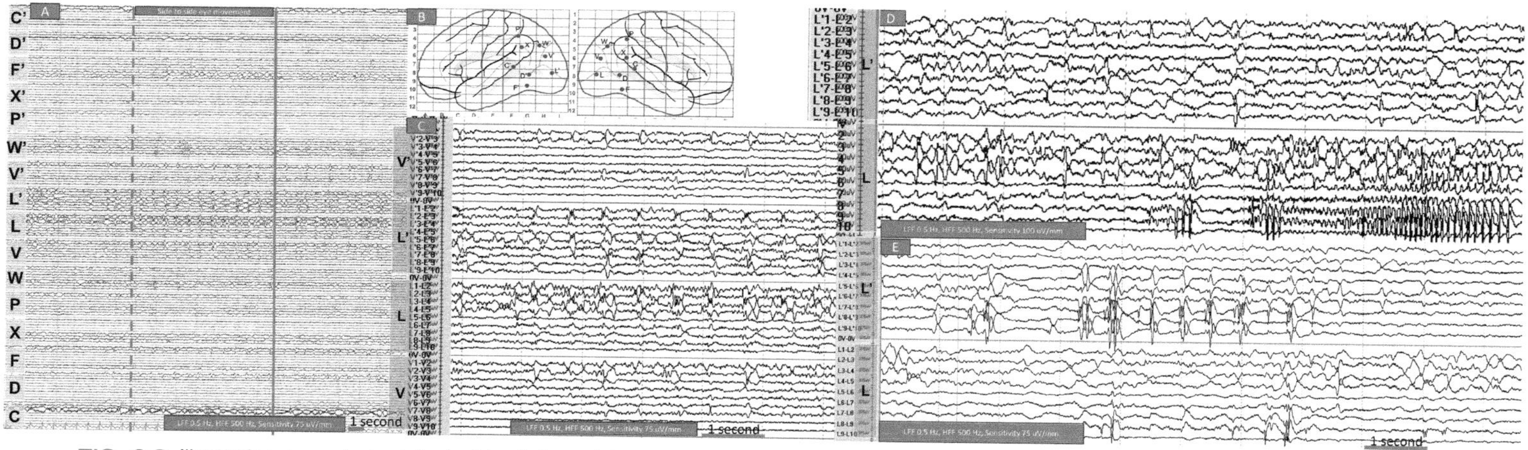


FIG. 6.3 Illustrating normal physiological lambda activity concurrently with pathological fast activity and polyspikes within the same electrode contacts in the posterior occipital head regions. Panel A: Background activity underwent changes following the activation procedure of side-to-side movement (*blue dashed line* marks the start of the activation procedure, and the blue solid line marks its conclusion). This demonstrated alterations in background activities in the bilateral posterior cortex symmetrically (*left*: V′ L′ electrode, *right*: V L electrodes - with electrode locations described in panel B: Talairach grid). Zoomed-in details were depicted in panel C. Panel C: Despite the symmetrical placement of L and L′ electrodes, the lambda activity was more pronounced over the left lateral occipital cortex compared to the right occipital cortex (indicated by the blue dash line pointing to the start of the side-to-side eye movement). Panels D and E show abnormal polyspikes interictal activity in the lateral contacts of the L electrode in the right lateral occipital cortex and independent spike wave in the lateral contacts of the L′ electrode in the left lateral occipital cortex following tapering off the antiepileptic medications.

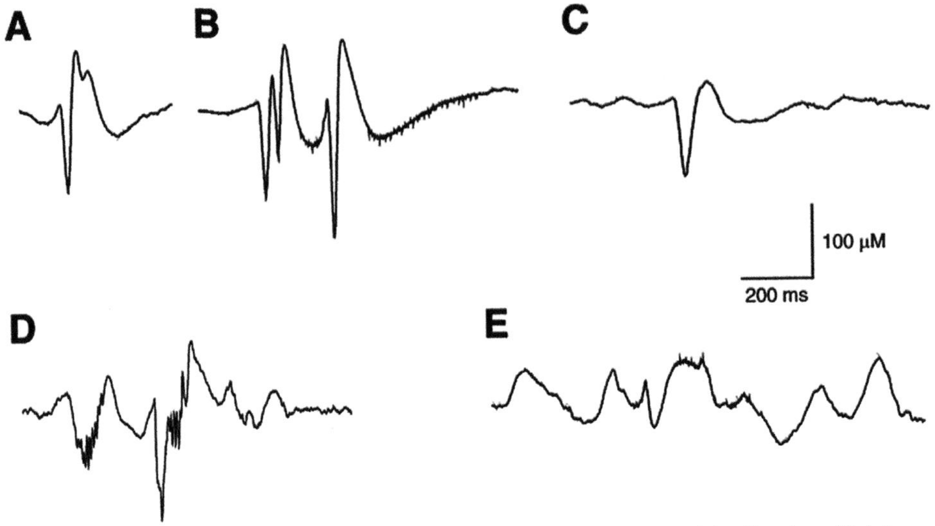


FIG. 6.4 Interictal epileptic discharge (IED) patterns recorded in human partial epilepsies with intracranial electrodes. (A) Interictal spike; (B) Group of interictal spikes from neocortical dysplasia, (C) Sharp wave from a lesional partial epilepsy; (D) Fast activity (brushes) riding on a spike recorded from a Taylor type II focal cortical dysplasia; (E) Paroxysmal slow activity superimposed to slow spikes recorded in a lesional partial epilepsy. (With permission from De Curtis M, Jefferys JGR, Avoli M. Interictal epileptiform discharges in partial Epilepsy. In: Noebels JL, Avoli M, Rogawski M, Olsen RW, Delgado-Escueta A V, eds. Jasper's basic mechanisms of the epilepsies. Fourth ed. Bethesda (MD):National Center for Biotechnology Information (US); 2013:213–227)

remains localized in the left mesial temporal structures (Fig. 6.8). As elucidated earlier, not all seizures manifest with localized onsets. It is not uncommon to observe fast activities transitioning across multiple networks concurrently (Fig. 6.9) or diffusely involving multiple networks simultaneously (Fig. 6.10). Two patients with mesio-lateral temporal lobe epilepsy are illustrated in Figs. 6.9 and 6.10. In Fig. 6.9's patient, two distinct synchronized preictal discharges are identified in the mesial temporal and lateral temporal networks. Subsequently, fast discharges concurrently intrude over both mesial and lateral temporal structures. In Fig. 6.10s patient, the preictal spikes synchronize between mesial and lateral temporal networks with simultaneous rapid discharges. This demonstrates the challenge of determining primary localization, especially in the patient illustrated in Fig. 6.10 and reflects the limitation of the conventional visual analysis of the SEEG.

The identification of EZ based upon the visual inspection of intracranial EEG required highly qualified experts due to the complexity of SEEG methodology.[42] In order to improve SEEG interpretation, several signal processing methods and pipelines are available for both interictal and ictal periods, but unfortunately, the use of signal processing techniques is still uncommon in day-to-day clinical practice.[42–45] Due to the scope of this chapter, the details on the pipelines will not be developed in detail, but it has been demonstrated that not only the frequency of multiple complex components during the interictal-ictal transition has to be considered.[42–45] Discriminating between different types of fast activities is difficult, even questionable, through visual analysis. Time-frequency analysis (TFA) is the most appropriate tool for differentiating between them. An electrical biomarker of the epileptogenic zone has been identified using TFA with a support vector machine for classification. Confirming that preictal spiking and fast activity with flattening are the three constitutive elements of this fingerprint, the narrow-band feature of the HFA is a critical discriminating factor. This time-frequency pattern can differentiate the epileptogenic zone from areas of propagation. It is demonstrated that analyzing fast activity alone can overestimate the EZ.[46]

On the other hand, there are seizures without any onset of fast activity at the interictal and ictal transition. Similar to interictal patterns, various types of interictal and ictal transition, i.e., seizure onset patterns (SOPs), have been reported (Fig. 6.11). However, the limitation lies in the discrepancy in defining SOPs between

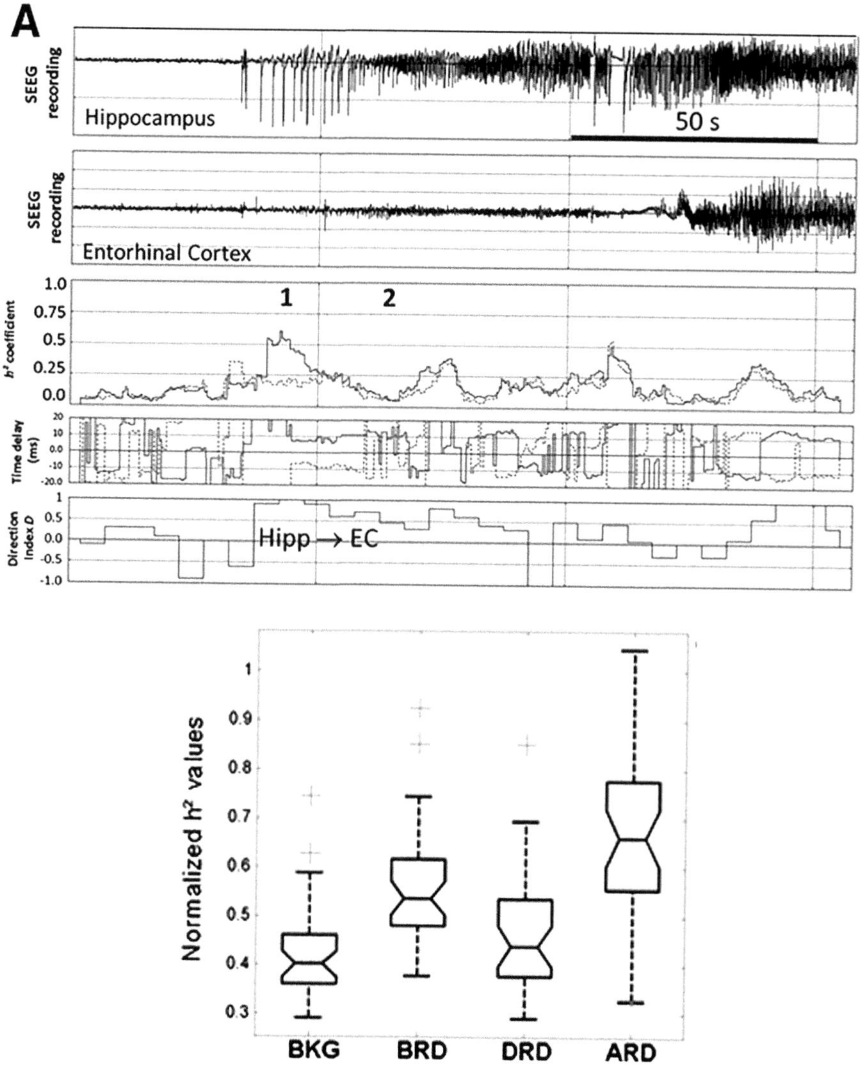


FIG. 6.5 The phenomenon of synchronization/desynchronization during focal (here, temporal lobe) seizures. (A) Upper part: functional coupling between entorhinal cortex and hippocampus in a patient with mesial temporal lobe seizures is studied using nonlinear regression (h2). An increase of synchrony (1) during the phase of preictal spiking is observed as measured by the h2 coefficient between the two structures. The direction index D indicates that the activity in the hippocampus is leading (positive values) the activity recorded in the entorhinal cortex. Note that the rapid discharge is associated with a decrease in correlation (indicated as two in the figure). Lower part: Box plot performed on normalized values of nonlinear correlations h2 values averaged from interactions between entorhinal cortex, amygdala, and hippocampus in SEEG recorded mesial temporal lobe seizures. The values are obtained in the BKG (background, interictal), BRD (before rapid discharge), DRD (during rapid discharge), and ARD (after rapid discharge) periods. h2 values measured before the rapid discharge(BRD) are significantly higher than those measured during background activity (BKG) and during the rapid discharge itself (DRD). (With permission from Bartolomei F, Lagarde S, Wendling F et al. Defining epileptogenic networks: Contribution of SEEG and signal analysis. *Epilepsia*. 2017; 58(7):1131–1147. https://doi.org/10.1111/epi.13791.)

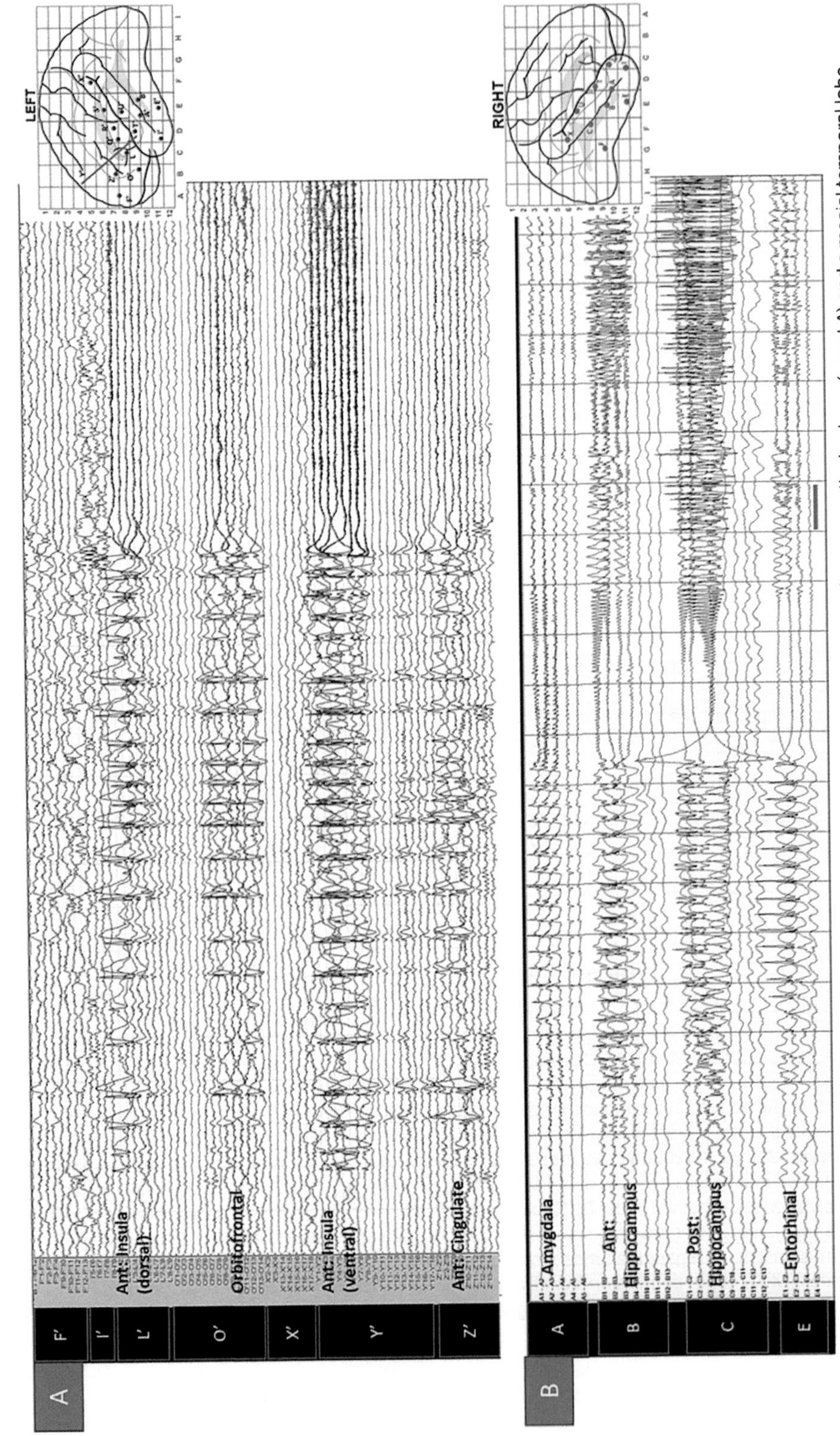


FIG. 6.6 Showing a comparison of synchronous preictal spikes/fast activity sequence in a neocortical seizure (panel A) and a mesial temporal lobe seizure (panel B). Figure 6B demonstrates the emergence of synchronous spikes in the mesial temporal network, encompassing the amygdala, hippocampus, and entorhinal regions, followed by a transition to fast activity. A similar pattern of preictal synchronization is evident in the anterior perisylvian network, involving the insula, orbitofrontal, and anterior cingulate areas, ultimately transitioning to fast activity (Fig. 6.6A).

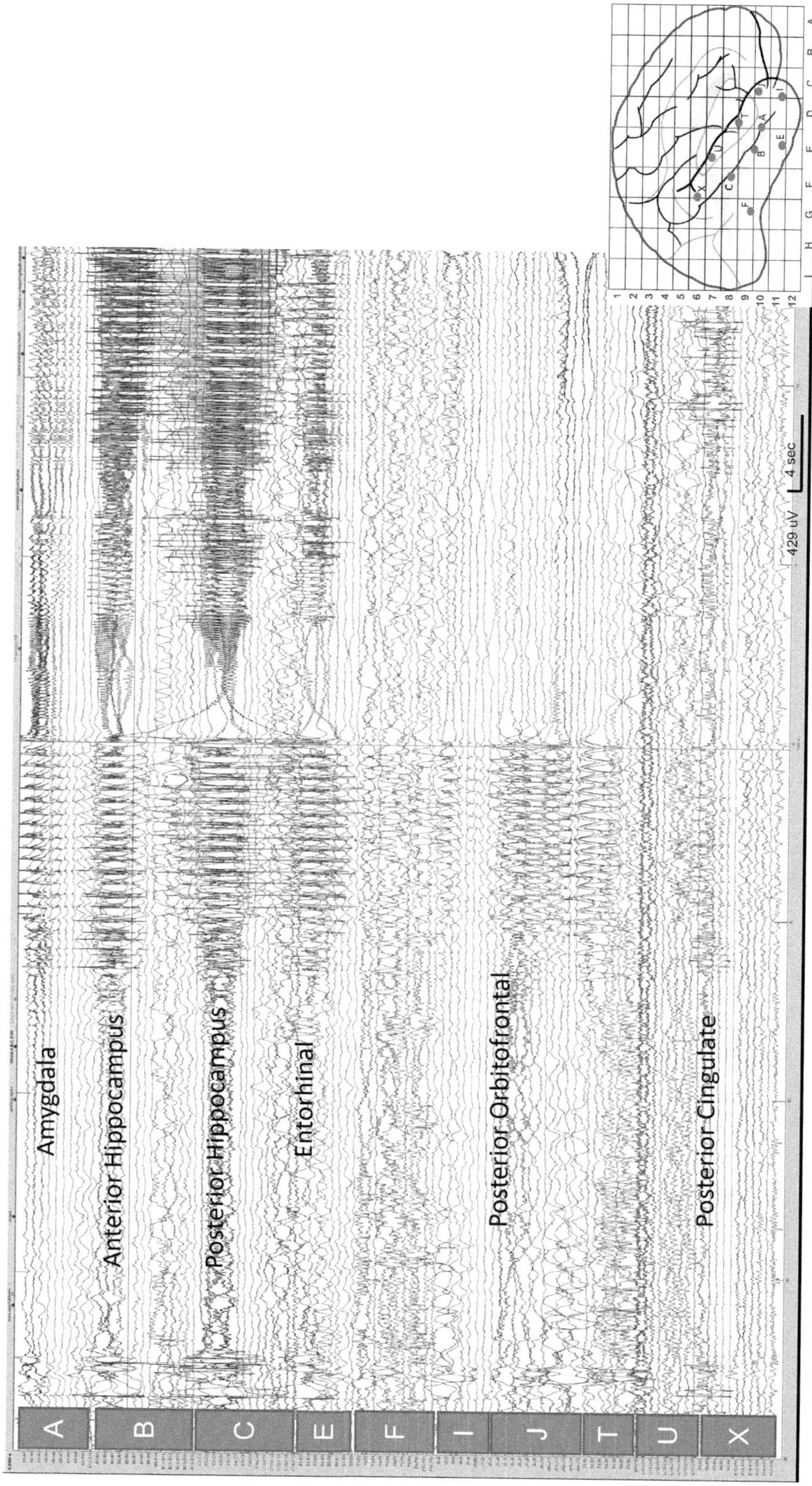


FIG. 6.7 Illustration of the right mesial temporal lobe epilepsy, showcasing synchronized preictal discharges localized within the mesial temporal structures, transitioning to fast activity.

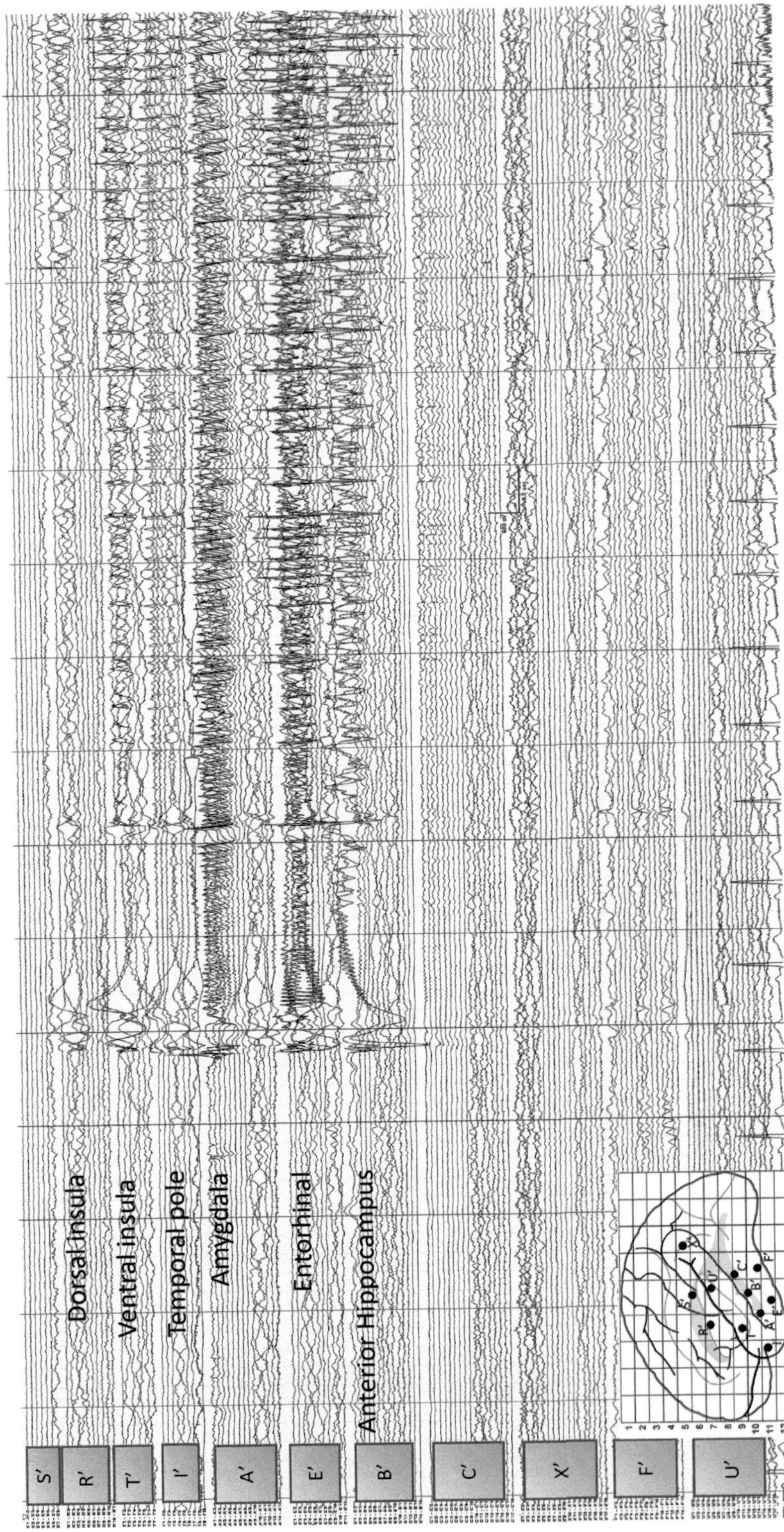


FIG. 6.8 Illustrating a patient with confirmed left mesial temporal lobe epilepsy, showcasing synchronized preictal discharges extended further beyond the left mesial temporal lobe structures involving the left temporal pole as well as the left anterior insular regions with fast activity transition only localized in the left mesial temporal structures.

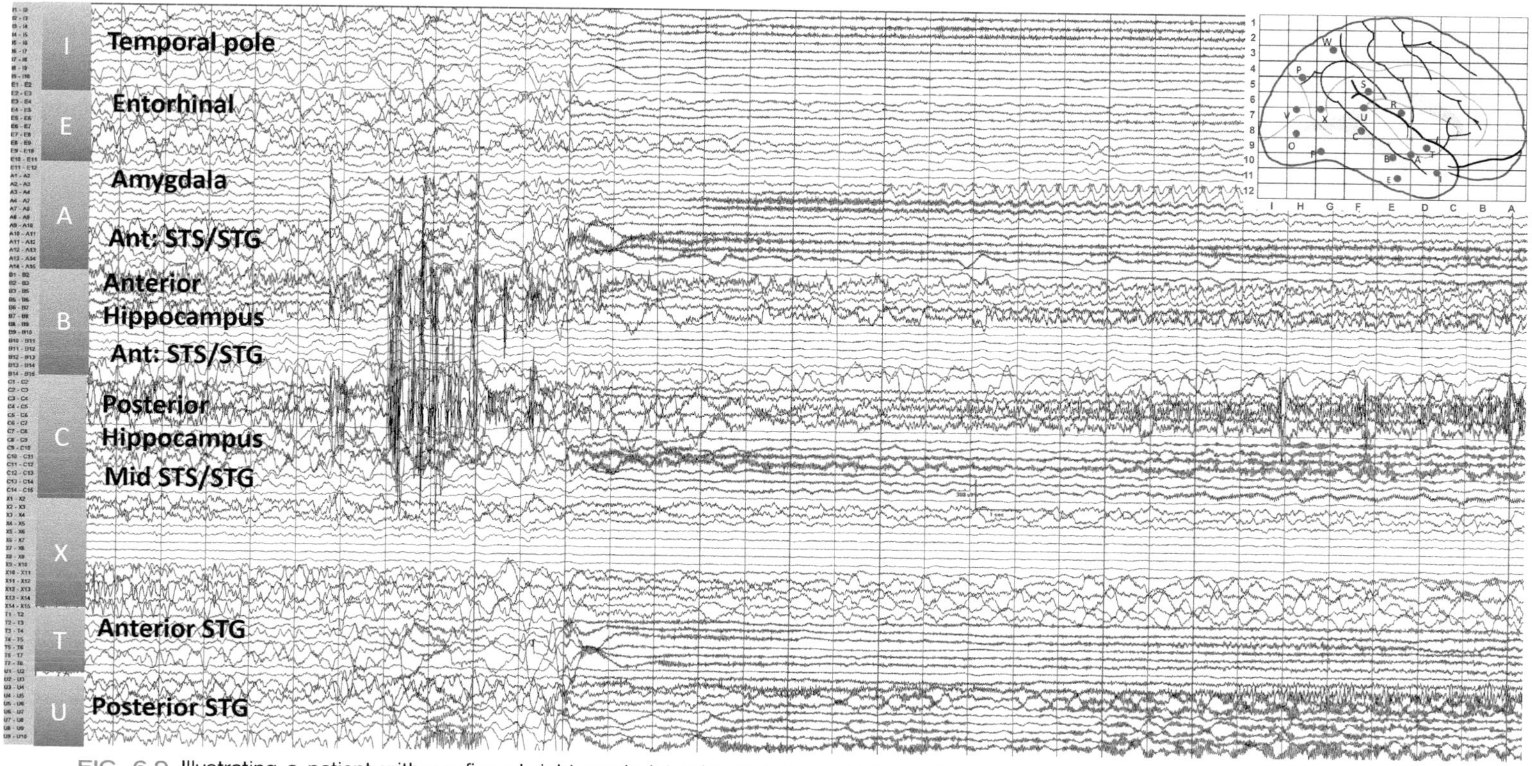


FIG. 6.9 Illustrating a patient with confirmed right mesio-lateral type temporal lobe epilepsy, showcasing two distinct synchronized preictal discharges are identified in the mesial temporal and lateral temporal networks. Subsequently, fast discharges intrude semi-simultaneously over both mesial and lateral temporal structures with different frequency of fast activities.

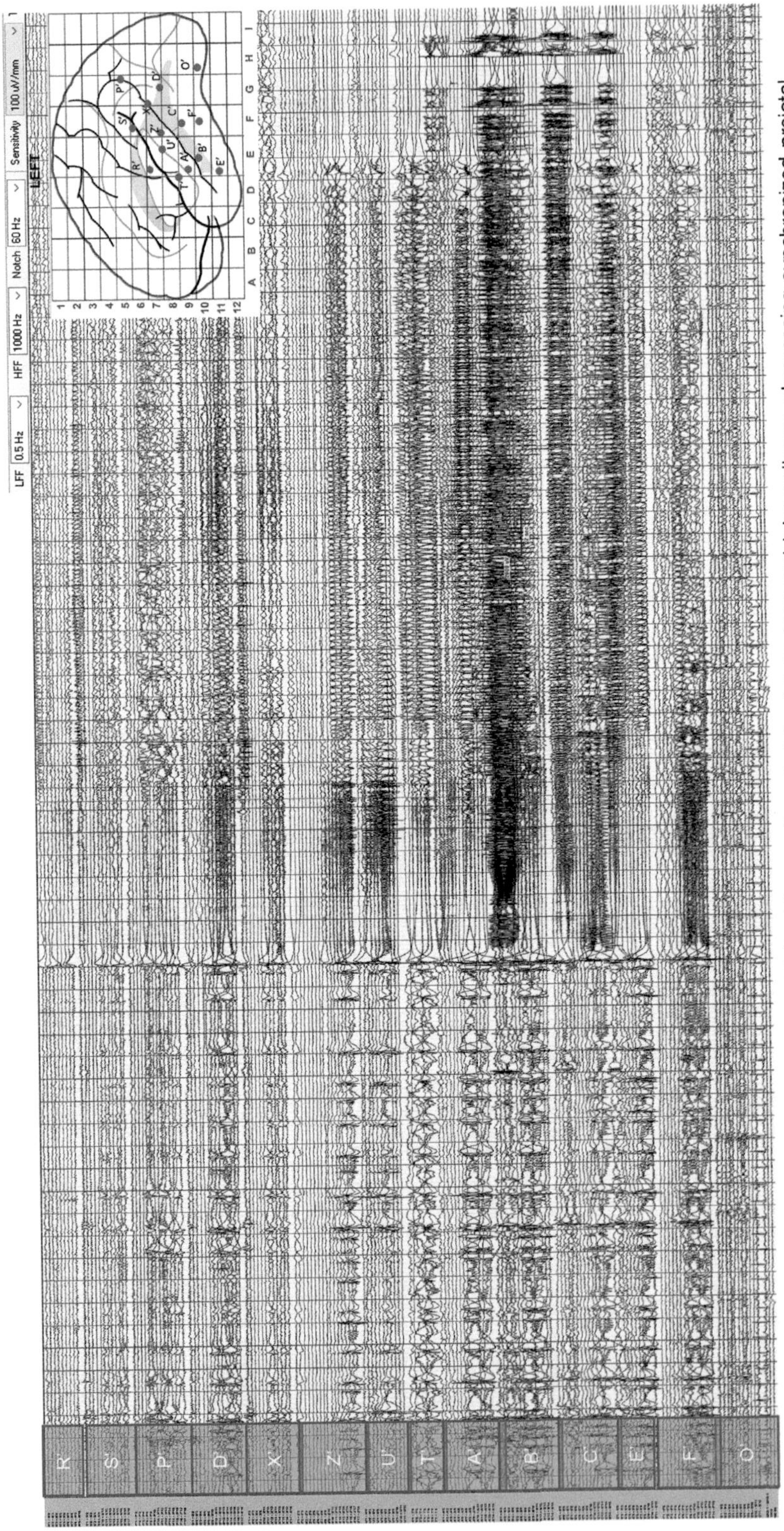


FIG. 6.10 Illustrating a patients with confirmed left widespread mesio-lateral type temporal lobe epilepsy, showcasing synchronized preictal discharges over mesial temporal and lateral temporal networks with simultaneous rapid discharges.

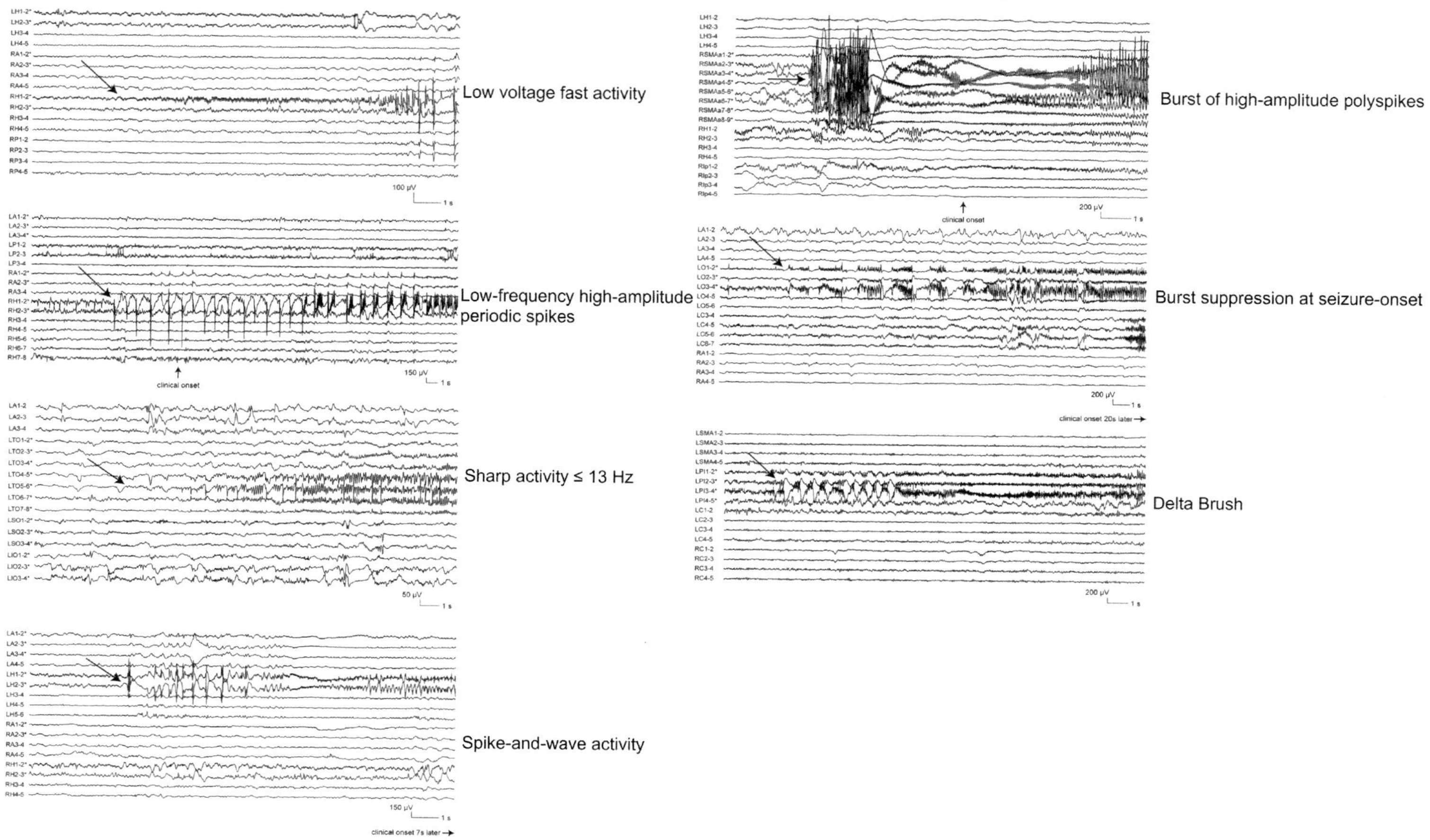


FIG. 6.11 Panel A: Low-voltage fast activity at seizure-onset. Panel B: Low-frequency high-amplitude periodic spikes at seizure-onset. Panel C: Sharp activity at $\leq$13 Hz at seizure-onset. Panel D: Spike-and-wave activity at seizure-onset. Panel E: Burst of high-amplitude polyspikes at seizure-onset. Panel F: Burst suppression at seizure-onset. Panel G: Delta brush at seizure-onset. (With permission from Perucca P, Dubeau F, Gotman J. et al. Intracranial electroencephalographic seizure-onset patterns: Effect of underlying pathology. *Brain*. 2014; 137(Pt 1):183–196. https://doi.org/10.1093/brain/awt299)

different groups.[47–51] Nonetheless, the relationship between the SOP in relation to mesial temporal lobe epilepsy and neocortical epilepsy has been analyzed in the recent meta-analysis by Singh et al.[52] LVFA is reported as a neocortical ictal rhythm, whereas low-frequency repetitive spikes SOP as a mesial temporal ictal rhythm, especially in mesial temporal sclerosis (MTS).[52] Sinusoidal theta and delta activities are reported as propagation rhythms and are associated with poor surgical outcome.[47–52] Consequently, it is important to clarify the type of SOP as each pattern has different basic cellular mechanisms of pathophysiology,[53] and numerous studies have explored the correlations between SOP and seizure outcome.[5,16,42,45,47–50]

Although overall agreement is that low voltage fast activity at the SOZ is associated with a good postoperative seizure outcome following the resection of the SOZ regardless of the temporal or extratemporal localization, one should keep in mind that there is no absolute guarantee that resection of the regions producing LVFA will result in 100% seizure freedom.[47–51] In particular, not having LVFA SOP is not a predictor of poor surgical outcome and SOP pattern has no absolute relationship in defining EZ. Not just the location of the EZ, the relationship between the seizure onset patterns (SOPs) and the underlying pathology has been studied. Although it is agreed that all pathologies can be associated with multiple SOPs, LVFA seems predominant in vascular pathologies and cavernoma and bursts of polyspikes followed by LVFA in malformations of cortical development.[47–51]

It is important that ictal data have to be considered together with preictal and interictal data in addition to the clinical symptoms with the emergence of the semiology in relation to the anatomo-clinico-electrical relationship (not illustrated in this chapter), which changes across both spatial and temporal distribution across the seizure.[51,54,55] Thus, it is important to analyze the SOZ in SEEG in both temporal transition from interictal to preictal and to ictal, as well as the spatial extent.[2,16,42,56]

## CONCLUSION

SEEG is considered the gold standard and the only current operational methodology to delineate the EZ and adjacent functional cortex to plan a safe and effective resection. The core of the SEEG implantation strategy is the concept of anatomo-electro-clinical correlations. The concept of SOZ in SEEG is not an absolute time mark to be measured as an astatic time point but to be analyzed in the context of preictal and interictal data in addition to the clinical symptoms with the emergence of the semiology in relation to the anatomo-clinico-electrical relationship which changes across in both spatial and temporal distribution across the seizure. The complexity of seizure onset frequency gamma activity in the epileptogenic zone has specific time-frequency features that allow it to differentiate it from regions of propagation, and thus, not only the spatial synchronic features but also the diachronic features are needed to be analyzed.

## REFERENCES


1. Talairach J, Bancaud J, Bonis A, Szikla G, Tournoux P. Functional stereotaxic exploration of epilepsy. *Confin Neurol.* 1962;22:328–331. https://doi.org/10.1159/000104378.
2. Bancaud J, Talairach J, Bonis A. La stéréoencéphalographie dans l'épilepsie. In: *Informations Neuro-Physio-Pathologiques Apportées Par L'investigation Fonctionnelle Stéréotaxique.* Paris: Masson; 1965.
3. Leblanc R. Epilepsy surgery. Published by. In: Lüders HO, Comair YG, eds. *C$292.53 Approx.* 2nd ed. Vol 28. Lippincott Williams & Wilkins; 2001:1060. https://doi.org/10.1017/s0317167100019296. Lippincott Williams & Wilkins.
4. Rosenow F, Lüders H. Presurgical evaluation of epilepsy. *Brain.* 2001. https://doi.org/10.1093/brain/124.9.1683.
5. Chauvel P, Gonzalez-Martinez J, Bulacio J. Presurgical intracranial investigations in epilepsy surgery. In: *Handbook of Clinical Neurology.* Vol 161. 2019:45–71. https://doi.org/10.1016/B978-0-444-64142-7.00040-0.
6. Penfield W. Epileptogenic lesions. *Acta Neurol Psychiatr Belg.* 1956;56(2):75–88.
7. Jasper HH, Arfel-capdeville G, Rasmussen T. Evaluation of EEG and cortical electrographic studies for prognosis of seizures following surgical excision of epileptogenic lesions. *Epilepsia.* 1961;2:130–137. http://www.ncbi.nlm.nih.gov/pubmed/14451406.
8. Rasmussen T. Characteristics of a pure culture of frontal lobe epilepsy. *Epilepsia.* 1983;24(4):482–493. https://doi.org/10.1111/j.1528-1157.1983.tb04919.x.
9. Rasmussen T. Localizationsal concepts in epilepsy: past, present and future. *Stereotact Funct Neurosurg.* 1987;50(1–6):355–358. https://doi.org/10.1159/000100739.
10. Penfield W, Jasper H. Epilepsy and the functional anatomy of the human brain. *South Med J.* 1954;47(7):704. https://doi.org/10.1097/00007611-195407000-00024.
11. Talairach J, Bancaud J. Lesion, "irritative" zone and epileptogenic focus. *Confin Neurol.* 1966;27(1):91–94. https://doi.org/10.1159/000103937.
12. Bancaud J, Geier S, Talairach J, Scarabin JM, E.E.G. et S.E.E.G. *DANS LES TUMEURS CEREBRALES ET L'EPILEPSIE.* Paris: Edifor; 1973.
13. Zijlmans M, Jacobs J, Kahn YU, Zelmann R, Dubeau F, Gotman J. Ictal and interictal high frequency oscillations in patients with focal epilepsy. *Clin Neurophysiol.* 2011;122(4):664–671. https://doi.org/10.1016/j.clinph.2010.09.021.

14. Bartolomei F, Trébuchon A, Bonini F, et al. What is the concordance between the seizure onset zone and the irritative zone? A SEEG quantified study. *Clin Neurophysiol.* 2016;127(2):1157–1162. https://doi.org/10.1016/j.clinph.2015.10.029.
15. Frauscher B, Von Ellenrieder N, Zelmann R, et al. Atlas of the normal intracranial electroencephalogram: neurophysiological awake activity in different cortical areas. *Brain.* 2018;141(4):1130–1144. https://doi.org/10.1093/brain/awy035.
16. Bartolomei F, Nica A, Valenti-Hirsch MP, Adam C, Denuelle M. Interpretation of SEEG recordings. *Neurophysiol Clin.* 2018;48(1):53–57. https://doi.org/10.1016/j.neucli.2017.11.010.
17. Peter-Derex L, von Ellenrieder N, van Rosmalen F, et al. Regional variability in intracerebral properties of NREM to REM sleep transitions in humans. *Proc Natl Acad Sci U S A.* 2023;120(26):e2300387120. https://doi.org/10.1073/pnas.2300387120.
18. Latreille V, von Ellenrieder N, Peter-Derex L, Dubeau F, Gotman J, Frauscher B. The human K-complex: insights from combined scalp-intracranial EEG recordings. *Neuroimage.* 2020;213:116748. https://doi.org/10.1016/j.neuroimage.2020.116748.
19. Von Ellenrieder N, Gotman J, Zelmann R, et al. How the human brain sleeps: direct cortical recordings of normal brain activity. *Ann Neurol.* 2020;87(2):289–301. https://doi.org/10.1002/ana.25651.
20. Klimes P, Peter-Derex L, Hall J, Dubeau F, Frauscher B. Spatio-temporal spike dynamics predict surgical outcome in adult focal epilepsy. *Clin Neurophysiol.* 2022;134:88–99. https://doi.org/10.1016/j.clinph.2021.10.023.
21. De Curtis M, Jefferys JGR, Avoli M. Interictal epileptiform discharges in partial epilepsy. In: Noebels JL, Avoli M, Rogawski M, Olsen RW, Delgado-Escueta AV, eds. *Jasper's Basic Mechanisms of the Epilepsies.* 4th ed. Bethesda (MD: National Center for Biotechnology Information (US); 2013:213–227. https://doi.org/10.1093/med/9780199746545.003.0017.
22. Kooi KA. Voltage-time characteristics of spikes and other rapid electroencephalographic transients: semantic and morphological considerations. *Neurology.* 1966. https://doi.org/10.1212/wnl.16.1.59.
23. Bourien J, Bartolomei F, Bellanger JJ, Gavaret M, Chauvel P, Wendling F. A method to identify reproducible subsets of co-activated structures during interictal spikes. Application to intracerebral EEG in temporal lobe epilepsy. *Clin Neurophysiol.* 2005. https://doi.org/10.1016/j.clinph.2004.08.010.
24. Lai N, Li Z, Xu C, Wang Y, Chen Z. Diverse nature of interictal oscillations: EEG-based biomarkers in epilepsy. *Neurobiol Dis.* 2023. https://doi.org/10.1016/j.nbd.2023.105999.
25. Tassi L, Colombo N, Garbelli R, et al. Focal cortical dysplasia: neuropathological subtypes, EEG, neuroimaging and surgical outcome. *Brain.* 2002. https://doi.org/10.1093/brain/awf175.
26. Sklenarova B, Zatloukalova E, Cimbalnik J, et al. Interictal high-frequency oscillations, spikes, and connectivity profiles: a fingerprint of epileptogenic brain pathologies. *Epilepsia.* 2023;64(11):3049–3060. https://doi.org/10.1111/epi.17749.
27. Guth TA, Kunz L, Brandt A, et al. Interictal spikes with and without high-frequency oscillation have different single-neuron correlates. *Brain.* 2021;144(10):3078–3088. https://doi.org/10.1093/brain/awab288.
28. Chauvel P, Buser P, Badier JM, Liegeois-Chauvel C, Marquis P, Bancaud J. [The "epileptogenic zone" in humans: representation of intercritical events by spatio-temporal maps]. *Rev Neurol (Paris).* 1987.
29. Badier JM, Chauvel P. Spatio-temporal characteristics of paroxysmal interictal events in human temporal lobe epilepsy. *J Physiol Paris.* 1995. https://doi.org/10.1016/0928-4257(96)83642-4.
30. Khambhati AN, Bassett DS, Oommen BS, et al. Recurring functional interactions predict network architecture of interictal and ictal states in neocortical epilepsy. *eNeuro.* 2017. https://doi.org/10.1523/ENEURO.0091-16.2017.
31. Tomlinson SB, Wong JN, Conrad EC, Kennedy BC, Marsh ED. Reproducibility of interictal spike propagation in children with refractory epilepsy. *Epilepsia.* 2019. https://doi.org/10.1111/epi.14720.
32. Azeem A, von Ellenrieder N, Hall J, Dubeau F, Frauscher B, Gotman J. Interictal spike networks predict surgical outcome in patients with drug-resistant focal epilepsy. *Ann Clin Transl Neurol.* 2021. https://doi.org/10.1002/acn3.51337. Published online.
33. Lagarde S, Roehri N, Lambert I, et al. Interictal stereotactic-EEG functional connectivity in refractory focal epilepsies. *Brain.* 2018. https://doi.org/10.1093/brain/awy214. Published online.
34. Wyllie E. *Wyllie's Treatment of Epilepsy: Principles and Practice.* 6th ed. 2015.
35. De Curtis M, Avoli M. Interictal epileptiform discharges in partial epilepsy: neurobiologic mechanisms based on clinical and experimental evidence. *Epilepsia.* 2010; 51(SUPPL. 5):22. https://doi.org/10.1111/j.1528-1167.2010.02808.x.
36. Truccolo W, Donoghue JA, Hochberg LR, et al. Single-neuron dynamics in human focal epilepsy. *Nat Neurosci.* 2011;14(5):635–643. https://doi.org/10.1038/nn.2782.
37. Lange HH, Lieb JP, Engel J, Crandall PH. Temporo-spatial patterns of pre-ictal spike activity in human temporal lobe epilepsy. *Electroencephalogr Clin Neurophysiol.* 1983; 56(6):543–555. https://doi.org/10.1016/0013-4694(83)90022-6.
38. Lévesque M, Ragsdale D, Avoli M. Evolving mechanistic concepts of epileptiform synchronization and their relevance in curing focal epileptic disorders. *Curr Neuropharmacol.* 2018. https://doi.org/10.2174/1570159x17666181127124803.
39. De Curtis M, Avanzini G. Interictal spikes in focal epileptogenesis. *Prog Neurobiol.* 2001. https://doi.org/10.1016/S0301-0082(00)00026-5. Published online.

40. De Curtis M, Avoli M. GABAergic networks jump-start focal seizures. *Epilepsia*. 2016. https://doi.org/10.1111/epi.13370.
41. Bartolomei F, Lagarde S, Wendling F, et al. Defining epileptogenic networks: Contribution of SEEG and signal analysis. *Epilepsia*. 2017. https://doi.org/10.1111/epi.13791. Published online.
42. Grinenko O, Li J, Mosher JC, et al. A fingerprint of the epileptogenic zone in human epilepsies. *Brain*. 2018; 141(1):117–131. https://doi.org/10.1093/brain/awx306.
43. Andrzejak RG, David O, Gnatkovsky V, et al. Localization of epileptogenic zone on pre-surgical intracranial EEG recordings: toward a validation of quantitative signal analysis approaches. *Brain Topogr*. 2015;28(6):832–837. https://doi.org/10.1007/s10548-014-0380-8.
44. Bartolomei F, Lagarde S, Wendling F, et al. Defining epileptogenic networks: Contribution of SEEG and signal analysis. *Epilepsia*. 2017;58(7):1131–1147. https://doi.org/10.1111/epi.13791.
45. Li J, Grinenko O, Mosher JC, Gonzalez-Martinez J, Leahy RM, Chauvel P. Learning to define an electrical biomarker of the epileptogenic zone. *Hum Brain Mapp*. 2020;41(2):429–441. https://doi.org/10.1002/hbm.24813.
46. Li J, Grinenko O, Mosher JC, Gonzalez-Martinez J, Leahy RM, Chauvel P. Learning to define an electrical biomarker of the epileptogenic zone. *Hum Brain Mapp*. 2020. https://doi.org/10.1002/hbm.24813.
47. Xu C, Zhang X, Yan X, et al. Multiple ictal onset patterns underlie seizure generation in seizure-free patients with temporal lobe epilepsy surgery: an SEEG study. *Acta Neurochir*. 2021;163(11):3031–3037. https://doi.org/10.1007/s00701-021-04960-7.
48. Di Giacomo R, Uribe-San-Martin R, Mai R, et al. Stereo-EEG ictal/interictal patterns and underlying pathologies. *Seizure*. 2019;72:54–60. https://doi.org/10.1016/j.seizure.2019.10.001.
49. Perucca P, Dubeau F, Gotman J. Intracranial electroencephalographic seizure-onset patterns: effect of underlying pathology. *Brain*. 2014;137(1):183–196. https://doi.org/10.1093/brain/awt299.
50. Lagarde S, Bonini F, McGonigal A, et al. Seizure-onset patterns in focal cortical dysplasia and neurodevelopmental tumors: relationship with surgical prognosis and neuropathologic subtypes. *Epilepsia*. 2016;57(9):1426–1435. https://doi.org/10.1111/epi.13464.
51. Lagarde S, Buzori S, Trebuchon A, et al. The repertoire of seizure onset patterns in human focal epilepsies: determinants and prognostic values. *Epilepsia*. 2019. https://doi.org/10.1111/epi.14604.
52. Singh S, Sandy S, Wiebe S. Ictal onset on intracranial EEG: do we know it when we see it? State of the evidence. *Epilepsia*. 2015. https://doi.org/10.1111/epi.13120.
53. Avoli M, De Curtis M, Gnatkovsky V, et al. Specific imbalance of excitatory/inhibitory signaling establishes seizure onset pattern in temporal lobe epilepsy. *J Neurophysiol*. 2016. https://doi.org/10.1152/jn.01128.2015.
54. Chauvel P, McGonigal A. Emergence of semiology in epileptic seizures. *Epilepsy Behav*. 2014;38:94–103. https://doi.org/10.1016/j.yebeh.2013.12.003.
55. Holtkamp M, Sharan A, Sperling MR. Intracranial EEG in predicting surgical outcome in frontal lobe epilepsy. *Epilepsia*. 2012. https://doi.org/10.1111/j.1528-1167.2012.03600.x.
56. Chauvel P. The epileptogenic zone: a critical reconstruction. In: *A Practical Approach to Stereo EEG*. 2020. https://doi.org/10.1891/9780826136930.0010.

CHAPTER 7

# The Extent of an Epileptogenic Zone: Application of Signal Processing Methods

STEPHEN THOMPSON, MD

## INTRODUCTION AND DEFINITIONS

The delineation of an effective surgical strategy depends on an accurate delineation of the epileptogenic zone (EZ); this is not a trivial matter. Whereas the EZ has been defined theoretically as "the area of cortex that is indispensable for the generation of epileptic seizures," recognized *post hoc* by the attainment of a seizure-free outcome and distinct from the seizure-onset zone (SOZ),[1] Bancaud and Talairach developed an earlier operational definition.[2] Here, "primary organization" is foremost, this referring to the spatio-temporal dynamic structure of the ictal discharge.[3] Stimulation-induced seizures (see chapter elsewhere in this book) are crucial to informing this organizational construct, but the question raised in this chapter is whether data from spontaneous seizures alone are sufficient for defining the EZ extent.

According to SEEG methodology, additional zones are understood. The most relevant for consideration here is the "primary" irritative zone (IZ), the cortical region(s) that display interictal abnormalities epileptiform (spikes or *pathological* high frequency oscillations [HFOs]) which colocalize—by definition—with the EZ; remote irritative regions are referred to as "secondary."[4,5] An important line of investigation is whether the primary IZ, and thus the EZ, can be defined independent of ictal data.[6–8] Identification of such a biomarker, especially if measurable noninvasively, would considerably simplify the presurgical workup. To date, the most robust biomarker, HFOs, has not proven adequate for this task.[9]

Various signal processing methods may be used to supplement visual analysis. These may be broadly categorized into time-frequency methods, which aim to depict the frequency content of a signal as a function of time, and connectivity methods, which aim to describe various interareal relationships. An important caveat with connectivity measures is that most techniques assume linearity and stationarity of the time series, conditions that do not hold for ictal data,[10] though nonlinear methods may be appropriately employed.[11] Connectivity measures will not be discussed in this chapter.

## THE DILEMMA OF FAST ACTIVITY

Low-voltage fast activity (LFVA) has long been considered a hallmark of the EZ,[12] and surgical outcomes are improved when it is demonstrated on intracranial recordings.[13] As discussed below, seizure-onset patterns (SOPs) that contain LFVA are prognostically favorable.[14] A vexing dilemma is whether all (early) fast activity is equally localizing of the EZ, and if not, how to discriminate these. For example, the temporal-plus epilepsies were identified as a distinct electroclinical entity because of the surgical failure in patients for whom regions of "very fast propagation" were not included in the resection.[15] Yet, the presence of fast activity in the insula per se is not a determinant of surgical prognosis[16], that is, not all patients with (early) fast activity in the insula have a temporo-perisylvian epilepsy.[17] Moreover, fast activity at onset is frequently encountered in homotopic cortical regions contralateral to the EZ, especially in mesial frontal cortices.[18–20] Discriminating "primary" from "propagated" fast activity remains a challenge, and methods that rely solely on fast activity risk inaccurate localization of the EZ.

## THE DILEMMA OF LATENCY

Latencies are often assumed to denote epileptogenicity, and the boundaries of the SOZ are defined by latency.[21] Yet, the temporal criterion (e.g., one second[7]) that

The Fundamentals of Stereoelectroencephalography. https://doi.org/10.1016/B978-0-443-10877-8.00004-8

demarcates this boundary is inherently arbitrary, and most studies broaching this question have utilized a subdural approach.[22] Moreover, while there are clearly measurable latencies in mesial temporal seizures,[23] neocortical seizures more typically demonstrate quasi-simultaneous onset across multiple regions. Indeed, "network organization" is the more common observation.[14] Further, when one considers the microdomain (where seizures truly start), activity may be late to appear in the macrodomain.[24] This important scale consideration aside, temporal sampling (the time when activity is recorded) is inherently dependent on spatial sampling; one must also always consider the "missing electrode."[5] To posit a relevance in sub-second relative latencies across channels is to posit a perfect spatial sampling. Therefore, how seizures start—SOPs/dynamics—may be more important than when seizures start (relative latencies). Primary organization may be more important than "early spread."[2]

## TIME–FREQUENCY TECHNIQUES

Methods exist for measuring and quantifying the frequency content of a time series. The most often employed, and utilized in the methods described below, are short-time Fourier transform, continuous wavelet transform (CWT), and Hilbert transform. The mathematical basis for these will not be elaborated, but each serves to capture the amount of frequency content (magnitude/power) as a function of time.[25] Thus, one may quantify the frequency changes (spectral dynamics) that occur with time; these are displayed as a spectrogram (or scalogram for the CWT).

Analysis is typically done on bipolar channels to eliminate extraneous common mode signals; however, this demands an important consideration. As bipolar recordings are inherently susceptible to in-phase cancellation, amplitude, and thus magnitude/power cannot be used to directly compare spectral content across channels. Furthermore, high frequencies are of inherently lower amplitude (the so-called 1/f spectrum[26]). Thus, to adequately quantify high frequencies and compare spectral content across channels, some form of normalization is required, most often against a "baseline" of interictal data.

## QUANTIFICATION OF FAST ACTIVITY AND LATENCY: EPILEPTOGENICITY INDEX

The Epileptogenicity Index (EI) was introduced to quantify the emergence of fast activity in temporal lobe epilepsies.[23] First, an energy ratio of the power within the high- and low-frequency bands is defined as a function of time: $ER = (E\beta + E\gamma)/(E\theta + E\alpha)$. This serves to capture the transition to LVFA. Second, a change-point algorithm (CUSUM) is used to indicate when this ratio deviates. Essentially, a penalty term is introduced to negatively offset the ER, which is then cumulatively summed. A detection threshold is set to identify the inflection point of this cumulative sum. Both detection terms are adjustable, and the process is thus semi-automated. The detection time is used to scale the ER. Finally, the values are normalized such that the highest channel is 1. Using this methodology (Fig. 7.1), Bartolomei et al. quantified the relative epileptogenicity of structures within the temporal lobe in a cohort of patients. Structures with an $EI > 0.3$ were considered highly epileptogenic. In a subsequent study, temporal lobe networks were identified by a clustering algorithm (k-means) according to relative epileptogenicity by structure.[27] At the group level, there was an association between the number of structures with high epileptogenicity ($EI > 0.3$) and seizure-free surgical outcome.

The EI methodology has since been applied to multiple epilepsy etiologies[28–30] and anatomic types.[31–33] More recently, EI has been used as a surrogate for the EZ extent, finding that interictal HFO rate was inadequate (low sensitivity) to define the EZ,[6] and that surgical outcomes were improved when the EZ ($EI > 0.4$) was completely removed.[34] It is unclear what portion of these complete-resection patients had a temporal lobe resection, or what portion had a "focal organization," itself associated with improved surgical outcomes.[14]

The EI was defined and optimized for temporal lobe epilepsies, but its performance in extratemporal lobe epilepsy has been questioned. The problem arises in seizures with a quasi-simultaneous onset across multiple cortical regions. In this situation, the latency term effectively drops out of the calculation, and EI thus depends solely on the ER. A recent study demonstrated that further scaling the ER by the Euclidean distance between contacts, essentially penalizing propagation, outperformed standard EI in term of conforming to the resection bed in seizure-free patients, especially in neocortical epilepsies.[35] This modified method also implicated areas outside of the resection in patients with poor surgical outcome (EZ incompletely resected). Obviously, the Euclidean distance between contacts carries little biological relevance, which the authors acknowledge.

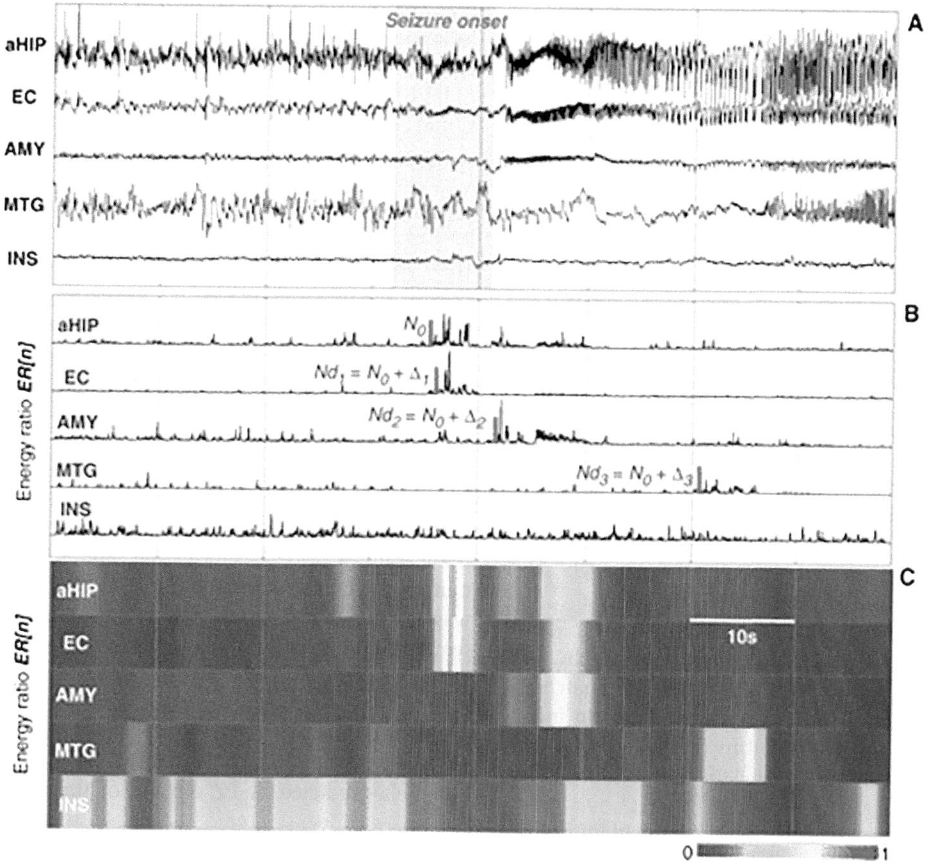


FIG. 7.1 Application of Epileptogenicity Index (EI) to a mesial temporal onset seizure. (A) There is a latency in the appearance of fast activity between the mesial temporal structures (anterior hippocampus [aHIP], entorhinal cortex [EC], amygdala [AMY]) and middle temporal gyrus (MTG). (B/C) ER is calculated as a function of time, and a detection algorithm is used to capture when this changes (*red bars*). The relative latencies (Δ) are used to scale the summated ER, to produce a final EI by channel (not shown; cf. Fig. 7.3).

## MAPPING FAST ACTIVITY: EPILEPTOGENICITY MAPPING

A related method relying on fast activity was introduced by David et al.[36] This utilized an approach, statistical parametric mapping (SPM), usually applied to functional imaging data, and was accordingly named epileptogenicity mapping (EM). Power in the fast frequency band (60–100 Hz) was quantified by CWT, normalized against a baseline, and using the spatial positions of electrodes, linearly interpolated to produce a statistical map after thresholding (SPM). Given the inherently spatial approach, comparison of the EM to resection volumes is feasible. As mentioned above, EM was applied to a cohort of temporal lobe patients, mapping the early (<10 seconds) involvement of the insula; this carried no prognostic significance.[16]

A more heterogeneous, mostly extratemporal, cohort was recently published,[37] comparing the EM with the postoperative resection mask. While the "FASTectomy" ratio was higher in seizure-free patients at the group level, this was achieved with only a partial resection of fast activity (mean 28%). Discrimination was not achieved at the patient level: some non-seizure-free patients showed higher resection ratios than seizure-free patients. That is, EM alone cannot be used to direct surgical planning. As with EI, this method appears to poorly discriminate between primary and propagated fast activity. Both methods also assume that only fast activity is relevant for EZ localization.

## CONSIDERATION OF SLOW FREQUENCY: QUANTIFIED FREQUENCY ANALYSIS INDEX

Ictal infraslow activity (baseline shift/DC shift) has recently gained interest in SEEG analysis.[38,39] Gnatkovsky et al.[40] developed a method that combined three quantitative parameters: 1. fast activity power (>80 Hz) 2. slow polarization shift (SPS), the integral of the smoothed time series after application of a moving average filter, and 3. flattening, intended to capture the transition to low voltage that occurs with LFVA. These three parameters were combined into a single index score. Unlike the above, this method was applied to monopolar (i.e., referential) data, presumably because infraslow activity (SPS) is better quantified in a referential montage.[38] The analytic window was set as the entire seizure. A threshold index score was found to separate EZ from non-EZ contacts in a retrospective cohort. Applied prospectively, QFAI agreed with visual evaluation in 12 of 14 patients; the postoperative outcome was reported to be favorable though the follow up was short (2–14 months).

The above three quantitative approaches were compared in a small study of four patients.[41] In the three seizure-free patients, QFAI most closely matched the surgical resection. Both EI and EM tended to indicate regions that were not within the EZ. The fourth case was not operated upon; here, the methods diverged greatly.

The QFAI method depends on the coincident emergence of ictogenic features: transition to fast activity, background suppression, and superimposed on baseline shifts. The analysis is applied to the entire seizure, not merely the period of onset. Infraslow activity shows late localizing value, with a second prominent phase at seizure termination,[38,42] which may account, in part, for why this method outperforms EI/EM. Furthermore, the relevance of SOPs/dynamics becomes evident, not merely the tracking of fast activity.

## SEIZURE ONSET PATTERNS/DYNAMICS: TRANSITION MATTERS

Recent studies have described a taxonomy of SOPs,[14,18] with common observations but some variability in terminology.[43] SOPs that *contain* LVFA, whether as the initial change or following a train of "preictal" spiking (or otherwise), convey a favorable surgical prognosis. Despite the appellation "preictal" these spikes are part of the seizure.[44] Facilitated by CWT scalograms, Wu et al. described these dynamics,[45] finding that patterns with greater transitional complexity better localized the EZ (seizure-free resection). Specifically, the occurrence of preictal spiking with superimposed fast activity (gamma/HFOs) followed by suppression was most localizing (all patterns contained LVFA by inclusion). Transitional patterns did not depend on the presence of lesion[34,45]; hence, the authors concluded that perilesional cortices with these dynamics were part of the primary organization of the seizure.

## FINGERPRINT OF THE EZ

The dynamics of the preictal–ictal transition were also considered by Grinenko et al.[46] A pattern of features unique to the EZ (seizure-free resection) was identified from baseline-normalized CWT scalograms. These were: 1. preictal spiking, 2. band-limited (vs. broadband) fast activity, and 3. coexisting suppression of lower frequencies at the time of LFVA. The fast activity bands were typically multiple and importantly, were not harmonically related.[47] These features were found to occur coincident in channels within the EZ; none of these features alone was localizing (Fig. 7.2). Moreover, neither the maximal frequency nor its timing (latency) was discriminating of the EZ at the patient level. Various feature characteristics (29 in total) were extracted, and a support vector machine (SVM)—a commonly used supervised machine learning algorithm—was trained to classify channels as EZ or not. This identified the EZ in 15 of 17 patients, with a false-positive rate (FPR; channels predicted as EZ outside of the resection) of 0.7%.

In a subsequent study, the earlier trained model was applied to a more heterogenous cohort, both seizure-free and not.[19] Here, the EZ was identified in a similar fraction of seizure-free patients, with an equally low FPR (0.6%). In the non-seizure-free patients, the "false-positive rate" was much higher (7.5%), implying that the EZ was incompletely resected (the EZ is not known in these patients). An analysis utilizing only fast activity was also done. This yielded an FPR of 33% in seizure-free patients, an observation reminiscent of the tendency of EI/EM to overestimate the EZ using fast activity (or ratio) only. Hence, the "fingerprint" in its entirety and not merely one feature, is of localizing salience. This image is also borne out over a time course well beyond seizure onset.

## EXAMPLE CASE

A patient with bilateral periventricular nodular heterotopia (PVNH) and a semiology of gelastic seizures was implanted. Electrodes targeted the nodular components, as well as cortical regions hypothesized relevant to her semiology, which was found to depend on the

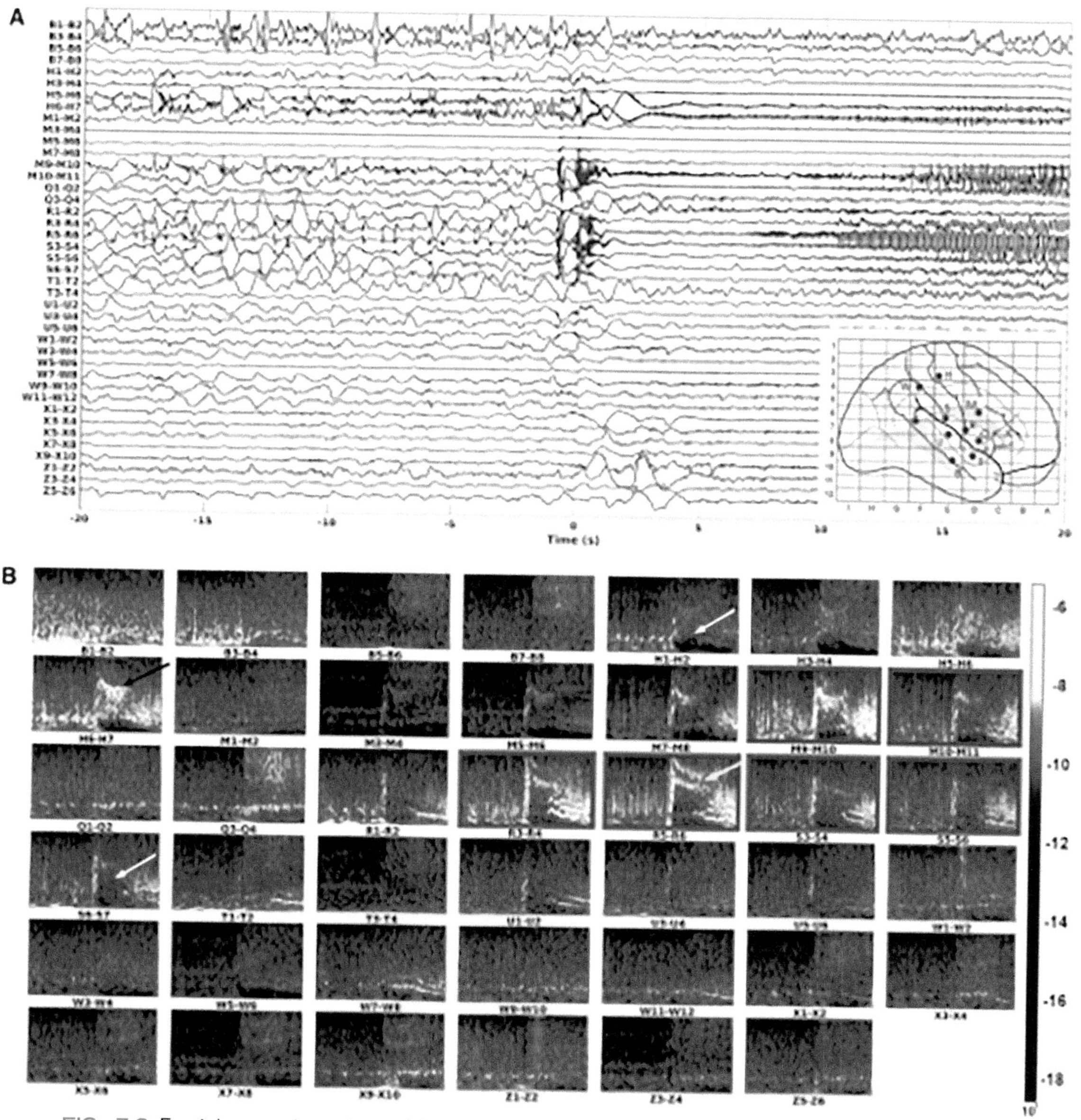

FIG. 7.2 Frontal opercular seizure, (A) abbreviated montage and (B) associated baseline-normalized scalograms. Channels in the seizure-free resection are outlined in blue. A pattern characterized by the combination of preictal spiking, band-limited fast activity, and suppression is found inside the resection (*yellow arrow*). Broadband fast activity (*black arrow*), and suppression without sustained fast activity (*white arrows*) are found outside the resection. It is the combination of features that is localizing of the EZ.

anterior cingulate.[48] Seizure onset was quasi-simultaneous across bilateral PNVH and cortical (frontal-cingulate) regions (Fig. 7.3). Utilizing the original trained model, the EZ was predicted in PVNH channels only. In contrast, by EI, the left (and not right) PVNH as well as other cortical regions were implicated (EI $> 0.3$). According to the definitions applied by Pizzo et al., this patient would be classified as "normo-heterotopic" by EI,[49] yet maintains a seizure-free outcome after bilateral PNVH ablation only. Interestingly, the HFO/spike detector (Delphos) used by Roehri et al.[6] was concordant with the fingerprint prediction

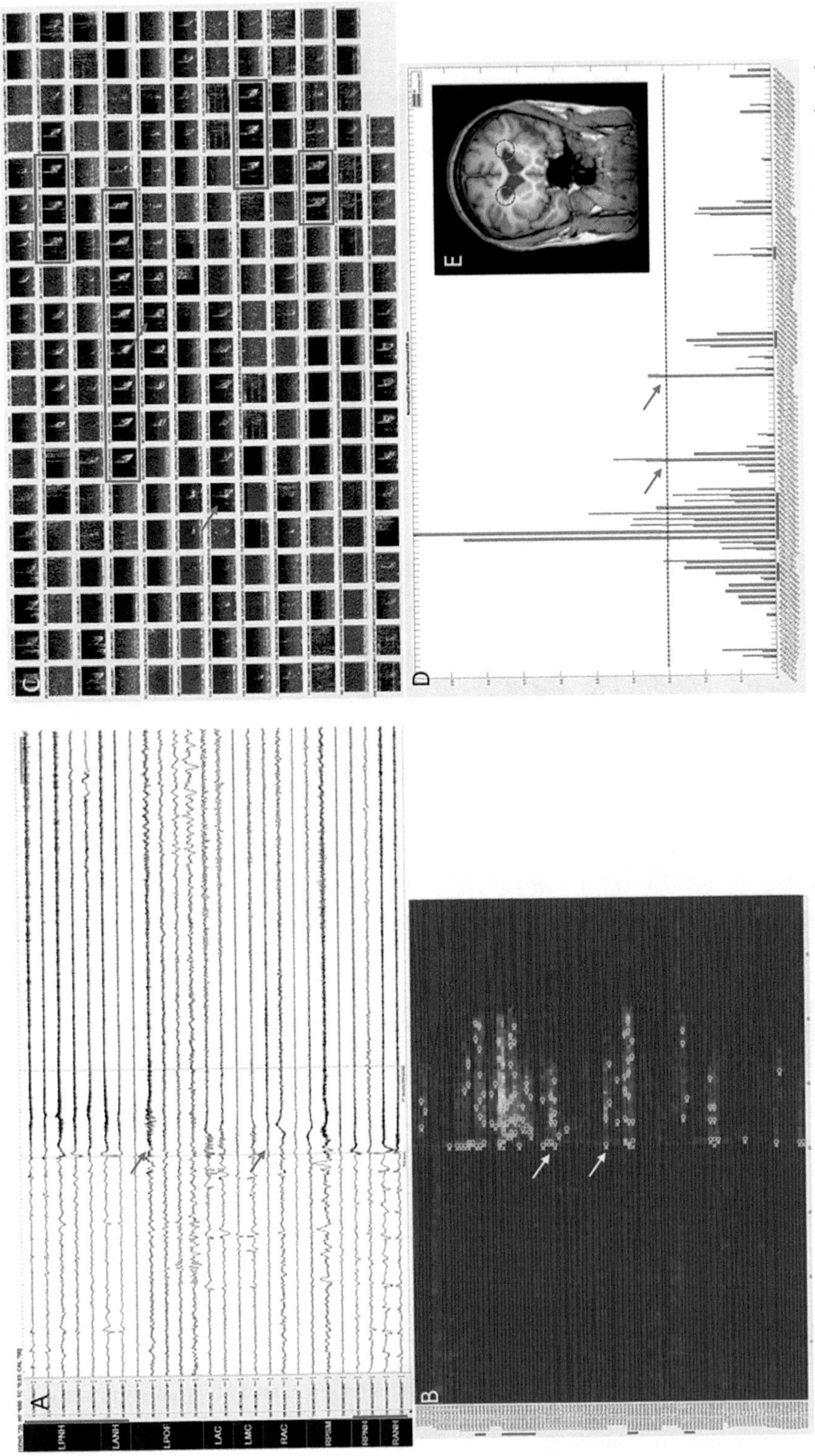


FIG. 7.3 Patient with bilateral PVNH. (A) Quasi-simultaneous onset on an abbreviated montage occurred across bilateral PVNH (*red bars*) and bilateral frontal-cingulate cortical regions (*AC*, anterior cingulate, *MC*, mid-cingulate, *POF*, Posterior orbitofrontal, *PSM*, Pre-SMA). *Arrows* indicate channels implicated by EI only. Note also the very active interictal spiking in PVNH channels; this did not appreciably change during transition into seizure. (B) Full montage with corresponding ER and channel detections. (C) Fingerprint prediction of EZ in PNVH channels only. Note the one outlying channel (LMC3-LMC4) was also sampling PVNH. (D) Summed ER and EI, with a threshold of 0.3 indicating channels with high epileptogenicity.[49] Only *left* PVNH channels are above threshold, as well as untreated cortical regions (*arrows*). E. Postablation MRI.

and not with EI. In this patient, it was adequate to define the primary IZ (not shown).

## REBOUND SYNCHRONIZATION: LATE "SEIZURE ONSET(S)"

The end of LFVA/suppression beacons the return of slow frequencies ("rebound"), which at the cellular level reflects the recovery of the excitatory pyramidal neurons.[44,50] It is theorized that an ictal "core" may be identified, distinct from the surrounding "penumbra," and that this is made evident by high gamma activity (80–150 Hz) phase-locked to lower frequencies (4–30 Hz).[51] Application of the Hilbert transform (HT) to these passbands allows for their phase-amplitude relationship (phase-locked high gamma [PLHG]) to be quantified as a function of time. This metric correlated with the hypersynchronous multiunit activity in microelectrode recordings[51] and thus serves a surrogate of the core. When applied to a large retrospective cohort of subdural-monitored patients, resection of "early" (first four channels) PLHG resulted in good outcomes; however, this did not differ statistically from resections based upon the clinical SOZ, though there was a trend to greater specificity with PLHG.[52] High gamma activity alone was not localizing.

This methodology was recently applied to a cohort of SEEG patients.[53] The formal phase-amplitude definition was relaxed, with high gamma activity (80–150 Hz) only visually correlated to slower rhythms. Like above studies, a late appearing "recruitment" was observed. This occurred in single or multiple "hubs" (brain regions). The authors tracked the sequential recruitment of hubs and asynchrony of seizure termination. All patients with a single hub, or in whom all recruited hubs were resected/ablated, had a good surgical outcome; those with incompletely removed hubs fared less well. There was an association between multiple hubs and an asynchronous termination. This was interpreted to imply the sequential recruitment of multiple independent seizure foci, each terminating uniquely. Regardless of the mechanism or theoretical model,[54] there may be prognostically relevant features within the course of propagation, though the number of treated patients was small.

## SLOWER MODES OF ONSET: FLY IN THE OINTMENT

All methods described thus far assume the presence of fast activity, however good outcomes are still possible, albeit less often, when slower SOPs are observed.[14] This included a minority of patients with dysplasia or neurodevelopmental tumors and slower SOPs, in whom the complete "SEEG-defined" EZ was resected.[55] In such cases, one would assume that the lesion—which was sampled—was at least part of the EZ. Not surprisingly, the above metrics perform poorly with slower onset patterns.[56,57] A recent extension of EI, connectivity EI, was proposed to address this problem.[58]

## SUMMARY AND PROPOSALS

The question of EZ extent is formidable, and time–frequency methods that approach it have been reviewed. When possible, these were vetted against surgical outcome. It has been argued that the definition of EZ operationalized by Bancaud and Talairach does not depend on surgical outcome,[6] that it is not the "what-to-remove area."[2] Yet, if an area is said to command the primary organization of the seizure, its removal should be expected to affect seizure control. For primary organization to have therapeutic relevance, it should be "indispensable for the generation of epileptic seizures."[1]

These terminological debates aside, how do we understand the distribution of ictal epileptiform activity within the cortex with respect to EZ extent? There is certainly merit in quantifying patterns of propagation, as these help define epileptogenic networks[27] and understand the emergence of semiology.[59] Arguably, methods that are limited to the analysis of fast activity (EI/EM) fail to distinguish between primary and propagated fast activity, especially in extratemporal or neocortical epilepsies, as judged by their performance against surgical outcomes at the patient level.[35,37] The risk is more of declaring an overly extensive EZ, and consequently withholding surgery, or misconstruing such cases as "regional" and offering palliative over potentially curative surgical therapy.[60]

The mechanisms of ictogenesis are complex and still debated[44,61]; it is unlikely that a single (macrodomain) feature will be uncovered adequate to define EZ extent. The proposed features are legion and heterogeneous: preictal spikes with embedded gamma/HFOs,[45,62] fast activity with coincident suppression,[40,46] baseline shifts,[38,40] and late phase-locked high gamma.[52,53] Whether some or all of these should be combined to describe a fuller "fingerprint" remains to be determined. This is not to mention interareal coupling/decoupling/recoupling.[63] Multidimensional analysis seems requisite, likely requiring a machine-learning approach. The historical priority has been on onset, but consideration of seizure in its entirety (somehow) may prove necessary to fully realize this goal.

## REFERENCES


1. Rosenow F, Lüders H. Presurgical evaluation of epilepsy. *Brain*. 2001;124(9):1683–1700. https://doi.org/10.1093/brain/124.9.1683.
2. Kahane P, Landre E, Minotti L, Francione S, Ryvlin P. The Bancaud and Talairach view on the epileptogenic zone: a working hypothesis. *Epileptic Disord*. August 2006;8(Suppl 2):S16–S26.
3. Chauvel P. In: Schuele SU, ed. *The Epileptogenic Zone: A Critical Reconstruction*. Springer Publishing Company; 2021:105–117.
4. Bettus G, Ranjeva JP, Wendling F, et al. Interictal functional connectivity of human epileptic networks assessed by intracerebral EEG and BOLD signal fluctuations. *PLoS One*. 2011;6(5):e20071. https://doi.org/10.1371/journal.pone.0020071.
5. Chauvel P, Gonzalez-Martinez J, Bulacio J. Presurgical intracranial investigations in epilepsy surgery. *Handb Clin Neurol*. 2019;161:45–71. https://doi.org/10.1016/B978-0-444-64142-7.00040-0.
6. Roehri N, Pizzo F, Lagarde S, et al. High-frequency oscillations are not better biomarkers of epileptogenic tissues than spikes. *Ann Neurol*. January 2018;83(1):84–97. https://doi.org/10.1002/ana.25124.
7. Cuello-Oderiz C, von Ellenrieder N, Sankhe R, et al. Value of ictal and interictal epileptiform discharges and high frequency oscillations for delineating the epileptogenic zone in patients with focal cortical dysplasia. *Clin Neurophysiol*. June 2018;129(6):1311–1319. https://doi.org/10.1016/j.clinph.2018.02.003.
8. Khoo HM, von Ellenrieder N, Zazubovits N, He D, Dubeau F, Gotman J. The spike onset zone: the region where epileptic spikes start and from where they propagate. *Neurology*. August 14, 2018;91(7):e666–e674. https://doi.org/10.1212/WNL.0000000000005998.
9. Zweiphenning W, Klooster MAV, van Klink NEC, et al. Intraoperative electrocorticography using high-frequency oscillations or spikes to tailor epilepsy surgery in the Netherlands (the HFO trial): a randomised, single-blind, adaptive non-inferiority trial. *Lancet Neurol*. November 2022;21(11):982–993. https://doi.org/10.1016/S1474-4422(22)00311-8.
10. Bartolomei F, Lagarde S, Wendling F, et al. Defining epileptogenic networks: contribution of SEEG and signal analysis. *Epilepsia*. July 2017;58(7):1131–1147. https://doi.org/10.1111/epi.13791.
11. Wendling F, Chauvel P, Biraben A, Bartolomei F. From intracerebral EEG signals to brain connectivity: identification of epileptogenic networks in partial epilepsy. *Front Syst Neurosci*. 2010;4:154. https://doi.org/10.3389/fnsys.2010.00154.
12. Bancaud J, Talairach J. *La Stereo-Electroencephalographie Dans L'epilepsie*. Masson; 1965.
13. Singh S, Sandy S, Wiebe S. Ictal onset on intracranial EEG: do we know it when we see it? State of the evidence. *Epilepsia*. October 2015;56(10):1629–1638. https://doi.org/10.1111/epi.13120.
14. Lagarde S, Buzori S, Trebuchon A, et al. The repertoire of seizure onset patterns in human focal epilepsies: determinants and prognostic values. *Epilepsia*. January 2019;60(1):85–95. https://doi.org/10.1111/epi.14604.
15. Barba C, Rheims S, Minotti L, et al. Temporal plus epilepsy is a major determinant of temporal lobe surgery failures. *Brain*. February 2016;139(Pt 2):444–451. https://doi.org/10.1093/brain/awv372.
16. Blauwblomme T, David O, Minotti L, et al. Prognostic value of insular lobe involvement in temporal lobe epilepsy: a stereoelectroencephalographic study. *Epilepsia*. September 2013;54(9):1658–1667. https://doi.org/10.1111/epi.12260.
17. Barba C, Minotti L, Job AS, Kahane P. The insula in temporal plus epilepsy. *J Clin Neurophysiol*. July 2017;34(4):324–327. https://doi.org/10.1097/WNP.0000000000000389.
18. Perucca P, Dubeau F, Gotman J. Intracranial electroencephalographic seizure-onset patterns: effect of underlying pathology. *Brain*. 2014;137(1):183–196.
19. Li J, Grinenko O, Mosher JC, Gonzalez-Martinez J, Leahy RM, Chauvel P. Learning to define an electrical biomarker of the epileptogenic zone. *Hum Brain Mapp*. February 1, 2020;41(2):429–441. https://doi.org/10.1002/hbm.24813.
20. Restrepo CE, Balaguera P, Thompson SA, et al. Safety and efficacy of bihemispheric sampling via transmidline stereoelectroencephalography. *J Neurosurg*. December 30, 2022:1–9. https://doi.org/10.3171/2022.11.JNS221144.
21. Luders HO, Najm I, Nair D, Widdess-Walsh P, Bingman W. The epileptogenic zone: general principles. *Epileptic Disord*. August 2006;8(Suppl 2):S1–S9.
22. Andrews JP, Ammanuel S, Kleen J, Khambhati AN, Knowlton R, Chang EF. Early seizure spread and epilepsy surgery: a systematic review. *Epilepsia*. October 2020; 61(10):2163–2172. https://doi.org/10.1111/epi.16668.
23. Bartolomei F, Chauvel P, Wendling F. Epileptogenicity of brain structures in human temporal lobe epilepsy: a quantified study from intracerebral EEG. *Brain*. July 2008;131(Pt 7):1818–1830. https://doi.org/10.1093/brain/awn111.
24. Weiss SA, Alvarado-Rojas C, Bragin A, et al. Ictal onset patterns of local field potentials, high frequency oscillations, and unit activity in human mesial temporal lobe epilepsy. *Epilepsia*. January 2016;57(1):111–121. https://doi.org/10.1111/epi.13251.
25. Bruns A. Fourier-, Hilbert- and wavelet-based signal analysis: are they really different approaches? *J Neurosci Methods*. August 30, 2004;137(2):321–332. https://doi.org/10.1016/j.jneumeth.2004.03.002.
26. Buzsaki G, Draguhn A. Neuronal oscillations in cortical networks. *Science*. June 25, 2004;304(5679):1926–1929. https://doi.org/10.1126/science.1099745.
27. Bartolomei F, Cosandier-Rimele D, McGonigal A, et al. From mesial temporal lobe to temporoperisylvian seizures: a quantified study of temporal lobe seizure networks. *Epilepsia*. October 2010;51(10):2147–2158. https://doi.org/10.1111/j.1528-1167.2010.02690.x.

28. Aubert S, Wendling F, Regis J, et al. Local and remote epileptogenicity in focal cortical dysplasias and neurodevelopmental tumours. *Brain*. November 2009;132(Pt 11):3072–3086. https://doi.org/10.1093/brain/awp242.
29. Sevy A, Gavaret M, Trebuchon A, et al. Beyond the lesion: the epileptogenic networks around cavernous angiomas. *Epilepsy Res*. May 2014;108(4):701–708. https://doi.org/10.1016/j.eplepsyres.2014.02.018.
30. Pizzo F, Roehri N, Catenoix H, et al. Epileptogenic networks in nodular heterotopia: a stereoelectroencephalography study. *Epilepsia*. December 2017;58(12):2112–2123. https://doi.org/10.1111/epi.13919.
31. Bartolomei F, Gavaret M, Hewett R, et al. Neural networks underlying parietal lobe seizures: a quantified study from intracerebral recordings. *Epilepsy Res*. February 2011;93(2–3):164–176. https://doi.org/10.1016/j.eplepsyres.2010.12.005.
32. Bonini F, McGonigal A, Wendling F, et al. Epileptogenic networks in seizures arising from motor systems. *Epilepsy Res*. September 2013;106(1–2):92–102. https://doi.org/10.1016/j.eplepsyres.2013.04.011.
33. Marchi A, Bonini F, Lagarde S, et al. Occipital and occipital "plus" epilepsies: a study of involved epileptogenic networks through SEEG quantification. *Epilepsy Behav*. September 2016;62:104–114. https://doi.org/10.1016/j.yebeh.2016.06.014.
34. Lagarde S, Scholly J, Popa I, et al. Can histologically normal epileptogenic zone share common electrophysiological phenotypes with focal cortical dysplasia? SEEG-based study in MRI-negative epileptic patients. *J Neurol*. August 2019;266(8):1907–1918. https://doi.org/10.1007/s00415-019-09339-4.
35. Parasuram H, Gopinath S, Pillai A, Diwakar S, Kumar A. Quantification of epileptogenic network from stereo EEG recordings using epileptogenicity ranking method. *Front Neurol*. 2021;12:738111. https://doi.org/10.3389/fneur.2021.738111.
36. David O, Blauwblomme T, Job AS, et al. Imaging the seizure onset zone with stereo-electroencephalography. *Brain*. October 2011;134(Pt 10):2898–2911. https://doi.org/10.1093/brain/awr238.
37. Job AS, David O, Minotti L, Bartolomei F, Chabardès S, Kahane P. Epileptogenicity maps of intracerebral fast activities (60-100 Hz) at seizure onset in epilepsy surgery candidates. *Front Neurol*. 2019;10:1263. https://doi.org/10.3389/fneur.2019.01263.
38. Thompson SA, Krishnan B, Gonzalez-Martinez J, et al. Ictal infraslow activity in stereoelectroencephalography: beyond the DC shift. *Clin Neurophysiol*. January 2016;127(1):117–128. https://doi.org/10.1016/j.clinph.2015.03.020.
39. Gnatkovsky V, Pelliccia V, de Curtis M, Tassi L. Two main focal seizure patterns revealed by intracerebral electroencephalographic biomarker analysis. *Epilepsia*. January 2019;60(1):96–106. https://doi.org/10.1111/epi.14610.
40. Gnatkovsky V, de Curtis M, Pastori C, et al. Biomarkers of epileptogenic zone defined by quantified stereo-EEG analysis. *Epilepsia*. February 2014;55(2):296–305. https://doi.org/10.1111/epi.12507.
41. Andrzejak RG, David O, Gnatkovsky V, et al. Localization of epileptogenic zone on pre-surgical intracranial EEG recordings: toward a validation of quantitative signal analysis approaches. *Brain Topogr*. 2015;28(6):832–837.
42. Jirsa VK, Stacey WC, Quilichini PP, Ivanov AI, Bernard C. On the nature of seizure dynamics. *Brain*. August 2014;137(Pt 8):2210–2230. https://doi.org/10.1093/brain/awu133.
43. Gotman J. Not just where, but how does a seizure start? *Epilepsy Curr*. Jul-Aug 2019;19(4):229–230. https://doi.org/10.1177/1535759719854756.
44. de Curtis M, Avoli M. GABAergic networks jump-start focal seizures. *Epilepsia*. May 2016;57(5):679–687. https://doi.org/10.1111/epi.13370.
45. Wu D, Zhang W, Lu H, Liu X, Sun W. Transitional pattern as a potential marker of epileptogenic zone in focal epilepsy - clinical observations from intracerebral recordings. *Epilepsy Res*. August 2021;174:106676. https://doi.org/10.1016/j.eplepsyres.2021.106676.
46. Grinenko O, Li J, Mosher JC, et al. A fingerprint of the epileptogenic zone in human epilepsies. *Brain*. January 1, 2018;141(1):117–131. https://doi.org/10.1093/brain/awx306.
47. Zhou H, Melloni L, Poeppel D, Ding N. Interpretations of frequency danalyses of neural entrainment: periodicity, fundamental frequency, and harmonics. *Front Hum Neurosci*. 2016;10:274. https://doi.org/10.3389/fnhum.2016.00274.
48. Caruana F, Avanzini P, Gozzo F, Francione S, Cardinale F, Rizzolatti G. Mirth and laughter elicited by electrical stimulation of the human anterior cingulate cortex. *Cortex*. October 2015;71:323–331. https://doi.org/10.1016/j.cortex.2015.07.024.
49. Pizzo F, Roehri N, Catenoix H, et al. Epileptogenic networks in nodular heterotopia: a stereoelectroencephalography study. *Epilepsia*. 2017;58(12):2112–2123.
50. Elahian B, Lado NE, Mankin E, et al. Low-voltage fast seizures in humans begin with increased interneuron firing. *Ann Neurol*. October 2018;84(4):588–600. https://doi.org/10.1002/ana.25325.
51. Weiss SA, Banks GP, McKhann Jr GM, et al. Ictal high frequency oscillations distinguish two types of seizure territories in humans. *Brain*. December 2013;136(Pt 12):3796–3808. https://doi.org/10.1093/brain/awt276.
52. Weiss SA, Lemesiou A, Connors R, et al. Seizure localization using ictal phase-locked high gamma: a retrospective surgical outcome study. *Neurology*. June 9, 2015;84(23):2320–2328. https://doi.org/10.1212/wnl.0000000000001656.
53. Tobochnik S, Bateman LM, Akman CI, et al. Tracking multisite seizure propagation using ictal high-gamma activity. *J Clin Neurophysiol*. November 1, 2022;39(7):592–601. https://doi.org/10.1097/wnp.0000000000000833.
54. Smith EH, Liou J-y, Davis TS, et al. The ictal wavefront is the spatiotemporal source of discharges during spontaneous

human seizures. *Nat Commun*. 2016/03/29 2016;7(1): 11098. https://doi.org/10.1038/ncomms11098.

55. Lagarde S, Bonini F, McGonigal A, et al. Seizure-onset patterns in focal cortical dysplasia and neurodevelopmental tumors: relationship with surgical prognosis and neuropathologic subtypes. *Epilepsia*. September 2016;57(9): 1426–1435. https://doi.org/10.1111/epi.13464.
56. Smith G, Stacey WC. The accuracy of quantitative EEG biomarker algorithms depends upon seizure onset dynamics. *Epilepsy Res*. Oct 2021;176:106702. https://doi.org/10.1016/j.eplepsyres.2021.106702.
57. Gollwitzer S, Valente I, Rodionov R, et al. Visual and semi-automated evaluation of epileptogenicity in focal cortical dysplasias - an intracranial EEG study. *Epilepsy Behav*. May 2016;58:69–75. https://doi.org/10.1016/j.yebeh.2016.03.009.
58. Balatskaya A, Roehri N, Lagarde S, et al. The "connectivity epileptogenicity index " (CEI), a method for mapping the different seizure onset patterns in StereoElectroEncephalography recorded seizures. *Clin Neurophysiol*. August 2020; 131(8):1947–1955. https://doi.org/10.1016/j.clinph.2020.05.029.
59. Chauvel P, McGonigal A. Emergence of semiology in epileptic seizures. *Epilepsy Behav*. September 2014;38: 94–103. https://doi.org/10.1016/j.yebeh.2013.12.003.
60. Ma BB, Fields MC, Knowlton RC, et al. Responsive neurostimulation for regional neocortical epilepsy. *Epilepsia*. January 2020;61(1):96–106. https://doi.org/10.1111/epi.16409.
61. Weiss SA, Staba R, Bragin A, et al. Interneurons and principal cell firing in human limbic areas at focal seizure onset. *Neurobiol Dis*. April 2019;124:183–188. https://doi.org/10.1016/j.nbd.2018.11.014.
62. Jmail N, Gavaret M, Bartolomei F, Benar CG. Despiking SEEG signals reveals dynamics of gamma band preictal activity. *Physiol Meas*. February 2017;38(2):N42–N56. https://doi.org/10.1088/1361-6579/38/2/N42.
63. Wendling F, Bartolomei F, Bellanger JJ, Bourien J, Chauvel P. Epileptic fast intracerebral EEG activity: evidence for spatial decorrelation at seizure onset. *Brain*. June 2003;126(Pt 6):1449–1459. https://doi.org/10.1093/brain/awg144.

CHAPTER 8

# Anatomo-electro-clinical Correlations

AILEEN MCGONIGAL, MBCHB, PHD • HUSSAM SHAKER, MD •
AMMAR KHEDER, MD • PATRICK CHAUVEL, MD

## INTRODUCTION

Jean Bancaud, who greatly contributed to the study of seizure semiology through his observations from the inception of the stereoelectroencephalographic (SEEG) era, commented that semiological expression of an epileptic seizure is similar to the arrangement of words in forming a meaningful sentence.[1] This statement highlights the difference between studying clinical signs occurring in the context of epileptic seizures and those arising in most other neurological conditions: in seizures (which by definition occur paroxysmally), there is an inherent temporal relation between the evolving signs, the nature of which is essential in order to make sense of the clinical picture. The metaphor of a meaningful sentence also conveys the notion that a certain "sense" exists in terms of the grouping and the evolution of clinical signs; semiological expression does not occur haphazardly but necessarily follows a sequence that is structured according to the effects of the epileptic discharge on functioning of brain networks.

Attempts to understand correlations between clinical symptoms/signs and brain electrical activity (i.e., using behavioral data to infer possible alterations in brain networks produced by epileptic discharges) must consider both the anatomical spread of seizure and the timescale over which changes occur.[2] Interpreting seizure semiology therefore implies not only studying discrete elements (individual symptoms and signs) but how they are assembled together, and over which time course. In the framework of epilepsy presurgical evaluation, the clinician's main goal is to formulate, and then prove or disprove, hypotheses of likely anatomical zone of seizure onset and early spread.

In this chapter, we will discuss (1) the relevance of semiologic analysis in conjunction with simultaneous EEG during the initial non-invasive phase of presurgical evaluation (*electroclinical correlations*), how this helps to formulate hypotheses of likely epileptogenic zone (EZ) and how it guides the clinician to decide upon an SEEG implantation strategy to confirm or refute these; (2) how to approach the key methodology of SEEG interpretation (*anatomo-electroclinical correlations*). We will highlight some common pitfalls and methodological challenges and will illustrate anatomo-electroclinical correlations using 2 case vignettes.

## FROM PHASE 1 TO SEEG: FROM ELECTROCLINICAL CORRELATIONS TO ANATOMO-ELECTROCLINICAL CORRELATIONS

The "Phase 1" non-invasive part of presurgical evaluation uses *electroclinical correlation*, i.e., careful study of seizure semiology and its surface EEG correlates, via review of all available recorded seizures. This important step, which is performed in conjunction with study of the ensemble of non-invasive data (patient history, neuroimaging, neuropsychology, etc.) is key to formulating hypotheses of likely cerebral organization of a specific patient's epilepsy. The surface-EEG based *electroclinical correlation* can be contrasted with SEEG-based *anatomo-electroclinical correlation*. The "*anatomo-*" part of this terminology becomes possible with SEEG due to the precise anatomic descriptors of the source of the electrical signal, based on intracerebral electrode contract positions, confirmed (nowadays) on post-implantation imaging, usually computerized tomography of electrodes in situ co-registered with the patient's pre-implantation magnetic resonance imaging. *Anatomo-electroclinical correlation* is the core methodology of SEEG interpretation. Its aim is to try to make clinical sense of the observed signal changes on SEEG in conjunction with concomitant semiologic features, in order to extrapolate the likely seizure onset and propagation dynamics underlying the clinical expression. SEEG interpretation cannot meaningfully be done without this careful reference to semiologic output, and no amount of quantitative tools for SEEG signal analysis (interictal or ictal) can be a substitute for this

The Fundamentals of Stereoelectroencephalography. https://doi.org/10.1016/B978-0-443-10877-8.00008-5

core methodology that is grounded in expert study of the patient's habitual seizure-related symptoms and signs. Apart from other aspects, semiologic analysis can help to check that a major SEEG electrode sampling error has not occurred. Going back to the Phase 1 and comparing the original electroclinical correlations with SEEG data can be a helpful last step to make sure that the conclusion following SEEG is compatible with the original non-invasive data.

### Importance of Phase I Semiological Data Prior to SEEG

The quality of the interpretation of the ensemble of Phase 1 data, including seizure semiology, will help in (1) optimally choosing candidates for SEEG (i.e., patients with focal, drug-resistant epilepsy in whom surgical decision making will be significantly altered by SEEG results, in a way that could benefit outcome, such that the risk-benefit ratio for that specific patient is clearly in favor of proceeding to invasive recording); and (2) optimally designing an implantation strategy to confirm/refute the main hypotheses. Decision making in these 2 steps largely determines the success or otherwise of the definition of the epileptogenic zone using SEEG via anatomo-electroclinical correlation. The quality of the electroclinical correlations derived from the Phase 1 thus directly shapes the robustness of the anatomo-electroclinical correlations of the SEEG.

Prior to getting to the point of SEEG and tackling anatomo-electroclinical correlations, detailed background knowledge of the particular patient's seizure semiology is very important. Starting with the Phase 1, interpretation of the video-EEG will ideally have been done by a clinician who knows the full case. In particular, it is important to be as familiar as possible with the semiologic history since onset of epilepsy (since patterns can evolve over time and with treatment changes), especially whether subjective symptoms have been reported at any time in the epilepsy history (see Clinical Vignette 1), and their precise description as provided by the patient. It is also important to know whether a single seizure type is described by the patient and their family, or whether different types occur (either variations of severity or clearly distinct semiologic patterns). These aspects will be important in correctly interpreting what is eventually recorded at the time of SEEG, both for spontaneous and stimulation-induced seizures.

## SEMIOLOGIC ANALYSIS: METHODOLOGICAL CONSIDERATIONS

Some basic methodological considerations can be discussed in terms of optimal conditions for semiological analysis as follows: (1) technical conditions of recording; (2) adequate ictal examination; (3) specialist expertise. These apply to all seizure recordings captured in the Epilepsy Monitoring Unit (EMU); since this chapter is on SEEG, we emphasize that all opportunities for capturing maximally useful seizure data should be prioritized, especially adequate ictal examination.

### Technical Conditions of Recording

Since semiological analysis is largely based on expert visual inspection of recorded video data, the information retrieved is dependent on both physical recording conditions (placement of patient in the camera field, quality of lighting, video resolution, etc.) and the observer's visual perception and ability to recognize and correctly interpret the signs. Video quality can be optimized through adequate technical parameters (such as including a close-up image of the patient's face, automated tracking of the head, and use of infra-red cameras for night-time filming). Placement of 2 different cameras recording simultaneously may allow better visualization depending on patient position,[3] but in most cases a single high density camera is sufficient if the seizure occurs while the patient is within the camera frame. With a wide-angle lens, the field is large enough to get the full body image, and HD camera allows for replay zooming with excellent resolution, for instance on the face.

### Ictal Examination

The quality of the clinical information obtained during the seizure can be greatly augmented by appropriate ictal examination, comprising evaluation of conscious level, language[4] and if required motor examination. This should be meticulously done during SEEG, with the healthcare team on stand-by to examine the patient at the very first sign of any seizure activity on the trace or clinically. Indeed, for some seizure types, it is essentially the ictal examination that reveals all relevant signs, such as a patient presenting a non-signaled seizure with loss of awareness and/or language dysfunction without motor features. Appropriate training in ictal examination for personnel who will be attending to the patient is an important component for optimal seizure recording. The key aspect of the ictal examination is the interaction between the examiner and the patient, to allow evaluation of awareness and language function, and the quality of this (depending on the individual questions to be answered for each patient's case) is influenced by the experience of the examiner in performing ictal testing. A standardized battery for ictal clinical testing has been proposed following a European study performed under the auspices of the ILAE[5] (see also chapters on stimulation in this book). Attaining optimal ictal examination requires specific training and ongoing practice of nurses, EEG technicians and medical staff. Lack of such training has indeed been identified as a major obstacle to obtaining good quality semiological data in many EMU[5].

The first step is to make that the patient is visible on camera (e.g., in camera field and if possible, facing the camera; remove bedsheets while protecting privacy), and then immediately test whether the patient is responsive by calling their name and asking simple commands. If the patient can respond, the examiner asks the patient what they can feel; simple naming tasks are given and orientation is checked. Audible commentary by the examining practitioner can be very helpful, for example mentioning out loud the presence of subtle signs that may be poorly visualized on video recording, such as skin color or pupillary change. Verbal memory can be tested by asking the patient to remember a word, or using recall of object naming as an episode that can be recalled by the patient afterward. If a trained person is not present to perform ictal testing, as a minimum any verbal interaction with a patient during a seizure (e.g., by a family member) can bring useful information. Depending on the clinical features of each case, other examination may be indicated, such as motor function, visual fields, proprioception or specific cognitive functions such as face recognition.

Post-ictal examination is also important (language recovery, memory of seizure, presence of focal deficit, etc.), and it may be during this period that the patient can give some description of early subjective symptoms experienced at seizure onset. Any symptoms mentioned by the patient should be carefully explored to achieve maximum descriptive detail, since the specific nature of a hallucination or visceral sensation could be an important clue as to localization of seizure onset. Stimulation studies require their own examination protocol (described in separate chapter on stimulation-induced seizures).

### The Importance of Specialist Expertise

Semiologic analysis in conjunction with concomitant electrophysiologic data very largely depends on clinician expertise and experience, at the individual and at the team level, because of the importance of pattern recognition.[2] As experience progresses, an important aspect is refined recognition of which semiologic patterns are robust with high specificity for certain brain regions, lobes or structures; and in contrast, which patterns have low specificity and relatively low predictive value (on their own) for localization. This last point is very important when using semiologic data to support hypotheses for subsequent SEEG implantation (discussed below in the section "Localizing value" of semiologic features: importance for SEEG hypotheses"). Equally, the correct interpretation of SEEG using anatomo-electroclinical correlations requires sufficient understanding of the different electrical seizure patterns, and pitfalls of SEEG including sampling limitations. The diagnostic framework of clinical acumen and electroclinical pattern recognition based on experience, and the "apprenticeship" process, are not yet replaceable by any other means of analysis of semiology or seizures, and this point is even more crucial for the more complex practice of SEEG compared to video-EEG.

## GENERAL TIPS FOR ANALYZING SEIZURE RECORDINGS

Seizures are viewed as video recordings (time-locked with electroencephalographic and other electrophysiologic data) that should allow sufficient time before the onset of the seizure, to determine, as far as possible, the precise moment at which the first clinical sign occurs. This may be obvious, such as a signaled aura or onset of motor signs, or may be very subtle, such as a slight change of facial expression. The clinical onset may be visible on the video, may be highlighted by an observer's recognition of the seizure (e.g., family member in the room), or can be another recorded change such as increased heart rate. This time-point can be annotated on the trace to facilitate comparison with the signal. Next, the sequence of signs should be carefully reviewed, often by more than one visualization of the video data to make sure that nothing has been missed, and again annotating key moments of the semiologic evolution is helpful for comparing with the signal. How best to describe semiologic signs can be challenging for rarer or subtle patterns; a general rule it is preferable to use standardized vocabulary[6] despite the limitations of this in some cases.

The full seizure period including the post-ictal phase should be reviewed; post-ictal signs may also provide important information (e.g., confusion, aphasia, visual field deficit, motor deficit, etc.). Visualizing seizure videos more than once, especially the early part of the seizure, can help in assessing the important features. Using video close-up on the face or specific body segments can be useful for looking at subtle changes (e.g., slight facial expression change), and it can sometimes be helpful to slow down the video playback speed (e.g., to study hyperkinetic movements) or speed it up (e.g., to review semiologic evolution in a prolonged seizure).

Since semiologic analysis is largely based on clinicians' pattern recognition, a seizure may immediately have recognizable features that we are drawn to. This however should not preclude detailed searching for other specific features that may be more or less obvious. It is useful to assess both isolated signs or groups of signs, and the overall "gestalt" of the semiology, and degree of reproducibility across recorded seizures from that patient. The order and time course of signs are very important, with more emphasis placed on early compared to late seizure signs for cerebral localization purposes, since the early signs are produced by earliest propagation (i.e., closest to the seizure onset zone). Attention should be paid to asymmetry of signs, which in some cases are very important for cerebral lateralization, although it is important to be aware of which asymmetric signs do not have consistent lateralizing value (e.g., head turning, eye blinking) versus those that do (contralateral dystonia, tonic contraction or clonic jerks).

If more than one seizure has been recorded, this allows assessment of degree of reproducibility in both semiology and electrical pattern. The degree of inter-seizure clinical similarity should be checked against the electrical pattern, and may again provide helpful information about propagation, since different semiologic evolution may reflect differences in seizure propagation even if onset of seizure discharge is similar. The most obvious and common example of this would be a patient who has both focal seizures and focal to bilateral tonic-clonic seizures, or focal seizures with and without impaired consciousness. Anti-seizure medication reduction should be done judiciously to try to record the most focal version of the patient's usual seizures, since rapid seizure propagation due to low ASM levels may make it harder to assess relevance of both semiologic and electrical features (e.g., seizures in clusters and/or focal to bilateral tonic clonic seizures).

## "LOCALIZING VALUE" OF SEMIOLOGIC FEATURES: IMPORTANCE FOR SEEG HYPOTHESES

Knowledge of the relative predictive power (specificity) of different semiologic features in understanding likely cerebral localization of seizures has to be built up over time. This occurs not just by reading literature and attending courses but through looking at as many videos as possible, of a large variety of seizures, in conjunction with discussion with specialist practitioners with large experience as mentioned earlier. When formulating hypotheses from Phase I data with a view to planning SEEG implantation, the specificity (or otherwise) of semiological features should be considered. The specificity of the semiologic features for a given patient is one component amongst the ensemble of non-invasive data that is used to judge whether a unifocal, spatially restrained and potentially surgical treatable zone of seizure organization is likely. To investigate predictors of focality of seizure onset on SEEG, a tool for clinicians called the 5-SENSE score, has been proposed, based on a composite of non-invasive data including "strongly localizing semiology".[7] Of course for this to be useful and correctly applied, the team needs to understand which semiologic features are "strongly localizing" and which are not; this is quite easy for some signs/patterns (and teams), much more difficult or even unknown for others. It should be remembered that this can be somewhat of a moving target since knowledge in this domain is always advancing. In addition, semiology (like EEG interpretation) is not an exact science and experts will not always agree on the significance or even the appearance and nomenclature of patterns, adding to the complexity of this area. Inter-observer agreement between experts can however be high even for complex semiologic patterns.[8] As research advances on seizure semiologic expressions and their neural correlates, clinical knowledge in this field can potentially benefit from more evidence-based data and be less prone to the risks of dogma.

As well as keeping in mind some individual clinical correlations that are usually fairly robust (e.g., déjà vu linked to peri-hippocampal structures; auditory hallucinations linked to lateral temporal neocortex; visual hallucinations linked to occipital cortex, clonic jerks linked to contralateral motor cortex), it can be helpful to think in terms of systems based on *clusters of semiologic features* being correlated to *clusters of connected brain structures* (i.e., networks). As such, one approach is to think about the patient's semiology in broad terms of "motor system," "sensory system," "memory system," "autonomic system," "emotional system," "consciousness system," and so on, and consider the groups of connected anatomic structures that underlie these general brain functions. This can allow the clinician to look at the bigger picture of possible anatomic correlates and avoid being too rapidly confined to a narrow set of choices, which is very important when trying to decide on optimal SEEG electrode implantation strategy. For example, a rising epigastric sensation (within the larger group of sensations termed abdominal aura[9]), is considered to be an autonomic sign and may occur with focal seizures involving any structure within or projecting to the central autonomic network (which is usually considered to comprise amygdala, anterior insula, anterior cingulate and their closely connected structures,[10] i.e., structures related to the limbic system). When epigastric sensation is reported at seizure onset, especially with a rising character, the balance of probabilities of localization is most often in favor of a role for mesial temporal structures because of their particularly frequent involvement in focal epileptic seizures[9,11,12] but all other semiologic features of the seizure should be considered in their sequence (as well as imaging data etc.), bringing additional clues to primarily temporal or extra-temporal organization.[13] This is why it is often appropriate in SEEG exploration to sample some structures that are anatomically connected to the main hypothesized region of seizure onset, as alternative hypotheses that could potentially produce a similar clinical picture. As such, in a case undergoing SEEG of suspected mesial temporal seizures with epigastric rising sensation as first clinical feature, it would be typical to decide to implant not only the mesial temporal structures but the anterior insula and often the orbitofrontal cortex, which could be alternate seizure routes potentially capable of producing similar semiology. Confirming or refuting the role of these different structures in seizure organization lends robustness to surgical decision making and can help predict likelihood of seizure freedom after surgical therapy.[14]

## HOW DOES ELECTRICAL SEIZURE ONSET AND SPREAD INFLUENCE SEMIOLOGIC OUTPUT?

Not only the presence of different semiologic features, but the timing of their appearance relative to each other and relative to electrophysiologic data are very important. In general, most weight is placed on symptoms/signs occurring at seizure onset or in the early part of the seizure, as these will likely reflect brain activity changes most directly linked to electrical seizure onset. Some seizures evolve gradually with a stepwise appearance of semiologic features, which if present tend to be intuitively and technically more straightforward for the stereo-electroencephalographer to compare with the equivalent timepoint on the electrical trace. Many focal seizures can show progressive semiologic evolution over seconds or even minutes, for example, an insulo-opercular seizure beginning with feeling of buccal sensation progressing to facial contraction then facial clonus evolving over 30–60 s. If SEEG sampling is optimal or at least sufficient, it will often be possible to see a relation between different signs emerging and changes in SEEG activity, which may be spatial (spreading to other structures), temporal (frequency, amplitude of discharge), and most often both (e.g., oro-alimentary automatisms associated with opercular seizure discharge propagation in a temporal lobe seizure as shown in Clinical Vignette 1).

However, some seizures on SEEG do not show such an evident stepwise progression either semiologically or electrographically, or both. These are always more challenging to interpret, in which the repertoire of possible semiologic features can also be wide and the discharge may appear synchronized over various distributed structures from onset. This could be for example a frontal lobe seizure with a semiologic picture of hyperkinetic behavior, complex tonic posturing and vocalization displaying simultaneous SEEG onset across widespread prefrontal and premotor structures; or a parietal lobe seizure presenting with sensory symptoms, tonic limb signs and head version, showing synchronous SEEG seizure activity in parietal, precentral and premotor structures of the same hemisphere. In addition, the main seizure dynamics driving semiologic output in some cases (such as repetitive motor behaviors, altered awareness, emotional expression) may critically depend on activities in non-sampled structures included subcortical ones, albeit tightly linked to the cortical component of the seizure. We must therefore always keep in mind when interpreting SEEG that much of the brain participating in the seizure dynamic is inevitably not sampled-we have to try to "see" the seizure organization by extrapolating the information that we can obtain from the electrodes that are there, hopefully well-enough placed to allow this, helped by our knowledge of structural and functional anatomy (brain connectivity).

As the timing of appearance of different semiologic features may give essential information as to seizure propagation, it is usually very helpful to annotate these different time points onto the SEEG trace, to facilitate comparison with electrical activity. In particular, it is important to pay attention to the time difference (latency) between the first electrical change and the first semiologic feature, and whether this is subjective (signaled by the patient), objective (visible on video) or objective from another source (e.g., observed by witness, tachycardia observed on electrocardiogram). The time-lag between onset of electrical discharge and onset of semiologic features is important in any recording but becomes essential in SEEG, because appearance of clinical features of a spontaneous seizure that precedes obvious discharge usually indicates a problem of inadequate electrode sampling.[15]

Analyzing semiology of stimulated seizures triggered during SEEG of course brings very useful complementary information to spontaneous seizures, using the same principles of anatomo-electroclinical correlation, and this topic is discussed in a separate chapter in this book. It is worth mentioning here that some stimulation-induced seizures on SEEG may have somewhat different time relations, with clinical signs appearing relatively earlier with respect to electrical discharge compared to spontaneous seizures.[16] Ideally stimulated seizures will always be compared to spontaneous SEEG seizures in the same patient.

## "SIMPLE" ANATOMO-ELECTROCLINICAL CORRELATIONS—EXAMPLE OF A MESIAL TEMPORAL SEIZURE

To illustrate the simpler and relatively straightforward end of the spectrum of anatomo-electroclinical correlations, the example will be taken here of a prototypical mesial temporal seizure of predominantly hippocampal onset. However, many seizures studied on SEEG will be much more complex than the recognizable pattern described below. In addition, temporal seizures as a group are not necessarily simple in their organization and many different patterns and sub-groups have been characterized using SEEG group-level data.[17–20]

*Seizure onset:* In this hypothetical seizure, the discharge starts in the hippocampus with repetitive high amplitude spikes followed by low amplitude discharge. This type of ictal discharge is often completely asymptomatic for the patient with mesial temporal lobe epilepsy, and the seizure onset, which will be readily seen on SEEG, would most often not be visualizable at this same point on scalp EEG. This is known from clinical experience in comparing SEEG and video-EEG seizures in the same patients, and also demonstrated in studies using simultaneous SEEG/EEG.[21]

*Early spread network:* Perhaps after 10 s or so, the hippocampal discharge starts to spread spatially and temporally (i.e., in its frequency and amplitude) to involve other closely connected structures (e.g., amygdala, anterior insula, entorhinal cortex). This is often the point at which the patient may signal their aura, that is, the first subjective semiologic manifestation, which if reported indicates that the patient feels something but remains aware and able to communicate, a clinical observation that itself yields additional semiologic information. Thus, the semiologic production related to seizure onset depends on the "seizure onset zone" (SOZ) (in this case, hippocampus, to which seizure onset was limited according to this SEEG example) but also the "early spread network" (the connected structures in which seizure discharge first spreads to, and the temporal features of the electrophysiologic relationship to the SOZ). The original sense of the epileptogenic zone (EZ) as conceived by Bancaud takes into account both SOZ and early spread network underlying the initial semiologic expression, in both its spatial and temporal aspects.[22]

The clinical manifestations of this "early spread network" activity for a given patient's seizure will tend to reflect the specific structures involved and how their activity is linked to that of the seizure onset. For example, a seizure that spreads predominantly from hippocampus to amygdala and/or anterior insula might manifest as feeling of fear ± autonomic signs, whereas hippocampal seizure onset that is synchronous with or rapidly spreads to involve entorhinal cortex might be more likely to manifest as a feeling of déjà vu. The same seizure onset beginning in hippocampus and rapidly engaging lateral temporal neocortex would be more likely to be associated with impairment of consciousness, critically dependent on discharge frequency.[23] However, a direct one-to-one relationship between structure and sign usually cannot be inferred outside of primary cortical areas, even in the relatively "simple" case of the mesial temporal seizure described here, and as a general rule it is more useful to think in terms of mapping clusters of signs onto clusters of connected brain structures.

*Later propagation:* Next in our prototypical example, let's say the seizure discharge then further spreads spatially and temporally (at this point likely with a lower frequency, higher amplitude recruiting spike discharge, synchronized across the various involved anatomic structures). This spread may be from mesial temporal structures into temporal pole, lateral temporal cortex, basal temporal cortex, opercular regions, insula, posterior cingulate, orbitofrontal cortex, as well subcortical structures such as hypothalamus and basal ganglia, and/or contralateral homologous anatomical structures, i.e., any of the usual connected structures related to hippocampus, which may be more or less co-engaged in different patients' seizure propagation patterns.

During this propagation phase (which might be taking place over a 30–90 s time window in this prototypical mesial temporal example), other signs will emerge that constitute further objective semiology for that patient's seizure. Again the clinical manifestations of the seizure will depend on the specific seizure dynamics and spatiotemporal propagation pattern, which will be prone to recur in a stable pattern across seizures for each patient[24,25] and may reflect changes in connectivity underlying those particular propagation patterns.[2] This helps to explain why patients tend to have a reproducible core semiologic signature, even if semiologic variations can occur according to various other influences including environmental conditions, antiseizure medications, psycho-physical state of the patient at the time of the seizure, and so on.[2]

The semiologic expression of this later phase of seizure propagation will depend on both the specific anatomic structures involved (e.g., predominantly basal or lateral temporal spread, vs. operculo-insular spread, vs. frontal spread, vs. contralateral spread) and the time-scale relationship between these structures' involvement and the original seizure onset (e.g., low voltage fast discharge vs. rhythmic spike discharge; degree of synchronization between structures; delay (latency) after which each new structure becomes involved; etc.). For example, mesial temporal seizures predominantly spreading to temporal and extra temporal cortex and thalamus, with abnormally increased synchronization of the rhythmic discharge across these structures, may be predisposed to manifest altered consciousness.[23,26] (Initial/early ictal loss of consciousness is uncommon in typical mesial temporal seizures and is more usually a feature of lateral or mesio-lateral temporal lobe seizures[17]). Mesial temporal seizures spreading to opercular cortex with a rhythmic theta band discharge are more likely to manifest chewing automatisms, if theta band coherence is present between temporal and opercular regions[27] (see also Fig. 8.6). On the other hand, mesial temporal seizures spreading to temporal pole and/or orbitofrontal cortex with a low voltage fast discharge are more likely to manifest complex motor behaviors that may display hyperkinetic features.[28] Mesial temporal seizures with prominent basal ganglia spread would probably be more prone to display contralateral dystonia, which has not so far been explicitly documented on SEEG (since limited electrophysiologic data on basal ganglia correlations with semiology have been documented) but would be in keeping with data from functional neuroimaging of dystonia in temporal lobe seizures.[29,30] Mesial temporal seizures that progress to secondary generalization with head version and facial contraction most likely do so via perisylvian spread to precentral and premotor cortex, although specific propagation patterns of focal to bilateral generalized tonic clonic seizures remain incompletely known.[31]

Thus a common focal seizure onset pattern, in this case from hippocampus, may display a variety of propagation patterns and thus a corresponding variety of anatomo-electroclinical correlations. This example can be seen as "simple" since the semiologic repertoire of mesial temporal seizures is both fairly limited and well known[17] and the SEEG dynamics of mesial temporal seizure production are also well characterized,[32,33] including their propensity to be reproducible for a given patient.[24,25] See also Clinical Vignette 1 for an example of anatomo-electrical correlations of a different mesial temporal seizure type, characterized by amygdalar onset.

### What About More Complex Anatomo-electroclinical Correlations?

The above scenario of a prototypical mesial temporal seizure seems fairly intuitive when trying to understand links between spatiotemporal seizure discharge and semiologic expression. However, a misleading aspect of SEEG work is to assume that seizures "should" be very focal (as in, with a seizure onset limited to one or possibly two electrodes) and that anatomo-electroclinical correlations "should" be explicit. In fact, fairly often in SEEG practice, patients may not have such a clear-cut seizure organization, even when an appropriate implantation has been performed based on expert interpretation of non-invasive data. Complex seizure types are very likely to be encountered by stereo-electroencephalographers, so it is best to be prepared for intrinsic differences between simple and more complex anatomo-electroclinical patterns. The difficulties can arise from semiologic challenges, complex SEEG signal patterns, sub-optimal electrode sampling, or any combination of these.

In terms of semiology, the interpretation of complex semiologies should be somewhat anticipated on SEEG following the patient's Phase I video-EEG recording of habitual seizures. Hyperkinetic or other complex motor patterns are always more difficult to interpret than seizures with simpler motor signs. (In addition hyperkinetic seizures during SEEG can create management issues if movements are very agitated or violent, as there can be a risk of electrode damage and/or harm to the patient). Difficulties can also present when clinical features are subtle and difficult to assess (e.g., some seizures with no motor or other clear objective features, perhaps also inadequately interrogated for consciousness/language features), or when initial symptoms are non-specific and poorly defined, or fluctuating. The ictal examination is key here; stimulation studies can also be helpful in more clearly revealing semiologic features and their electrophysiologic correlates.

In terms of electrophysiologic pattern and relation to semiology, some very complex semiologic patterns can still have a clearly defined and focal seizure onset pattern and spread (e.g., a prefrontal seizure starting with a "silent" orbitofrontal or frontopolar discharge that expresses with complex motor behavior only during the early propagation phase involving cingulate and dorsolateral frontal cortex; see also Case Vignette 2 for an example of a frontal lobe seizure). As a general rule, propagation patterns of seizures with complex motor semiology (as opposed to elementary motor signs) will tend to be more widespread, as they arise within more densely connected regions, thus facilitating rapid, multi-directional propagation,[34] because of the connectivity pattern of heteromodal cortex.[2]

A main challenge arises when seizure patterns on SEEG look very widespread in a synchronized (simultaneous) fashion from the outset across many brain regions, which can potentially occur for any lobar localization, perhaps especially for frontal and posterior cortex seizures. In its most extreme from this can appear like a "generalized" epileptic seizure pattern at seizure onset, for example, as described in some frontal seizures.[35] This can raise the question for stereoelectroencephalographers of whether the seizure onset is genuinely characterized by a widespread synchronization, or whether the true seizure onset has been missed through electrode sampling error. Here, the relation of signal to semiology is very important in resolving this question, since semiologic features preceding the earliest SEEG changes will indicate inadequate electrode sampling; in addition the semiologic expression may provide clues as to the likely degree of focality (or not) of the recorded seizure. (The use of SEEG signal analysis tools in conjunction with semiologic data can also help to make more sense of widespread fast activity, see other chapters for more discussion of this). It is worth reiterating here that a crucial component of SEEG methodology is patient selection, as mentioned earlier: some widespread ictal patterns on SEEG are the end result of sub-optimal patient selection (e.g., patient with pre-existing "red flag" signs of a potentially widespread epilepsy organization, such as bilateral surface EEG abnormalities, normal MRI and PET, nonlocalizing semiology).

## Framework for Thinking About Semiology: Cortical Hierarchy

As a general rule, seizures involving associative cortical areas rather than primary cortical areas are prone to display a much greater repertoire of clinical features across patients and tend to involve more variable and widespread network patterns, both spatially and temporally.[34,36–38] This observation is most likely explained by the more complex cytoarchitecture and connectivity of associative cortical areas.[39] We can think of seizure discharge within primary cortex as primarily expressing elementary clinical signs with a more linear, "one-to-one" mapping of sign to brain region. This spatial specificity can still be modulated by temporal features of the electrical discharge, for example different seizure discharge frequencies determining the occurrence of either tonic or atonic signs from the same region of motor cortex.[40] On the other hand, seizures involving cytoarchitecturally higher level heteromodal cortex, because of its multi-level connectivity and integrative role,[39] will tend to arise within co-involved connected structures from the early spread phase. As such these seizures will be clinically expressed as more elaborate behaviors or symptoms, made up of complex combinations of signs, determined by the specific anatomic networks involved (i.e., constrained by connectivity) and influenced by many temporal aspects of electrical discharge (e.g., latency between structures, frequency, synchrony, coherence, phase lag) (Fig. 8.17). This explains why we may not be able to visually see obvious correlations between individual semiologic features with SEEG activity in individual anatomic structures in such seizures, even if such correlations nevertheless exist at the sub-visual level of analysis.[41] We know however that patient group level correlates can be demonstrated by mapping clusters of signs to clusters of connected brain structures,[2,42] and as such even complex ictal behaviors and symptoms show relation to cortical seizure organization as assessed by standard visual analysis of SEEG, for many sublobar localizations of seizures. This last point is important because pathophysiologic mechanisms of semiologic production, especially complex ictal behaviors, are poorly understood for the most part, and almost certainly involve inhibitory as well as activating effects of cortical and subcortical circuitry in different seizure types at the epileptogenic network level.[2] As such, we should not really expect to fully understand all of the semiological correlates from individual SEEG electrode signal in such cases, at least not in a step by step way throughout the duration of the seizure discharge. Nevertheless, cortical signal-semiology correlations can be demonstrated even for complex patterns in which a main subcortical driving dynamic is present yet tightly linked to cortical seizure discharge, such as ictal rhythmic body rocking.[41] This example serves to highlight the intricate relations between the epileptogenic zone and the emergence of semiology,[43] in which the cortical seizure onset activity is perhaps inevitably and reproducibly "hooked" to the network underlying semiologic outflow, whether this is simple or complex, focal or widespread. This serves as a working framework in which we can aim to better stratify the specificity of relation of behavior (semiology) to brain activity, that is, better define the predictive power of different semiologic patterns for cerebral localization of seizures.

## CONCLUSION

Electroclinical correlations of the Phase 1 non-invasive data are key to correct diagnosis, classification and localization of epilepsy. These pave the way for optimal anatomo-electroclinical correlations during SEEG. We recall that semiology and EEG have been considered as "inseparable" sources of data with regards to seizure classification.[2,44] This is because seizure semiologic expression and its corresponding brain electrical activity (constrained by structural and functional connectivity) can be seen as two modalities expressing the same underlying dynamic system operating within a network that alters reproducibly with each seizure. The electrical activity is the causal mechanism of the semiologic expression, but not necessarily in a linear and transparent way. In the context of presurgical evaluation, the degree of specificity of semiological patterns in relation to certain brain systems/regions/structures that may be involved in initial seizure organization carries great weight when deciding whether clear hypotheses of unifocal, spatially constrained EZ exist, and thus largely influences decision to proceed (or not) to SEEG, and implantation strategy. In other words, as clinician-electroencephalographers, we need to be able to recognize when we can predict likely cerebral correlates from other data with some certainty, and we also need to "know when we don't know." This important question requires ongoing clinical research to better understand the stratification of specificity of different semiologic signs and patterns.

In patients proceeding to SEEG, the process of anatomo-electroclinical correlation is the core methodology for data interpretation. Much progress has been made on elucidating granular spatial (sublobar) correlations at group level as well as putative mechanisms underlying some semiologic expression,[2] but many unknowns remain. SEEG is the only available method allowing distributed, multi-lobar sampling and millisecond signal capture that is time-locked with clinical seizure expression, and as such is currently the best available tool for improving knowledge of seizure patterns, dynamics and anatomic correlates. In the future, artificial intelligence methods might optimize data obtained from video-recorded seizures, for example by allowing quantification of ictal movements[45] or eventually detecting subtle features that are hard for humans to see[46], which will be a very valuable tool for ongoing research and in the future could potentially help increase clinicians' accuracy in decision making. This is where further harnessing signal analysis of SEEG,[47–50] linked to video analysis techniques applied to seizure semiology,[46,51] ideally studying large datasets reflecting the large repertoire of semiologic expression, will be very important for making future progress in our recognition and understanding of complex seizure patterns, with important implications for clinical practice.

## CLINICAL VIGNETTE 1

31-year-old right-handed female, with no significant past medical history, presents with panic attack like symptoms for the last 5 years. Patient was diagnosed with focal epilepsy at age 26. Patient did not respond to two different antiseizure medications. Her seizures occur on daily basis, lasting up to 1 min.

### Semiology

Her seizures start with feeling rushed and anxious, they are characterized by a feeling of déjà vu; feeling as if she was in the same place before. Moreover, she tries not to talk during the seizure to avoid making her seizures worse. On examination, the patient has a flushed face then 10–15 s later she has rhythmic oro-alimentary movements. She also has tachycardia at the beginning of her seizures. Patient is able to follow commands during the seizures. There are no speech arrest or language deficit during or after seizures.

### Phase 1 Video-EEG

Patient had multiple typical seizures characterized by déjà vu and feeling anxious, lasting up to 60–90 s. There were no clear electroencephalogram (EEG) changes during these episodes. Two years later, patient was re-admitted to the epilepsy monitoring unit (EMU) and 13 habitual clinical seizures were detected. Interictal scalp EEG showed occasional spike and slow wave discharges in the right temporal region (sphenoidal) SP2>F8>T8 (Fig. 8.1). Ictally, EEG change was seen 9 s after the clinical onset. Patient was able to push seizure button for all of her seizures. The earliest EEG changes were seen in the right sphenoidal electrode Sp2 with low amplitude 8–12 Hz followed by rhythmic 2–4 Hz slow waves were seen in the right temporal chain (Sp2>F8>T8). Her first oro-alimentary movements co-occurred with high amplitude rhythmic 2–4 Hz 60–100 uV in Sp2>F8>T8 (Fig. 8.2). Postictally, the patient was able to communicate, repeat, and remember.

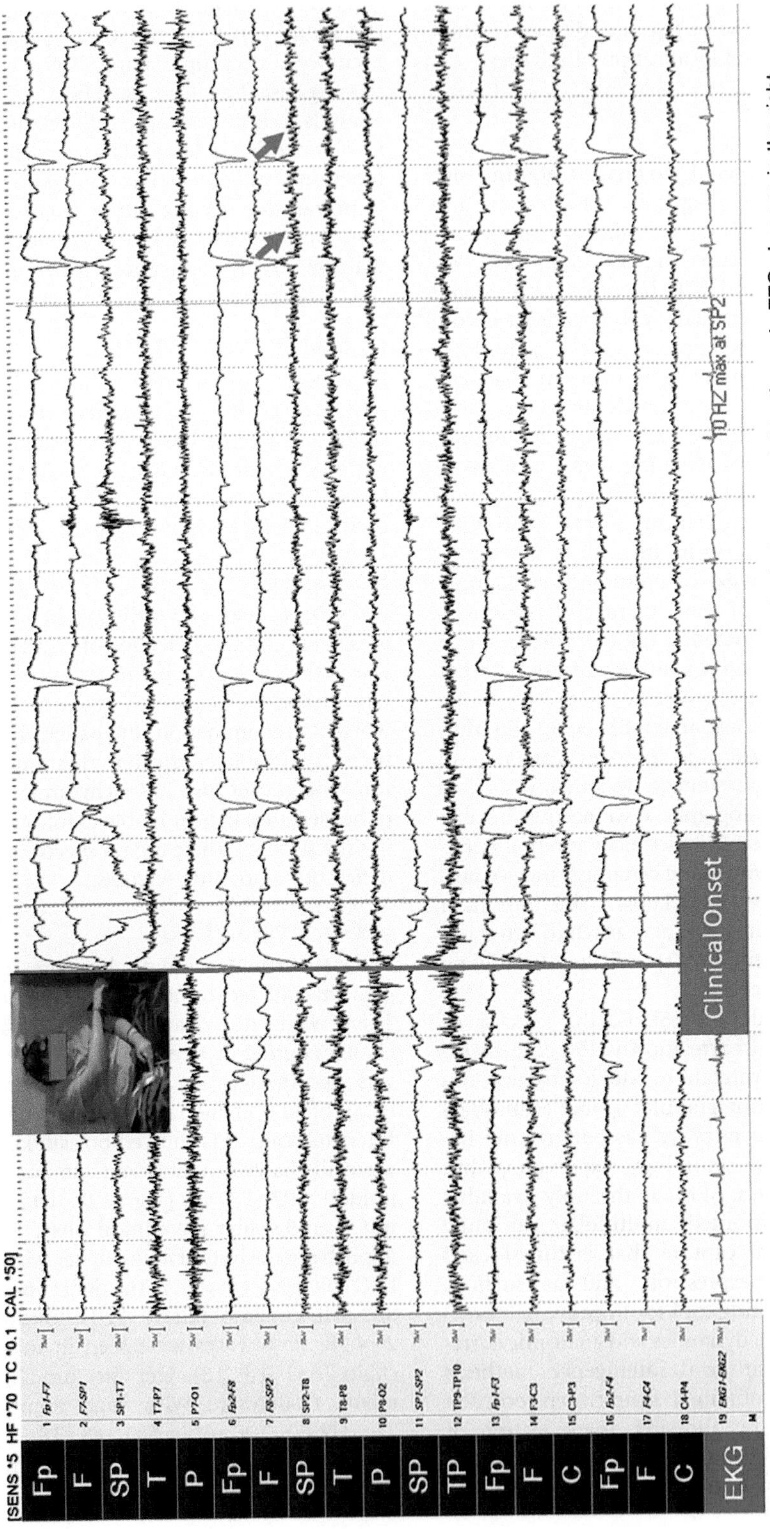


FIGURE 8.1 Scalp EEG (20 s page, bipolar montage with sphenoidal electrodes Sp1-Sp2). Arrows point to the early EEG changes in the right basal-mesial temporal region.

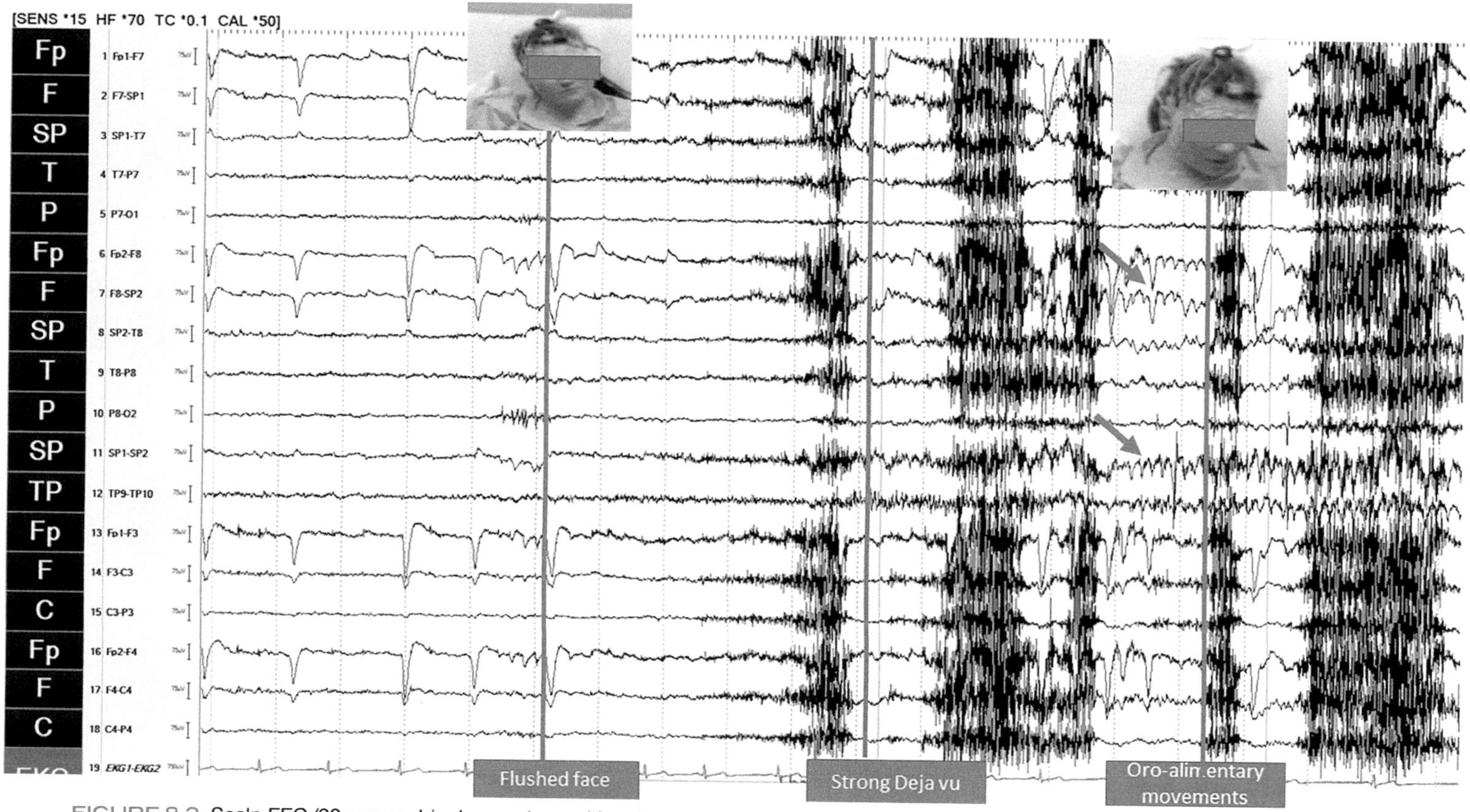


FIGURE 8.2 Scalp EEG (20 s page, bipolar montage with sphenoidal electrodes Sp1-Sp2). Arrows point to the EEG evolution with theta to delta rhythm. Oro-alimentary movements co-occurred with the high amplitude theta to delta rhythm in the right basal/mesial temporal region.

## Pre-surgical Workup

Brain MRI (3T) without gadolinium, with epilepsy protocol, was unremarkable. Ictal SPECT was achieved with late injection, 40 s, due to technical issues. SISCOM subtraction showed hyperperfused area in the right orbito-frontal region. Magnetoencephalogram (MEG) showed an interictal dipole cluster in the right mesial temporal and right insula region (Fig. 8.3).

Neuropsychological testing showed overall cognitive abilities that are in the low average to average range.

The case was discussed in patient management conference. Keeping in mind the anatomo-electro-clinical correlations, the decision was made to proceed with SEEG, and to target the first hypothesis: right amygdala-hippocampus and temporal pole. Our second hypothesis was organization within right perisylvian region given the autonomic features and oro-alimentary movements (Fig. 8.4).

## SEEG Data

*Interictal findings:* Abundant spikes in the right amygdala (A 1–5) and right temporal pole (1–5) with co-occurrence of spikes in the right hippocampus (B 1–4 and C 1–4) and entorhinal area (E1-4). Synchronized spikes/polyspikes were seen in the right mesial temporal structures and right temporal pole in sleep.

*Ictal data:* 15 clinical habitual seizures were recorded. These seizures were characterized by feeling anxious, flushed face, and whole-body numbness followed by oro-alimentary movements with preserved consciousness. SEEG showed earliest changes in the right amygdala (A 1–5) with transitioning from slow background to low

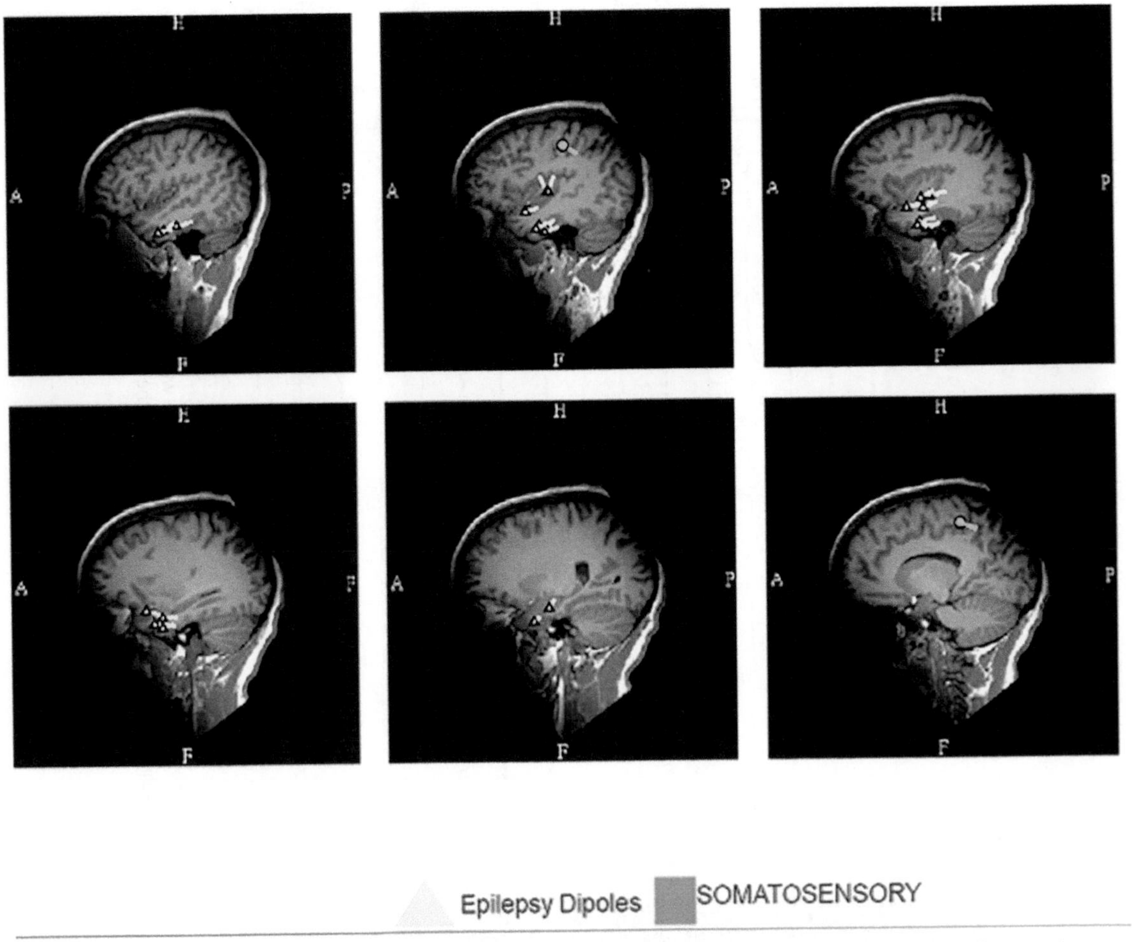


FIGURE 8.3 Magnetic source imaging (MSI) map co-registered with MRI brain T1 sagittal view T1. Scattered interictal dipoles in the right mesial temporal region and insula.

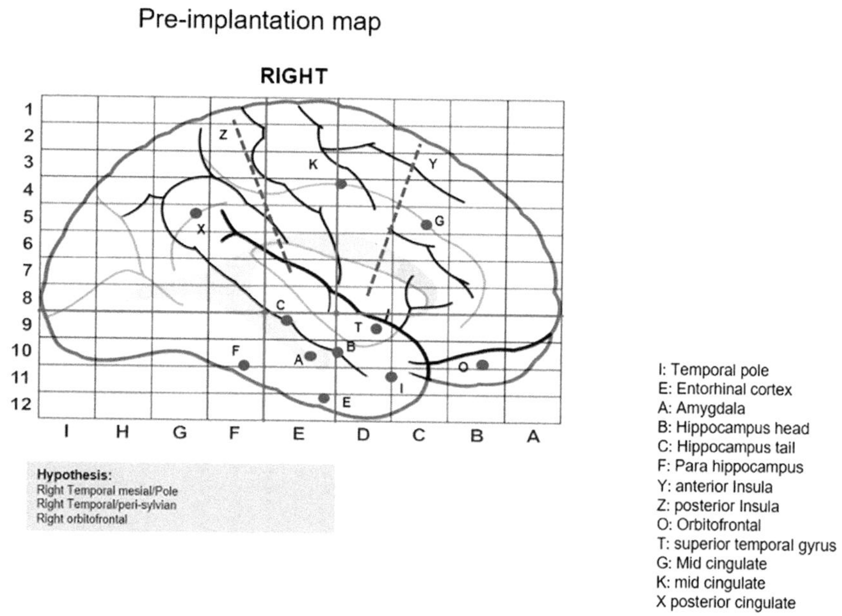


FIGURE 8.4 Pre-implantation map with Talairach grid and our hypotheses.

amplitude fast rhythm (Fig. 8.5). Temporal pole (I 1–5) and entorhinal also showed a clear change with faster rhythm in the temporal pole, arising 1–2 s after amygdala changes. Moreover, hippocampus head and tail were involved 7 s later with repetitive spikes. Later on, ictal rhythm was spread to the insula-operculum region (Y 2–6) with rhythmic 3–5 Hz followed by repetitive spikes. No motor movements were seen as long as the ictal pattern restricted to the mesial temporal structures, and that explains the absence of scalp EEG changes in the first 9 s of the clinical onset. The emergence of oro-alimentary movements co-occurred with the presence of rhythmic slow in the insula-operculum region (Y 2–6); Fig. 8.6. This rhythm in the peri-sylvian region was driven by the ictal generator in the mesial temporal region and translated clinically to well-organized rhythmic oro-alimentary movements. In comparison, to scalp EEG findings, this rhythmic slow, delta/theta discharge, is the first EEG change that was seen. In the absence of discrete lesion in the peri-sylvian region, this rhythmic slow is a good indicator of a spreading, rather than primary epileptogenic zone.

*Other findings:* Patient experienced high level of anxiety and became very emotional. Her neurological exam was normal. Her SEEG did not show ictal discharges but showed active interictal discharges in the mesial temporal and temporal pole. Patient responded very well to Ativan and her electrical activity improved.

*Stimulation data:* We were able to trigger habitual clinical seizure by stimulating the amygdala (50 Hz, 3 mA) and it activated mesial temporal and temporal pole.

### Conclusion

Based on the ensemble of data, we concluded that this patient's epileptogenic zone involves the right-sided amygdala and temporal pole. Patient underwent surgery and due to surgical difficulty, right temporal pole was removed with preserved amygdala and hippocampus (Fig. 8.7A). Patient overall did better but continued to have nocturnal episodes of flushed face and feeling nervous. 3 months later, patient underwent amygdala resection with preserved hippocampus (Fig. 8.7B). Pathology showed gliosis, and patient has been seizure-free for 1 year. Patient denied having any speech or memory issues, and her mood subjectively got better.

Tailored resection based on the accurate SEEG ictal data should be warranted. Standardized resection should be avoided if possible.

## CLINICAL VIGNETTE 2

The patient is a 16-year-old right-handed male who began experiencing seizures at the age of 4 years, evolving from staring episodes to generalized tonic-clonic and drop seizures. At age 5, he underwent a left

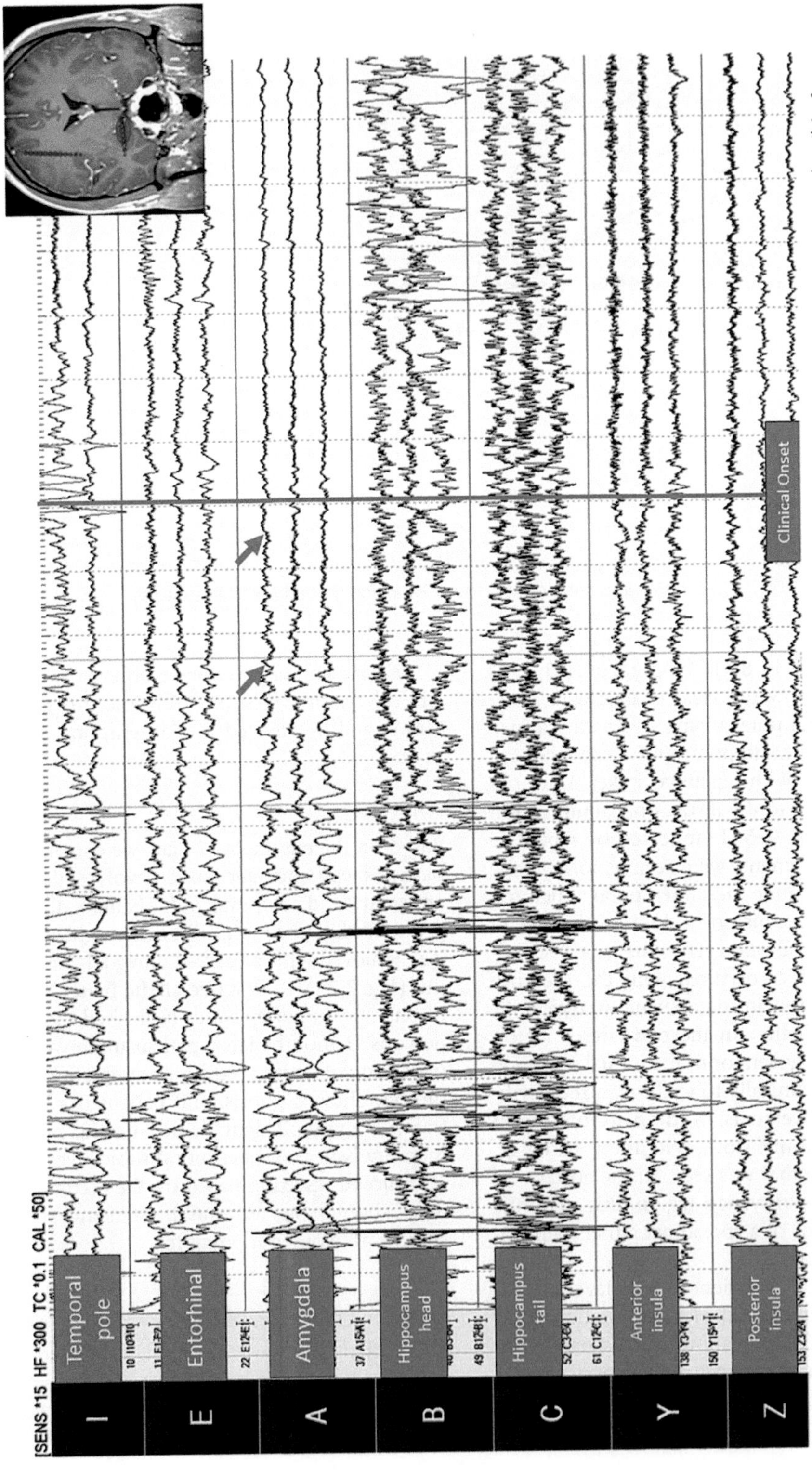


FIGURE 8.5 SEEG (bipolar montage, 20 s). Arrows point to the early SEEG background changes were seen in the right amygdala A (1–4) before the clinical onset, followed by changes in the basal temporal region E (1–4) and temporal pole I (1–4) with faster rhythm in I (1–5) temporal pole. Arrows point to the low amplitude fast activity in the amygdala A1-4. Post implantation MRI brain in the right upper corner with highlighted electrode of interest A one to four in the right amygdala.

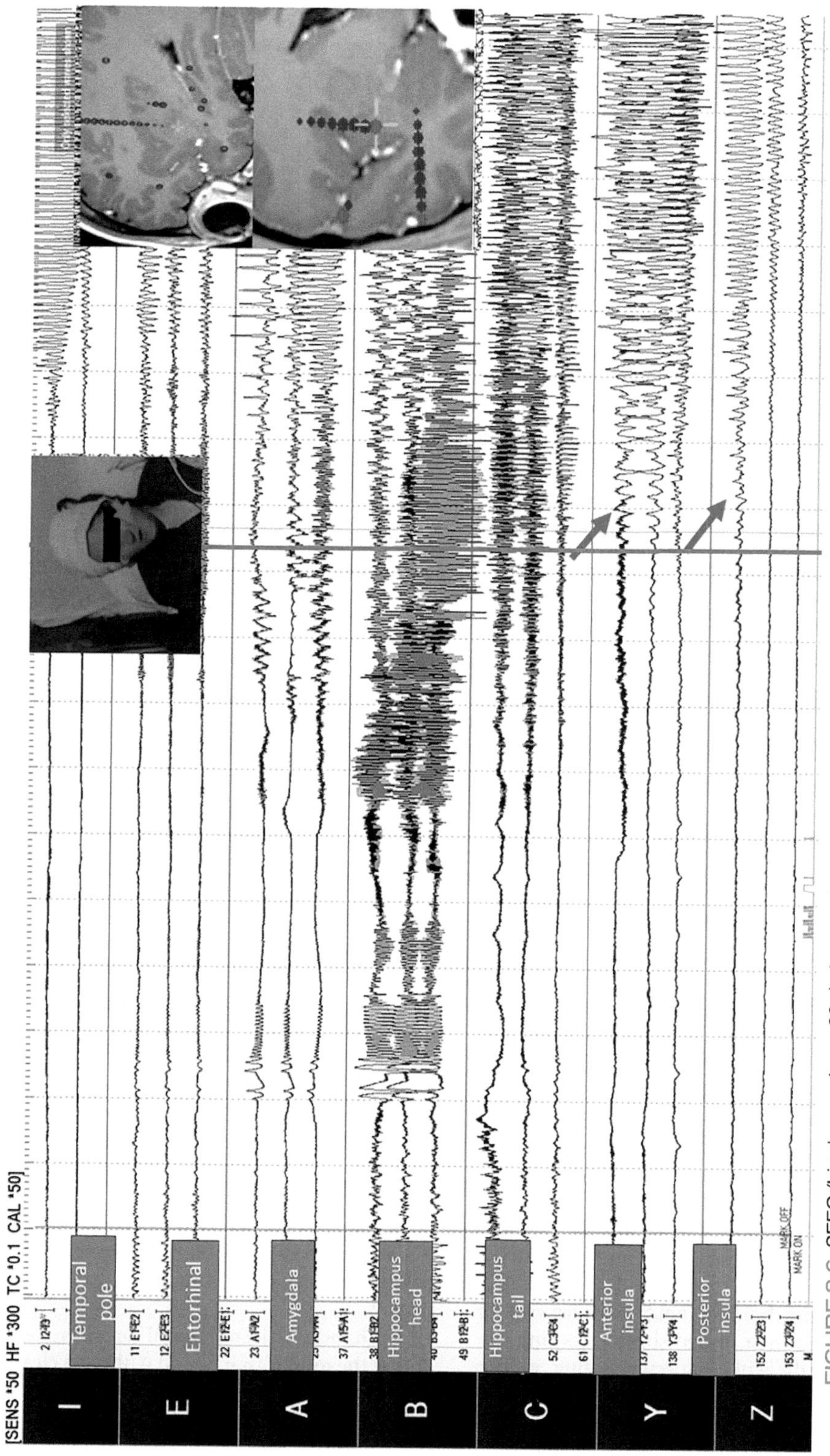


FIGURE 8.6 SEEG (bipolar montage, 20 s) shows seizure evolution. Arrows point to the rhythmic high amplitude slow rhythm in the right insula-operculum region. Arrow heads point to the first oro-alimentary movements. MRI brain on the right with oblique electrode Y in the right insula-operculum.

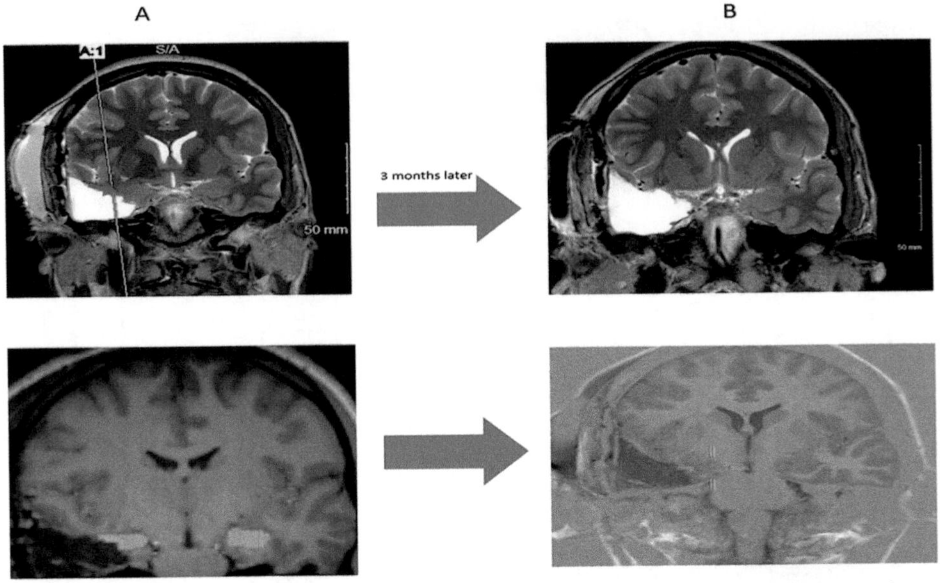


FIGURE 8.7 MRI brain 3T. T2 Blade coronal (on top) and T1 coronal (bottom) after the first procedure with resection of right temporal pole. Arrow points to the right amygdala. Hippocampi are highlighted in yellow. Second surgery with removal of right amygdala with preserved hippocampus (body and tail).

frontal resection following presurgical evaluation, which included intracranial monitoring at another medical center. Despite being initially seizure-free for a year, the seizures recurred, leading to refractory epilepsy despite adequate trials of various antiseizure medications. The initial pathology showed unremarkable findings. Subsequently, he underwent a second presurgical evaluation at another institution, but the proximity of the epileptogenic zone to eloquent areas hindered further surgical intervention. Seeking a second opinion, he presented to our institution.

### Seizure Semiology

The patient experienced one consistent seizure type. The aura preceding the seizure entailed a sensation that he was on the verge of experiencing a seizure, but articulating it proved challenging. Frequently, this prompted behaviors like seeking comfort through hugging or turning to family members, although the predictability of these actions has become inconsistent over time. Additionally, the patient engaged in breath-holding for approximately 1 minute during the aura. The patient's habitual seizure is characterized by sudden and uncontrolled movements involving holding onto whatever he is sitting on (whether a chair or bed sheets), rocking the body back and forth, with witnesses noting visible distress and gasping for air. Occasionally, unilateral facial twitching was observed without clear laterality, accompanied by cyanosis of the lips. The patient's arms exhibit a locked or rigid posture, and forced head-turning to one side is noted. Lateral clonic arm movements were observed before secondary generalization, with occasional urinary incontinence and tongue-biting.

In the postictal phase, the patient exhibited aphasia, confusion, and lethargy, lasting for up to 10 min.

The patient had daily seizures, occasionally occurring in clusters, with each seizure lasting less than 1 minute.

### Phase 1 Video EEG

The interictal EEG recordings revealed a multitude of abnormalities, with frequent spikes, sharp waves, and spike and polyspike and slow wave complexes distributed across various brain regions. Notably, C3 demonstrates a higher prevalence of these abnormalities compared to C4 and Cz. Similar findings were observed in the frontal regions (Fp1/F3/F7 and Fp2/F4/F8) and temporal regions (T3/T5/T4). Additionally, sporadic occurrences of spikes and spike-slow waves were noted in other areas, such as F4/F8, T4, P4/Pz, P4/T6, and O1. Intermittent focal slowing was identified in the left parietal region, adding complexity to the overall EEG pattern.

Six habitual electroclinical seizures were captured during the monitoring period without a clear EEG onset (Fig. 8.8). The ictal pattern was marred by muscle and movement artifacts with diffuse postictal EEG suppression and no lateralizing postictal patterns (Fig. 8.9).

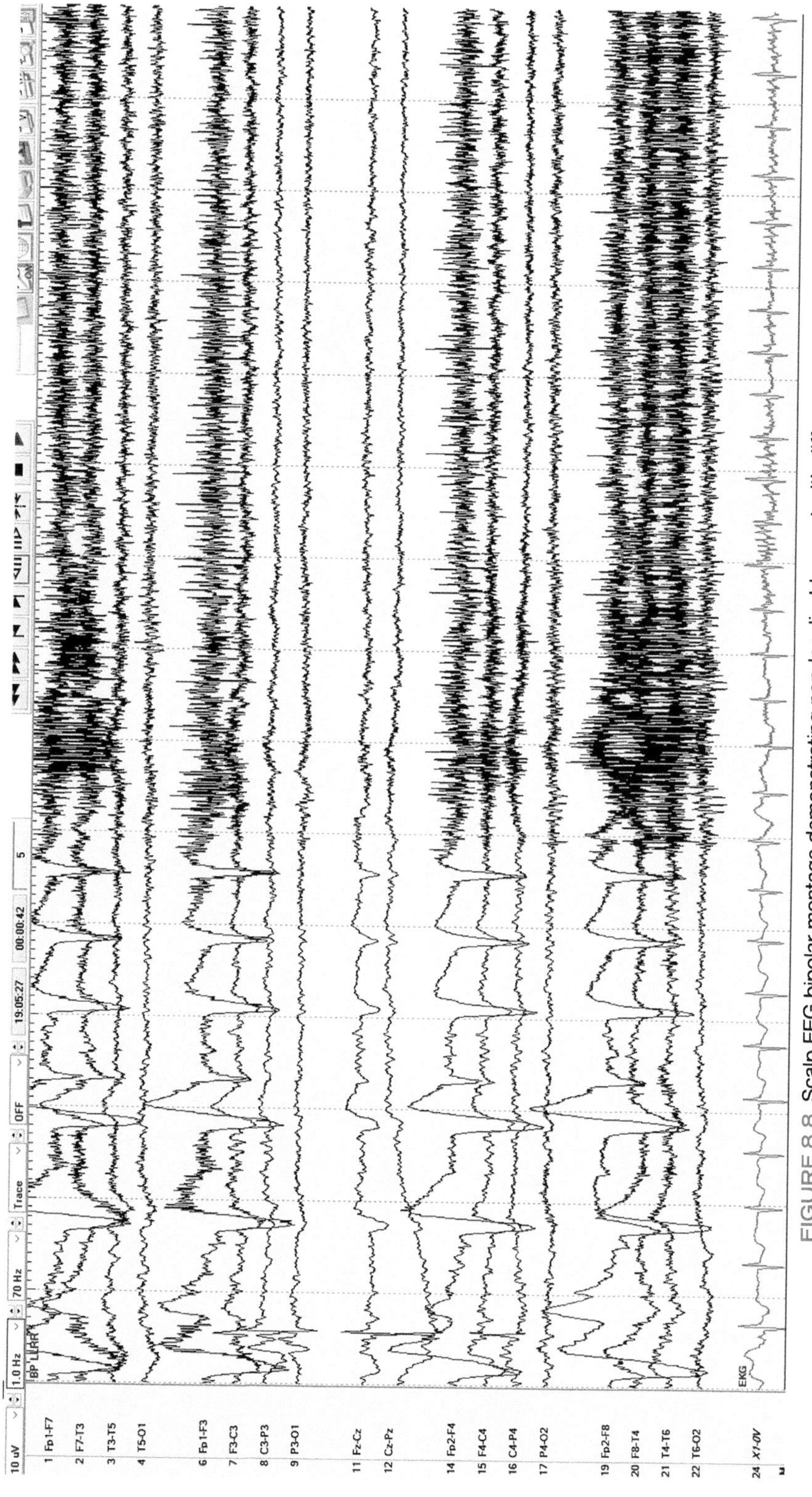


FIGURE 8.8 Scalp EEG bipolar montage demonstrating non-localizable onset with diffuse muscle artifact.

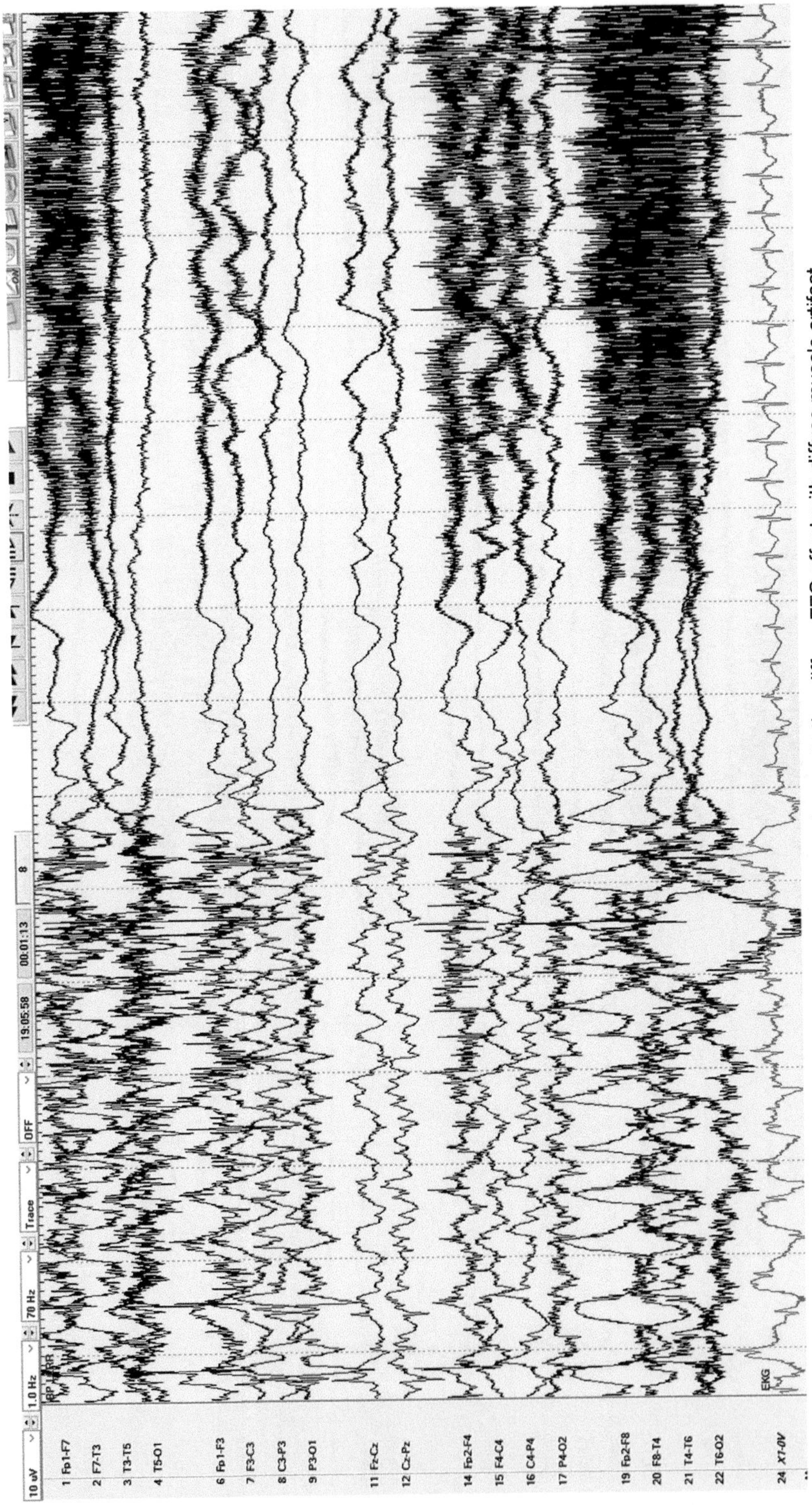


FIGURE 8.9 Scalp EEG bipolar montage demonstrating diffuse EEG offset with diffuse muscle artifact.

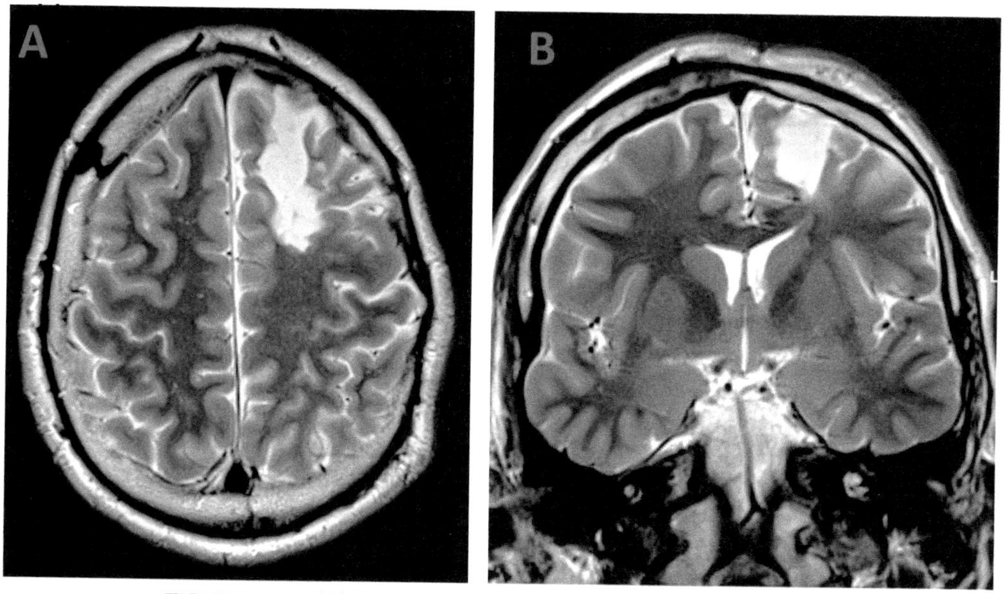


FIGURE 8.10 (A.) Axial and (B.) Coronal MRI images of prior resection.

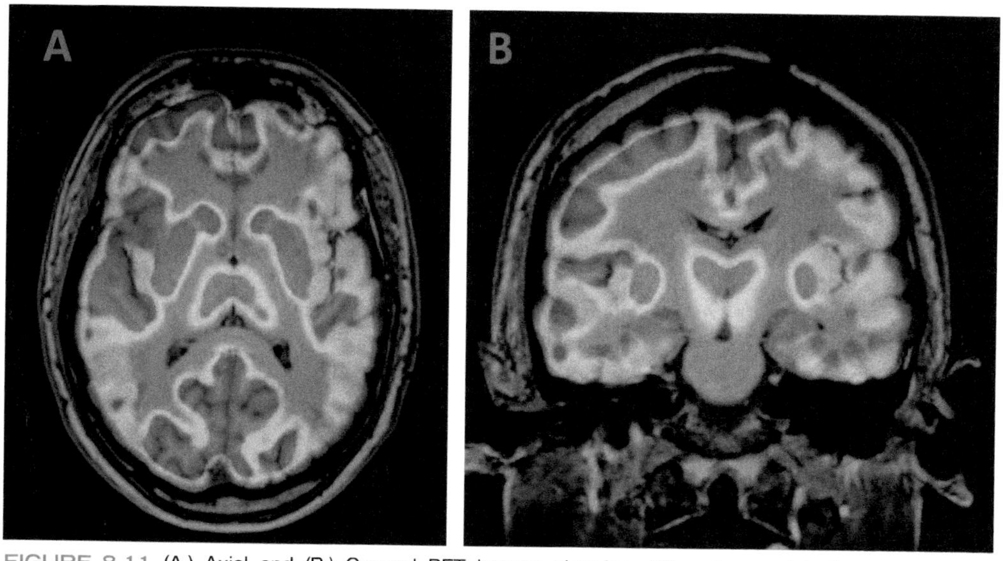


FIGURE 8.11 (A.) Axial and (B.) Coronal PET images showing diffuse hypometabolism over the left hemisphere.

## Presurgical Workup

MRI showed stable postoperative changes in the left frontal lobe. The prior resection involved the superior frontal sulcus and gyrus (Fig. 8.10). The hippocampi were symmetric.

FDG PET showed diffuse hypometabolic activity of the left cerebral hemisphere with sparing of the occipital poles (Fig. 8.11). fMRI using an auditory description decision paradigm demonstrated weak clusters of BOLD activation and was indeterminate for language lateralization.

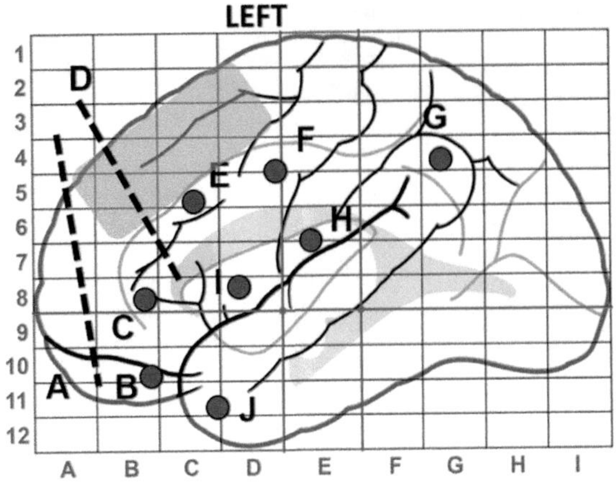


| Electrode | Target |
|---|---|
| A | Frontal resection margin |
| B | Orbitofrontal |
| C | Pregenual cingulate |
| D | Medial frontal |
| E | Premotor cortex → mid-cingulate |
| F | Primary Motor |
| G | Supramarginal → precuneus |
| H | Parietal operculum → posterior insula |
| I | Frontal operculum → anterior insula |
| J | Temporal pole |

FIGURE 8.12 Preimplantation map.

The neuropsychological evaluation demonstrated exceptionally low overall cognitive functioning with relatively stronger nonverbal compared to verbal abilities.

### Hypothesis Based on Phase 1 Data

The aura is nonspecific. Hyperkinetic semiology with integrated behavior, and gasping might be indicative of dorsolateral prefrontal cortex (DLPFC) involvement but is not specific and a similar pattern might also occur with predominantly orbitofrontal or cingulate seizure onset. The lack of lateralizing or localizing onset on EEG lend additional support to these latter anatomic hypotheses, which might be more likely than dorsolateral prefrontal cortex to not reveal a scalp EEG onset. Unilateral facial twitching suggests a spread to the face motor area, while the presence of cyanosis indicates potential disruptions in oxygenation, potentially due to the engagement of limbic structures or tonic contraction of the diaphragm. Clonic activity is likely mediated by involvement of the primary motor area. Put together and taking into account all the data including neuroimaging and previous surgical results, we hypothesized that the semiology might be related to the early involvement of the DLPFC with spread to the face motor area and then a march up in the primary motor area with wider serial and parallel spread leading to secondary generalization.

EEG, imaging and neuropsychological data were not strongly localizing.

The primary hypothesis was that the epileptogenic zone is within the DLPFC. Additional hypotheses were medial frontal with spread to DLPFC or parieto-frontal, or frontotemporal with temporal pole involvement.

### Electrode Map (Fig. 8.12)

A left hemispheric implantation was proposed using orthogonal trajectories sampling the lateral prefrontal, and opercular cortex as an entry point, and the medial frontal, the anterior and posterior insula, the cingulate cortex, Primary and Supplementary Motor Area (SMA) as targets. Both the medial parietal cortex and temporal pole were sampled as a potential area of interest that could give rise to hyperkinetic semiology.

### SEEG Data

The interictal SEEG showed abundant spikes in the left middle frontal gyrus (MFG). Polymorphic delta slowing was noted in the subgenual cingulate and anterior insula. There were frequent spikes at the anterior margin of the resection cavity, pars triangularis, and posterior cingulate. Three habitual seizures were captured. Electrographically, they were characterized by rhythmic spiking in the left MFG, then within a second, it spread to the anterior margin of the resection cavity, followed by low voltage fast activity (LVFA), which propagated to the inferior frontal gyrus and frontal operculum, remnant of medial superior frontal gyrus, and pars triangularis (Figs. 8.13 and 8.14).

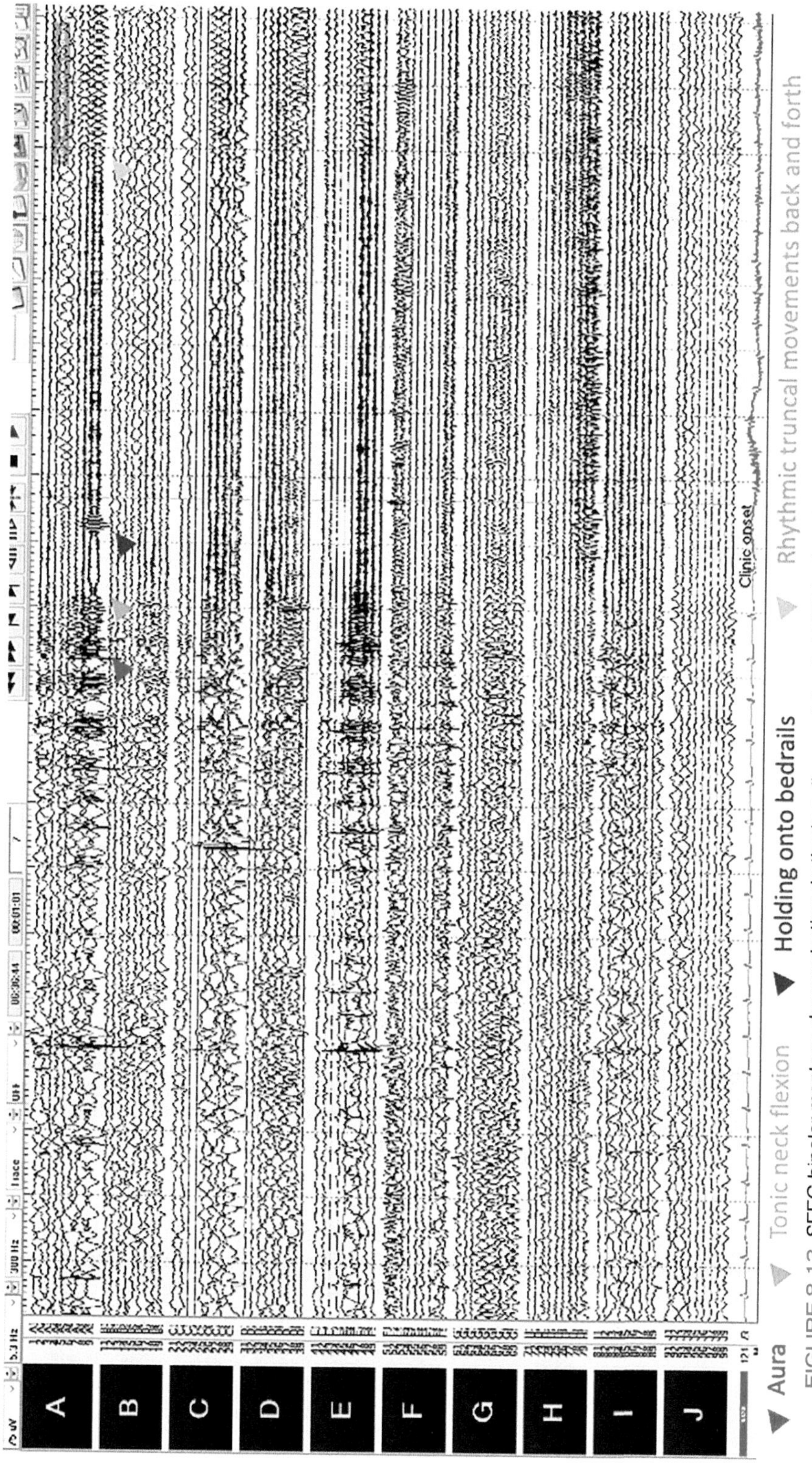

FIGURE 8.13  SEEG bipolar montage demonstrating rhythmic spikes evolving to LVFA in the middle frontal gyrus. The color arrows indicate the semiologic signs and symptoms observed.

▼ Aura    ▼ Tonic neck flexion    ▼ Holding onto bedrails    ▼ Rhythmic truncal movements back and forth

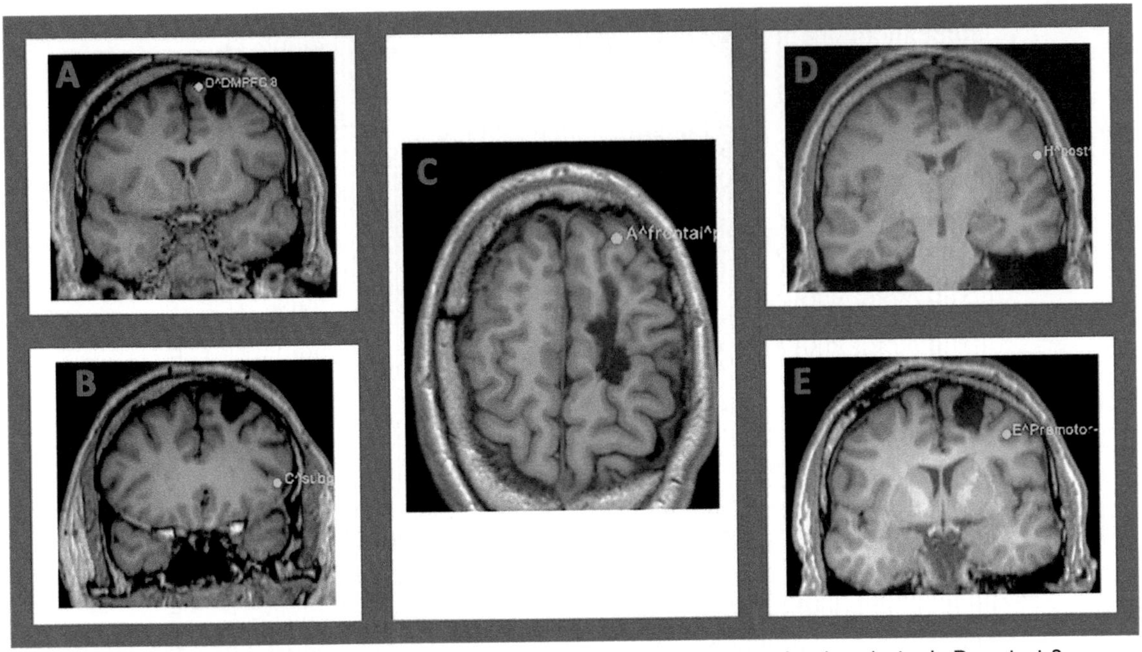


FIGURE 8.14 Coregistration of electrodes of interest. (A) coronal image showing electrode D contact 8. (B) coronal image showing electrode C contact 9. (C) Axial image showing electrode A contact 9. (D) coronal image showing electrode H contact 9. (E) coronal image showing electrode E contact 7.

Anatomo-electroclinical correlation revealed an aura linked to rhythmic spiking (RS) in the middle frontal gyrus (MFG) and the anterior and medial margins of the prior resection. RS evolved into an LVFA in the same region, characterized by tonic forward flexion of the neck. The LVFA swiftly propagated to multiple areas, including the cingulate cortex, dorsolateral prefrontal cortex (DLPFC), and operculum. During this progression, the patient gripped the bedrails, gasped for air, and exhibited asymmetric facial pulling to the right. As the activity frequency changed to 7–8 Hz, the patient began rocking his trunk back and forth. Subsequently, as the ictal discharges slowed in frequency, clonic movements were observed in the right arm whilst the left hand grabbed the bedsheets.

## Electric Stimulation (Fig. 8.15)

Habitual seizures were produced by stimulating the MFG (50 Hz, 300 us, 3 mA, 5 s).

## Recommendations

Based on the findings of the SEEG and the anatomo-electro-clinical correlation, the patient was recommended to undergo resection of the dorsal medial prefrontal cortex, the rest of the superior frontal gyrus including the superior frontal sulcus, middle frontal gyrus, and extend that resection to the frontal pole. Fig. 8.16 shows the MRI changes following the resection.

## Histopathology

Focal cortical dysplasia with balloon cells (ILAE type IIb).

## Outcome

Seizure-free Engel IA at 26 months and off antiseizure medication. The patient reported an improvement in mood and no adverse effect on cognitive function.

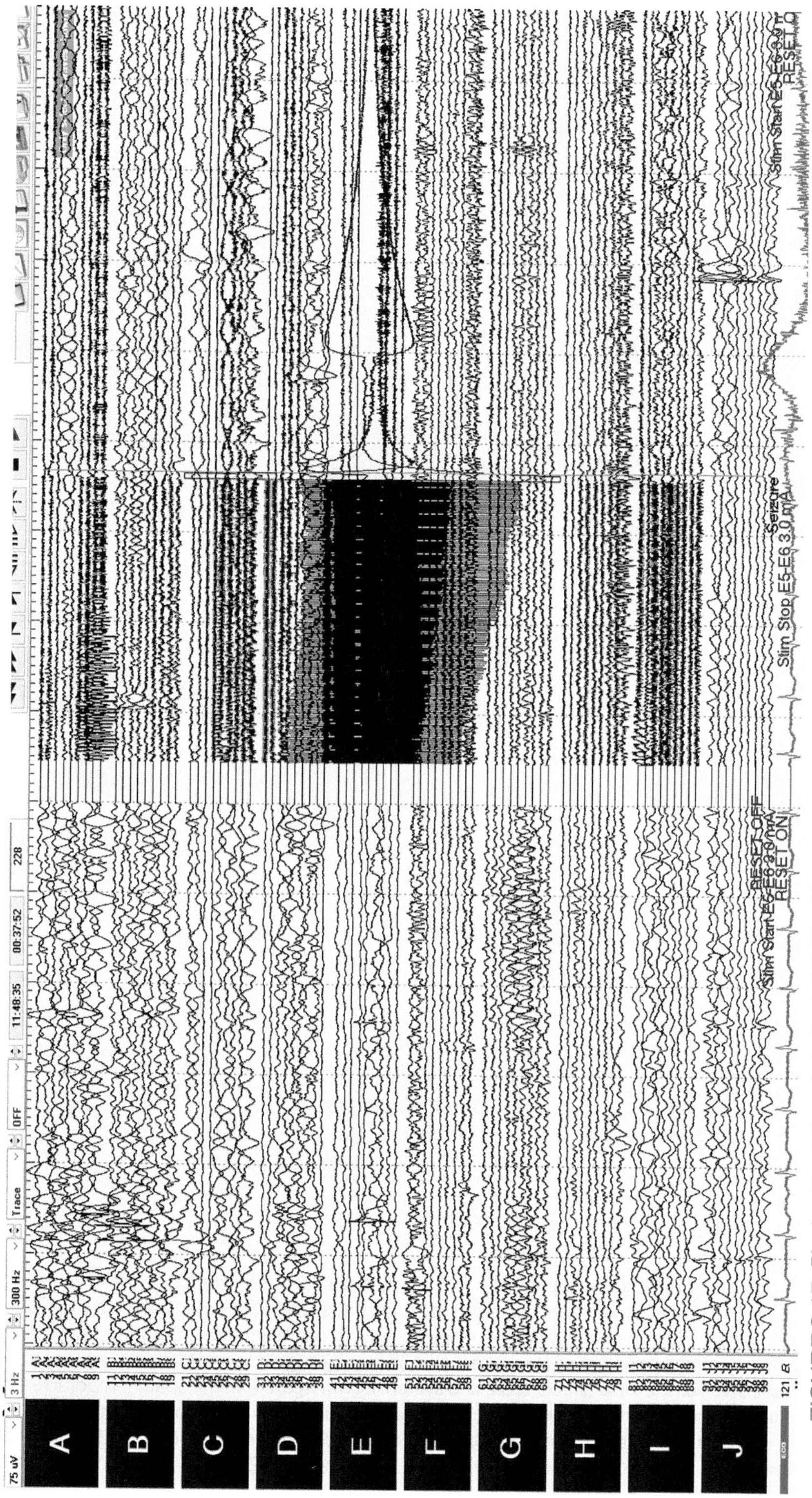


FIGURE 8.15 Bipolar stimulation of electrode E5-E6 middle frontal gyrus produced habitual electroclinical seizure (stimulation parameters: 50 Hz, 300 us, 3 mA, 5 s).

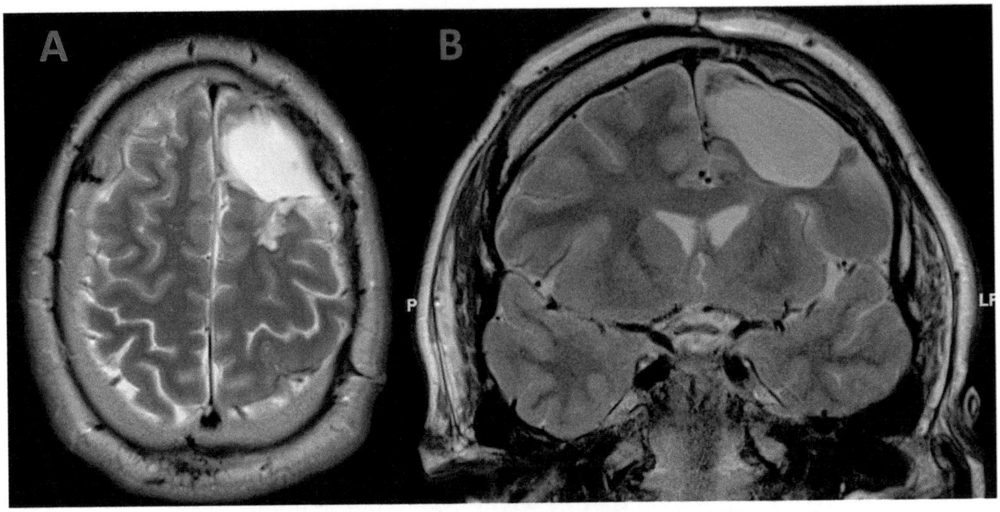


FIGURE 8.16 (A.) Axial and (B.) Coronal post-operative MRI images.

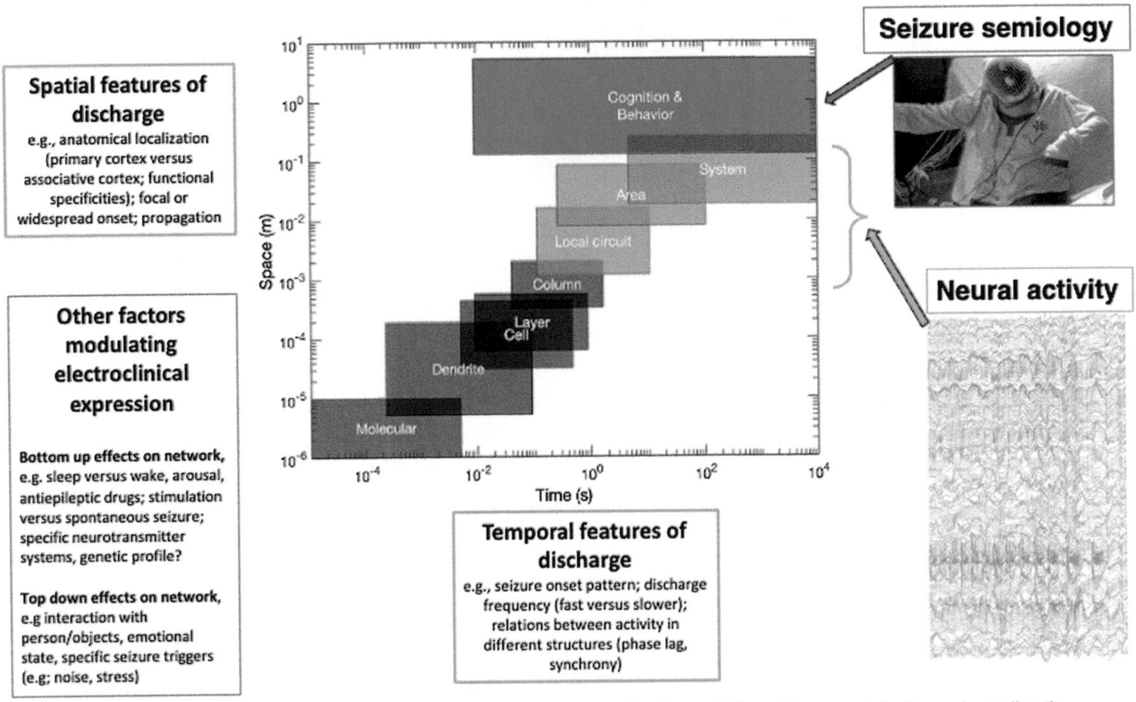


FIGURE 8.17 Use of a multi-scale framework to think about spatial and temporal features in epileptic seizure expression. The center panel illustrates temporal and spatial scales of organization in the nervous system. Both semiologic expression and cerebral epileptic activity can be mapped onto this spatiotemporal framework. Semiology involves the higher-level dimension shared by cognition and behavior, whereas cerebral electrical discharge involves the local circuit, area, and system levels. Apart from the spatiotemporal features of the seizure discharge, other factors influencing electroclinical expression can be bottom-up (driven by neuronal changes) or top-down (driven by environmental factors). (Reproduced with permission from McGonigal A, Bartolomei F, Chauvel P. On seizure semiology. Epilepsia. 2021 Sep;62(9):2019–2035; Adapted from Lytton et al.[52])

## ACKNOWLEDGMENTS

The authors thank all staff and patients from their Epilepsy Monitoring Units.

## REFERENCES

1. Chauvel P. *Contributions of Jean Talairach and Jean Bancaud to Epilepsy Surgery. Epilepsy Surgery*. 2nd ed. Philadelphia, PA: Lippincott Williams & Wilkins; 2001:35–41.
2. McGonigal A, Bartolomei F, Chauvel P. On seizure semiology. *Epilepsia*. 2021;62(9):2019–2035.
3. Hamandi K, Beniczky S, Diehl B, et al. Current practice and recommendations in UK epilepsy monitoring units. Report of a national survey and workshop. *Seizure*. 2017;50:92–98.
4. Trebuchon A, Lambert I, Guisiano B, et al. The different patterns of seizure-induced aphasia in temporal lobe epilepsies. *Epilepsy Behav*. 2018;78:256–264.
5. Beniczky S, Neufeld M, Diehl B, et al. Testing patients during seizures: a European consensus procedure developed by a joint taskforce of the ILAE–Commission on European Affairs and the European Epilepsy Monitoring Unit Association. *Epilepsia*. 2016;57(9):1363–1368.
6. Beniczky S, Tatum WO, Blumenfeld H, et al. Seizure semiology: ILAE glossary of terms and their significance. *Epileptic Disord*. 2022;1.
7. Astner-Rohracher A, Zimmermann G, Avigdor T, et al. Development and validation of the 5-SENSE score to predict focality of the seizure-onset zone as assessed by stereoelectroencephalography. *JAMA Neurol*. 2022;79(1): 70–79. https://doi.org/10.1001/jamaneurol.2021.4405.
8. Singh R, Giusiano B, Bonini F, et al. Characteristics and neural correlates of emotional behavior during prefrontal seizures. *Ann Neurol*. September 1, 2022;92:1052–1065. https://doi.org/10.1002/ana.26496.
9. Van Buren J. The abdominal aura a study of abdominal sensations occurring in epilepsy and produced by depth stimulation. *Electroencephalogr Clin Neurophysiol*. 1963;15(1):1–19.
10. Thijs RD, Ryvlin P, Surges R. Autonomic manifestations of epilepsy: emerging pathways to sudden death? *Nat Rev Neurol*. 2021;17(12):774–788. https://doi.org/10.1038/s41582-021-00574-w.
11. Alim-Marvasti A, Romagnoli G, Dahele K, et al. Probabilistic landscape of seizure semiology localizing values. *Brain Commun*. 2022;4(3). https://doi.org/10.1093/braincomms/fcac130.
12. Gil-Nagel A, Risinger MW. Ictal semiology in hippocampal versus extrahippocampal temporal lobe epilepsy. *Brain*. 1997;120(1):183–192.
13. Barba C, Barbati G, Minotti L, Hoffmann D, Kahane P. Ictal clinical and scalp-EEG findings differentiating temporal lobe epilepsies from temporal 'plus' epilepsies. *Brain*. 2007;130(7):1957–1967.
14. Barba C, Rheims S, Minotti L, et al. Temporal plus epilepsy is a major determinant of temporal lobe surgery failures. *Brain*. 2015;139(2):444–451. https://doi.org/10.1093/brain/awv372.
15. Bartolomei F, Nica A, Valenti-Hirsch MP, Adam C, Denuelle M. Interpretation of SEEG recordings. *Neurophysiol Clin*. 2018;48(1):53–57.
16. McGonigal A, Lagarde S, Trébuchon-Dafonseca A, Roehri N, Bartolomei F. Early onset motor semiology in seizures triggered by cortical stimulation during SEEG. *Epilepsy Behav*. 2018;88:262–267.
17. Maillard L, Vignal JP, Gavaret M, et al. Semiologic and electrophysiologic correlations in temporal lobe seizure subtypes. *Epilepsia*. 2004;45(12):1590–1599. https://doi.org/10.1111/j.0013-9580.2004.09704.x.
18. Bartolomei F, Cosandier-Rimele D, McGonigal A, et al. From mesial temporal lobe to temporoperisylvian seizures: a quantified study of temporal lobe seizure networks. *Epilepsia*. October 2010;51(10):2147–2158. https://doi.org/10.1111/j.1528-1167.2010.02690.x.
19. Kahane P, Bartolomei F. Temporal lobe epilepsy and hippocampal sclerosis: lessons from depth EEG recordings. *Epilepsia*. 2010;51:59–62.
20. Bartolomei F, Wendling F, Bellanger J-J, Régis J, Chauvel P. Neural networks involving the medial temporal structures in temporal lobe epilepsy. *Clin Neurophysiol*. 2001;112(9): 1746–1760.
21. Ferrand M, Baumann C, Aron O, et al. Intra-cerebral correlates of scalp EEG ictal discharges based on simultaneous recordings. *Neurology*. 2023;100.
22. Chauvel P. The epileptogenic zone: a critical reconstruction. In: Schuele SU, ed. *A Practical Approach to Stereo EEG*. Springer Publishing Company; 2020:105–120.
23. Arthuis M, Valton L, Régis J, et al. Impaired consciousness during temporal lobe seizures is related to increased long-distance cortical-subcortical synchronization. *Brain*. 2009; 132(Pt 8):2091–2101. https://doi.org/10.1093/brain/awp086.
24. Wendling F, Badier JM, Chauvel P, Coatrieux JL. A method to quantify invariant information in depth-recorded epileptic seizures. *Electroencephalogr Clin Neurophysiol*. June 1997;102(6):472–485.
25. Gnatkovsky V, Francione S, Cardinale F, et al. Identification of reproducible ictal patterns based on quantified frequency analysis of intracranial EEG signals. *Epilepsia*. 2011; 52(3):477–488.
26. Guye M, Régis J, Tamura M, et al. The role of corticothalamic coupling in human temporal lobe epilepsy. *Brain*. July 2006;129(Pt 7):1917–1928. https://doi.org/10.1093/brain/awl151.
27. Aupy J, Noviawaty I, Krishnan B, et al. Insulo-opercular cortex generates oroalimentary automatisms in temporal seizures. *Epilepsia*. 2018;59(3):583–594.
28. Vaugier L, Aubert S, McGonigal A, et al. Neural networks underlying hyperkinetic seizures of "temporal lobe" origin. *Epilepsy Res*. October 2009;86(2–3):200–208. https://doi.org/10.1016/j.eplepsyres.2009.06.007.
29. Newton MR, Berkovic SF, Austin M, Reutens DC, McKay W, Bladin PF. Dystonia, clinical lateralization, and regional blood flow changes in temporal lobe seizures. *Neurology*. 1992;42(2):371.

30. Dupont S, Semah F, Baulac M, Samson Y. The underlying pathophysiology of ictal dystonia in temporal lobe epilepsy an FDG-PET study. *Neurology.* 1998;51(5):1289–1292.
31. Marchi A, Giusiano B, King M, et al. Postictal electroencephalographic (EEG) suppression: a stereo-EEG study of 100 focal to bilateral tonic–clonic seizures. *Epilepsia.* 2019;60(1):63–73.
32. Bartolomei F, Wendling F, Vignal J-P, et al. Seizures of temporal lobe epilepsy: identification of subtypes by coherence analysis using stereo-electro-encephalography. *Clin Neurophysiol.* 1999;110(10):1741–1754.
33. Bartolomei F, Wendling F, Bellanger JJ, Régis J, Chauvel P. Neural networks involving the medial temporal structures in temporal lobe epilepsy. *Clin Neurophysiol.* September 2001;112(9):1746–1760.
34. Bonini F, McGonigal A, Trébuchon A, et al. Frontal lobe seizures: from clinical semiology to localization. *Epilepsia.* 2014;55(2):264–277.
35. Bancaud J, Talairach J, Morel P, et al. "Generalized" epileptic seizures elicited by electrical stimulation of the frontal lobe in man. *Electroencephalogr Clin Neurophysiol.* 1974;37(3):275–282.
36. Fayerstein J, McGonigal A, Pizzo F, et al. Quantitative analysis of hyperkinetic seizures and correlation with seizure onset zone. *Epilepsia.* 2020;61(5):1019–1026.
37. Pelliccia V, Avanzini P, Rizzi M, et al. Association between semiology and anatomo-functional localization in patients with cingulate epilepsy: a cohort study. *Neurology.* 2022;98.
38. Bartolomei F, Gavaret M, Hewett R, et al. Neural networks underlying parietal lobe seizures: a quantified study from intracerebral recordings. *Epilepsy Res.* 2011;93(2–3):164–176. https://doi.org/10.1016/j.eplepsyres.2010.12.005.
39. Mesulam M. The evolving landscape of human cortical connectivity: facts and inferences. *Neuroimage.* 2012; 62(4):2182–2189.
40. Maillard L, Gavaret M, Régis J, Wendling F, Bartolomei F. Fast epileptic discharges associated with ictal negative motor phenomena. *Clin Neurophysiol.* 2014;125(12): 2344–2348.
41. Zalta A, Hou J-C, Thonnat M, Bartolomei F, Morillon B, McGonigal A. Neural correlates of rhythmic rocking in prefrontal seizures. *Neurophysiol Clin.* 2020;50(5):331–338.
42. Wang H, McGonigal A, Zhang K, et al. Semiologic subgroups of insulo-opercular seizures based on connectional architecture atlas. *Epilepsia.* 2020;61(5):984–994.
43. Chauvel P, McGonigal A. *Emergence of Semiology in Epileptic Seizures.* Epilepsy & Behavior; 2014.
44. Gastaut H, Broughton RJ. *Epileptic Seizures: Clinical and Electrographic Features, Diagnosis and Treatment.* Charles C. Thomas Publisher; 1972.
45. Hou J-C, Thonnat M, Huys R, Bartolomei F, McGonigal A. Rhythmic rocking stereotypies in frontal lobe seizures: a quantified video study. *Neurophysiol Clin.* 2020.
46. Hou J-C, Thonnat M, Bartolomei F, McGonigal A. Automated video analysis of emotion and dystonia in epileptic seizures. *Epilepsy Res.* 2022;184:106953. https://doi.org/10.1016/j.eplepsyres.2022.106953.
47. Karimi-Rouzbahani H, McGonigal A. Generalisability of epileptiform patterns across time and patients. *Sci. Rep.* 2024 Mar 15;14(1):6293. https://doi.org/10.1038/s41598-024-56990-7.
48. Li J, Grinenko O, Mosher JC, Gonzalez-Martinez J, Leahy RM, Chauvel P. Learning to define an electrical biomarker of the epileptogenic zone. *Hum Brain Mapp.* February 1, 2020;41(2):429–441. https://doi.org/10.1002/hbm.24813.
49. Bartolomei F, Lagarde S, Wendling F, et al. Defining epileptogenic networks: contribution of SEEG and signal analysis. *Epilepsia.* 2017;58(7):1167–1528.
50. Gnatkovsky V, de Curtis M, Pastori C, et al. Biomarkers of epileptogenic zone defined by quantified stereo-EEG analysis. *Epilepsia.* February 2014;55(2):296–305. https://doi.org/10.1111/epi.12507.
51. Ahmedt-Aristizabal D, Armin MA, Hayder Z, et al. *Deep Learning Approaches for Seizure Video Analysis: A Review.* arXiv; 2023.
52. Lytton WW, Arle J, Bobashev G, et al. Multiscale modeling in the clinic: diseases of the brain and nervous system. *Brain Inform.* December 2017;4(4):219–230. https://doi.org/10.1007/s40708-017-0067-5.

CHAPTER 9

# Method of Direct Cortical Stimulation for Triggering Seizures

PATRICK CHAUVEL, MD • AGNÈS TRÉBUCHON, MD, PHD • AILEEN MCGONIGAL, MBCHB, PHD

Stereoelectroencephalography (SEEG)-based presurgical evaluation of epilepsies has a double objective: to localize the epileptogenic zone (EZ) and to specify a surgical plan. Direct electrical stimulations from the intracerebral electrodes are an essential technique to reach these goals. As such, they are an integral part of SEEG.

Stimulations have been performed to trigger seizures ever since SEEG has been practiced. In the beginning, the presurgical "stereotaxic functional investigation"[1] subscribed to the Penfield principles. The earliest sign or symptom of the patient's seizures induced by stimulation of a circumscribed area constituted a solid argument for localization. Also, until the mid 70ies SEEG was a 1-day investigation. If the patient did not present any spontaneous seizure during the time allotted for recording, it became necessary to provoke a seizure by stimulation or chemical activation.[2] Fifty years later, electrical stimulation still represents an indispensable tool to define the EZ.[3,4]

Electrical simulation (ES) has been used in ECoG to identify "eloquent" regions related to motor and cognitive functions. This procedure has been called "functional mapping". There is a growing body of evidence considering the usefulness of ES to map language cortex in patients undergoing resection of epileptogenic cortex in the language dominant hemisphere.[5–7] Electrical simulation producing a transient and functional impairment might predict which functions will be disturbed if the stimulated cortex were to be removed. However, the dispersed patterns of SEEG implantations hamper the possibility of a real mapping, so that the most reliable functional evaluation comes from a comparative behavioral analysis of spontaneous and electrically induced seizures. This is one of the major differences between subdural grids and intracerebral depth electrodes (SEEG) methods.

## RATIONALE

The concept of EZ in SEEG is quite different from that of seizure onset zone used in subdural grid recordings. Without entering into detail, one of its main ideas is that the EZ is defined by its specific capability to synchronize the epileptogenic network. Therefore, stimulation of any of its component areas can trigger the patient's seizure. It works as a validation of a method which, by nature, must tolerate a sampling bias.

Another difficulty for EZ localization through spontaneous seizures only is because of **neocortical seizure patterns**. Seizure onset in the neocortex can occur like quasi-simultaneous high frequency activities throughout a vast territory, possibly more extensive than the EZ. Whatever the signal processing applied, a cut-off frequency for epileptogenicity is impossible to define. Only stimulation will help discriminating between the involved areas and determine which ones are essential to activate the epileptogenic network according to its proper spatial-temporal pattern and to trigger seizures (Fig. 9.1).

Stimulation is the only way to decipher seizure organization in **infra- and peri-sylvian epilepsies**. Temporal or occipital epilepsies may present with different seizure subtypes depending on whether one or two (or more) elements of the ictal architecture are activated. For instance, in a patient one seizure can be only temporal, another one temporal/peri-sylvian, and another one with a peri-sylvian seizure onset remotely from the propagation network. A similar organization can be observed in occipital/temporal or occipital/temporal/peri-sylvian epilepsies. To determine what is the primary epileptogenic organization and discriminate it from spread, stimulation will unravel how its constitutive elements are linked and how each of them contributes to early and late clinical semiology. Contrary to the stimulation techniques used for

The Fundamentals of Stereoelectroencephalography. https://doi.org/10.1016/B978-0-443-10877-8.00013-9

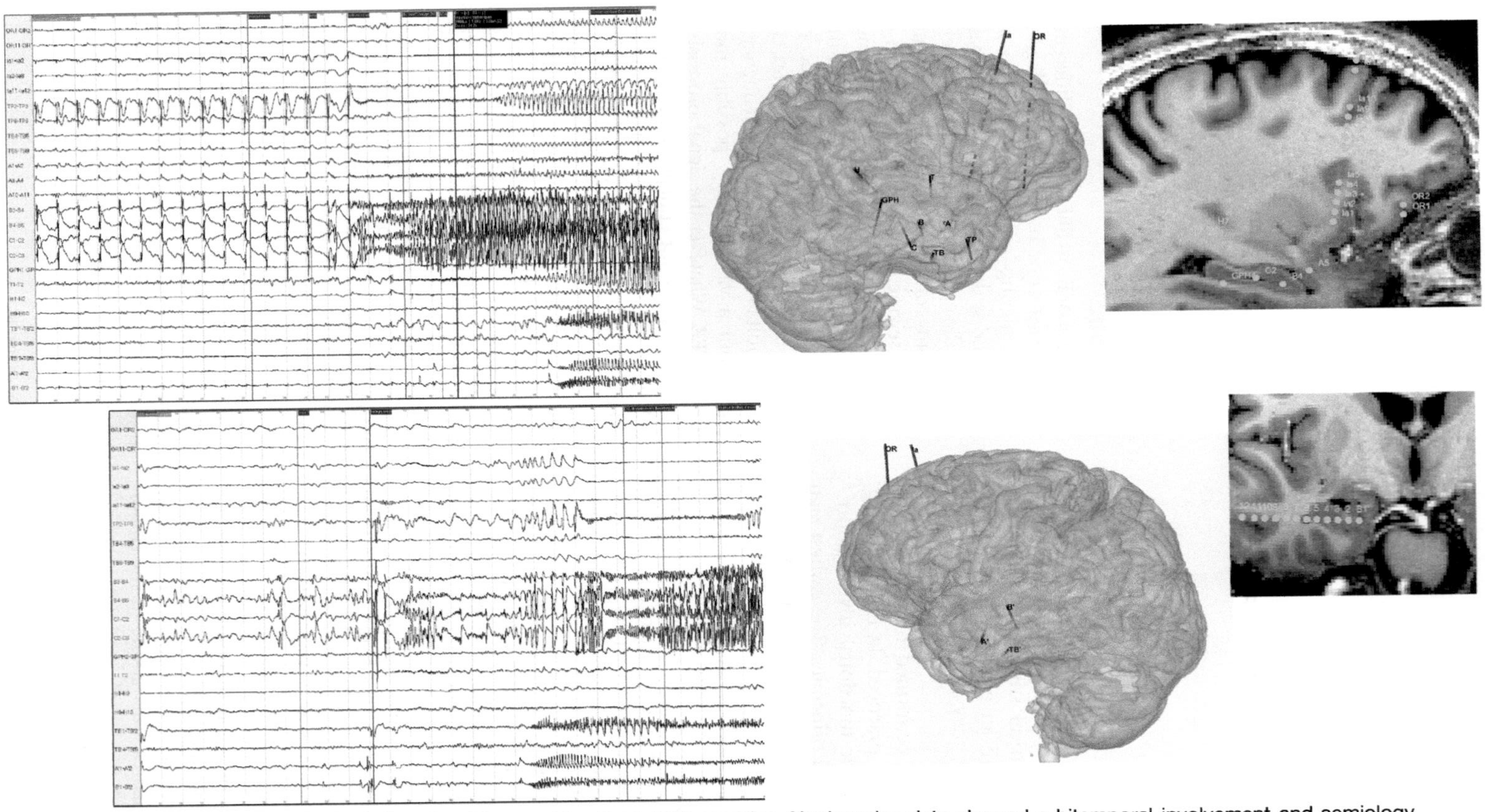

FIG. 9.1 Presurgical investigation of a 45-year-old patient, MRI negative. Noninvasive data showed a bitemporal involvement and semiology pointed to either both hemispheres or the left hemisphere (left manual automatisms and postictal aphasia). Hypometabolism was seen in both temporal lobes on FDG-PET. Top left panel: An LFS 1 Hz induced seizure after stimulation of right hippocampus (electrode B) with typical semiology; note the involvement of the insula (T1-2), the temporal pole (TP2-3) and 9 seconds later involvement of the left medial temporal structures (amygdala A′ and hippocampus B′). No seizure was induced by stimulations (LF and HF) on the left side. Bottom left panel: Right hippocampal onset spontaneous seizure. Note the similar SEEG pattern with an earlier involvement of the left side electrodes. Right panels: electrode positions.

functional mapping with subdural grids, after-discharges are utilized to differentiate nonepileptogenic from epileptogenic areas. Electrical and clinical criteria are analyzed to interpret the effect of the stimulation trials (see below).

## TECHNIQUES

The optimal time to perform stimulations depends on multiple individual factors during SEEG. Generally, stimulation sessions occur after some spontaneous seizures have been recorded. However, they may precede spontaneous seizure recordings in cases where the patient did not have any during the first week. Stimulations are performed in several sessions, each of them rarely exceeding 1 hour.

Stimulation is applied between two adjacent leads of one electrode. Single bipolar pulse or train stimuli are used. Single pulses (0.3–0.5 ms; 0.5–5 mA) are delivered pseudo-randomly or periodically (for instance 1/s) to stimulate the motor cortex, the hippocampus, or Heschl's gyrus because of their low threshold for after-discharges or seizures. The same is applicable to dysplastic cortex, especially when interictal activity is characterized by repetitive spiking intermingled or not with bursts of fast activities.[8,9] All other areas are stimulated by single pulses or by train (50 Hz; 0.5 ms; 0.5–4 mA; 1–5 seconds). Train stimulation (50 Hz) can also be used for motor cortex, hippocampus, and Heschl's gyrus once the risk of triggering generalized seizure (motor cortex, Heschl's gyrus) has been estimated or when single pulse stimulations were ineffective (hippocampus). Comparing the chance of obtaining after-discharges with stimulations of different frequencies and intensities, Motamedi et al. (2007) showed that higher frequency (100 vs. 50 Hz) and larger pulse width (1 vs. 0.2 ms) were more effective.[10] This is in good agreement with the fact that single pulses up to 3 ms duration were successfully used to obtain electroclinical responses in nonprimary motor areas, especially Supplementary Motor Area.[11,12]

There is no need to apply increasing intensities to measure a clinical or electrical threshold, the main goal being to obtain after-discharges and/or seizures. Repetition of stimulation at the same site exhausts the area stimulated leading to a refractory period of variable duration. This is in contrast with what has been reported with subdural grids, where after-discharges are "likely to occur when an electrode pair showed after-discharge (ADs) and was stimulated again, especially after short intertrial intervals or for longer duration."[13]

Obtaining an after-discharge is the test for cortical excitability. Pulse width and train frequency generally are kept constant throughout the whole stimulation procedure. The initial intensity may vary according to several factors[1]: level of current anti-seizure medication (ASM),[2] history of generalization (particularly when stimulating lateral premotor or precentral cortex),[3] area stimulated supposed to be part of the EZ (as indicated by already recorded spontaneous seizures),[4] type of structure stimulated (see above). Triggering of after-discharges needs to be prevented only during electrocorticography (ECoG) functional mapping.[14] Blum et al., studying properties of after-discharges from cortical electrical stimulation in focal epilepsies, stated that when ADs involved more than the stimulus site, they might inaccurately localize cortical function.[14] Interestingly, in the same work, no consistent relationship was noted between the site of stimulation elicited AD and that of spontaneous seizures. This observation made during ECoG paradoxically serves as a rationale for triggering seizures in SEEG.

In fact, the main objective of stimulations in SEEG is to find the site(s) from which stimulation is capable of synchronizing the epileptogenic network (or part of it) to induce an electro-clinical seizure. Consequently, the site(s) from which a local after-discharge without any electrical or ictal clinical features can be triggered is (are) considered as being outside the EZ. The EZ being structured as a neural network, the site location from which a seizure can be triggered does not define by itself the localization of a "focus" at this site. The way synchronization is produced between the areas involved through stimulating this site critically informs about the organization of the EZ. This is the reason why analysis of stimulation effects does not simply consist in identifying the areas from where a seizure could be triggered and concluding that EZ lies there. Interpretation is less straightforward. Its local and remote electrical effects must be carefully analyzed before reaching any conclusion. Puzzling situations are encountered when an ictal discharge is generated from the efferent network of the stimulated cortex. According to the afferent-tract targeting principle (further detailed below),[15,16] the optimal electrode placement is upstream to the target structure.

Frontal and parietal (supra-sylvian) epilepsies on the one hand, temporal and occipital (infra-sylvian) epilepsies on the other hand have different EZ organizations. It turns out that results of stimulation differ from one to the other. In supra-sylvian epilepsies, except for early symptoms ("auras") that can occur during stimulation time even without after-discharge, triggering a seizure is an all-or-none phenomenon. In the infra-sylvian epilepsies, parts of the typical seizure can be evoked from different sites of the network. The high excitability and the wide cortical efferent connectivity of the limbic system (especially hippocampus) adds another factor of complexity in interpreting results of stimulation. Chauvel et al. (1993) studied the conditions of obtaining seizures similar to the patients' spontaneous ones.[17] In medial temporal epilepsies, hippocampal onset seizures could be triggered by hippocampal or by amygdala stimulation as well, amygdala onset seizures by amygdala or hippocampus stimulation, and rarely by temporal neocortical stimulation. This should be paralleled with the fact that in lateral temporal epilepsies, except for superior temporal gyrus epilepsies, seizures are preferentially triggered from medial limbic regions. Therefore, any directly connected area can elicit a delayed after-discharge or ictal discharge in the hippocampus; conversely, the hippocampus can trigger a seizure in any efferent epileptogenic area. Hence, interpretation of stimulation in hippocampus-related areas must consider the network organization of the triggered discharge pattern, especially its frequency characteristics (fast activities) and its electrical and clinical similarity with spontaneous seizures.

According to the afferent-tract targeting principle, any electrical stimulation in the brain is more efficient for driving a downstream structure discharge than for eliciting a local excitatory effect. This fact explains a classical pitfall in stimulation interpretation in SEEG. Triggering a seizure from a given electrode does not necessarily mean that this electrode is in the epileptogenic zone. A usual observation is that the best way to trigger a seizure from the hippocampus is to stimulate amygdala and vice-versa (see Fig. 9.2). This is also true in the cortical motor system where a stimulation in a nonepileptogenic cortical motor area can remotely trigger a seizure from epileptogenic premotor and/or precentral cortex. The stimulation procedure in SEEG is not a binary approach. Interpretation of its effects requires a meticulous analysis of the frequency patterns and their spatial distribution in correlation with any induced behavior. Much emphasis has been put on the "reproducibility" of the spontaneous seizure to corroborate the EZ localization. Some of the earliest studies gave an estimation of the "concordance" between stimulation-induced and spontaneous seizures.[3,17–19] A total of 77%–90% were concordant in temporal epilepsies, and 86% in frontal epilepsies[17,20] (note that Chauvel et al. selected patients only with concordant seizures). Bernier et al. confirmed that obtaining an after-discharge is not a tool for localizing the EZ.[20]

## FALSE-POSITIVE, FALSE-NEGATIVE RESPONSES TO STIMULATION

As mentioned above, after-discharges are used to assess the excitability of a given area. If an after-discharge is not followed locally by an ictal discharge, its occurrence demonstrates that this area does not take part of the epileptogenic organization. Local, even local-regional hyperexcitability is not equivalent to abnormal functional coupling that characterizes an epileptogenic zone.[21] However, false-positive responses to stimulation of primary sensory or motor cortices or hippocampus can be observed because of low threshold properties of these cortices. Generalized seizures can also be triggered by stimulation of nonepileptogenic lateral premotor cortex or medial transverse temporal gyrus of Heschl, as these structures are short afferents to the motor systems.

False-negative results in stimulation during SEEG represent a more ambiguous situation. Their occurrence is variable from patient to patient and depends on several factors. Given the small volume of brain tissue subjected to the electric field of the bipolar stimulation (between two leads of one electrode), and the necessity to synchronize multiple areas involved in the EZ to trigger a seizure, one of the main reasons of stimulation failures is an electrode anatomical placement leading to an inability for the area(s) stimulated to establish a sufficient functional connectivity to trigger seizures. Two contingent factors generally influence the stimulation performance: (1) the time elapsed since the last seizure (or the last after-discharge in a stimulation session), and (2) a too high antiepileptic drug level (this happens very often when the stimulations are practiced after spontaneous seizures have been recorded and the patient has been put back on medications). A recent large study from two experienced centres reported that cortical stimulation for seizure provocation was performed on usual doses on anti-seizure medications (ASM), considered to reduce risk of atypical events.[9] However, systematic data and guidelines on this topic are lacking.

## PROGNOSTIC SIGNIFICANCE OF STIMULATION RESULTS

Recent works have looked at prognostic significance of seizures triggered by stimulation during SEEG, and

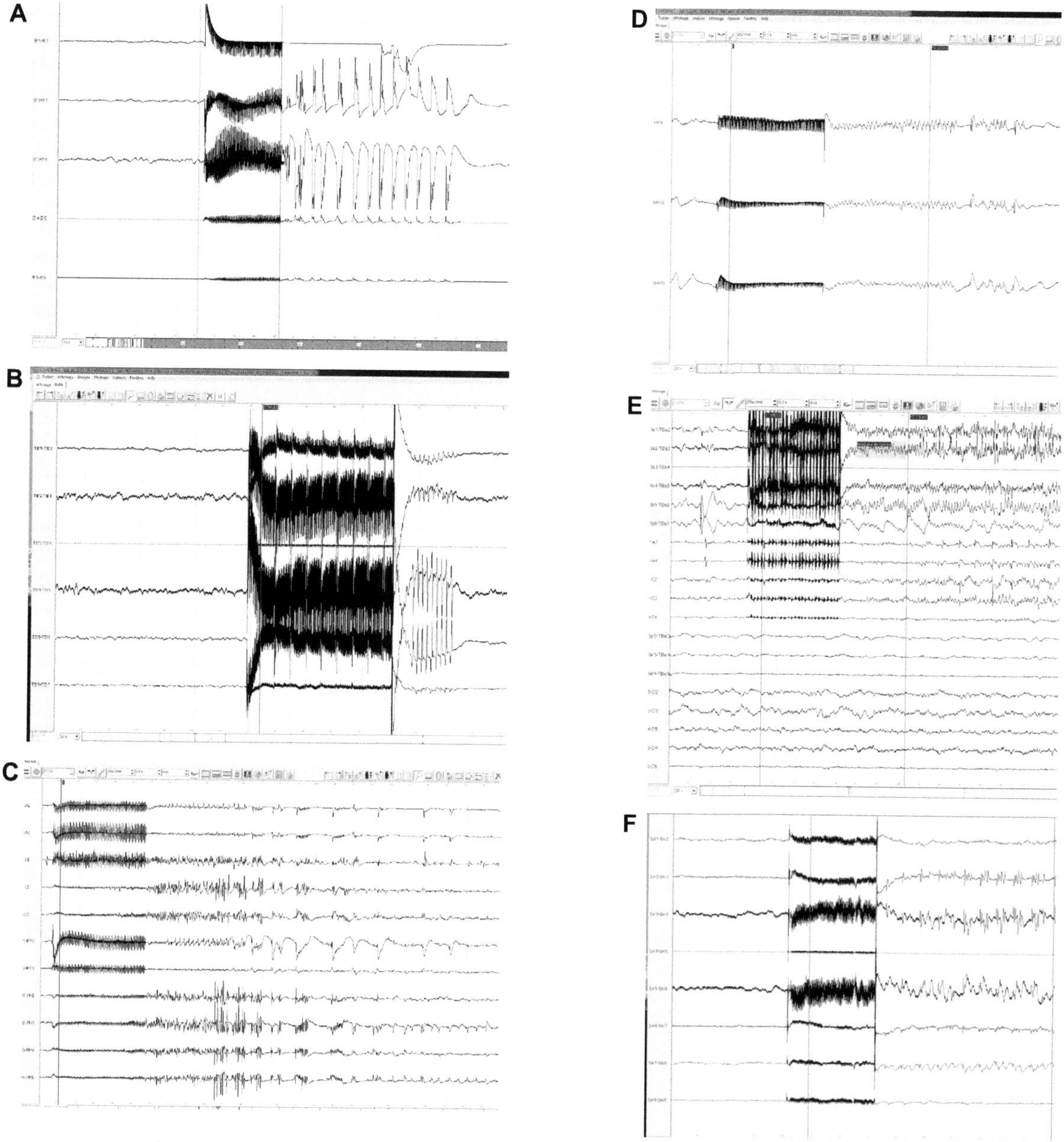

FIG. 9.2 Example of after discharge (AD). A and B poly spike after hippocampus (A) or rhinal (B) stimulation. (C) Complex after discharge in a network involving temporo-mesial structures (amygdala, hippocampus, pole and rhinal cortex. (D) Rhythmic alpha after discharge after stimulation of dorsolateral frontal cortex. (E) Rhythmic alpha AD + polyspike after stimulation of insular cortex. (F) Bursting polyspike AD after stimulation of premotor cortex.

also relative effects of high-frequency stimulation (HFS) (train) versus low frequency stimulation (LFS) (pulse) stimulation. Oderiz et al. studied 103 patients from two tertiary centers (Montreal, Canada and Grenoble, France) to investigate whether removal of the "seizure-onset zone resulting from cortical stimulation" was associated with a good surgical outcome.[9] The type of cortical stimulation, and electroclinical characteristics of stimulation-induced seizures (SIS), were studied; these authors reported on 1 Hz LFS and 50 Hz HFS stimulation protocols. Note that these authors excluded any stimulated auras without electrical correlate (discussed earlier), including only events with both clinical and electrical features similar to usual seizures. A clear difference was seen in efficacy between HFS and LFS, with a 54.9% response rate of HFS 50 Hz for triggering habitual electroclinical seizures, compared to a seizure response rate of 18.2% for 1 Hz LFS. The proportion of patients with stimulated seizures (from any stimulation protocol) was noted to be higher (70.5%) in patients who subsequently underwent surgical resection with good outcome (Engel class I), compared to patients with poorer outcome (in whom only 47.5% had stimulated seizures). This fact may reflect issues of sampling and/or more widespread epileptogenic zones (especially extra-temporal) in those cases who did not become seizure free following surgery; as described above, in the situation of a widespread neocortical EZ, it may not be possible to produce sufficient synchronization from stimulation of a single cortical region.[17] In the study by Cuello-Oderiz et al., the association of stimulated seizures and better surgical outcome was interpreted as evidence that stimulated seizures were as reliable as spontaneous seizures reliable for identification of the epileptic generator, in the context of SEEG.[9] In this study, 57.3% of patients had at least one electroclinical seizure induced, the majority being by HFS stimulation.[9] Interestingly, HFS stimulation was more likely to trigger a seizure in patients who had not presented a spontaneous seizure for at least 24 hours before, suggesting an effect of refractory period, in keeping with earlier observations (Chauvel et al., 1993),[17] discussed earlier in this chapter.

In a separate large study of 346 patients from two tertiary centers (Marseille, France and Milan, Italy), the relative effects of low frequency (up to 6 Hz) versus high frequency stimulation (50 Hz) were studied.[8] Earlier observations by Claudio Munari had highlighted a useful role for low frequency stimulation during SEEG, which, even if somewhat less effective in triggering seizures than high frequency stimulation, could potentially be more reliable since false positive responses are rare. Munari had also identified a prognostic value of LFS-induced seizures in temporal lobe epilepsy, showing an association with good surgical outcome.[22] Trebuchon et al. found that 68.2% of all 346 patients had some form of stimulation-induced electroclinical seizure[8] (i.e., slightly more than the 57.2% of SIS found in the study by Cuelleo-Oderiz et al.).[9] Overall, stimulation-induced seizures occurred more commonly with high frequency stimulation than with LFS: 70% of all triggered seizures were by HFS, and 40% by HFS alone.[8] On multi-variate analysis, seizure induction by LFS (but not HFS) was found to be an independent positive predictive factor for seizure outcome after surgery (along with lesional MRI and etiology). Interestingly, there was a significant effect of type of semiologic expression of LFS-induced seizures, since those cases in which LFS produced either complete habitual semiology or the habitual aura were more strongly associated with good surgical outcomes than those in which LFS produced some other fragment of habitual semiology.[8]

## CONCLUSION

To summarize, direct electrical stimulation represents an essential tool for unraveling the organization of the EZ. It provides controlled observation of seizures (per-ictal and postictal) with precise timing of clinical semiology providing temporal accuracy. Localization of its effects should be interpreted through the concept of an epileptogenic network: local effects with or without AD as outside of the EZ, or regional or multiregional as a function of its ability to synchronize, thus providing spatial accuracy. False-negative effects are more difficult to interpret than false-positive. False-positive effects should be analyzed considering the neural systems involved (temporal limbic vs. neocortical).

## REFERENCES


1. Techniques of stereotaxic exploration of the encephalic structures in MAN-(CORTEX, SUB-cortex, basal ganglia). In: Bancaud J, Dell M, eds. *Electroencephalography and Clinical Neurophysiology*. Elsevier Ireland Ltd Elsevier House, Brookvale Plaza, East Park Shannon, Co...; 1959.
2. Bancaud J, Talairach J. *La Stéréo-Électroencéphalographie Dans L'épilepsie: Informations Neurophysiopathologiques Apportées Par L'investigation Fonctionnelle Stéreotaxique*. Paris: Masson et Cie; 1965.
3. Kovac S, Kahane P, Diehl B. Seizures induced by direct electrical cortical stimulation—mechanisms and clinical considerations. *Clin Neurophysiol*. 2016;127(1):31–39.
4. Trébuchon A, Chauvel P. Electrical stimulation for seizure induction and functional mapping in stereoelectroencephalography. *J Clin Neurophysiol*. 2016; 33(6):511–521.
5. Hamberger MJ. Cortical language mapping in epilepsy: a critical review. *Neuropsychol Rev*. 2007;17:477–489.
6. Ojemann G, Ojemann J, Lettich E, Berger M. Cortical language localization in left, dominant hemisphere: an electrical stimulation mapping investigation in 117 patients. *J Neurosurg*. 1989;71(3):316–326.

7. Penfield W, Rasmussen T. *The Cerebral Cortex of Man; a Clinical Study of Localization of Function*. Oxford, England: Macmillan; 1950.
8. Trebuchon A, Racila R, Cardinale F, et al. Electrical stimulation for seizure induction during SEEG exploration: a useful predictor of postoperative seizure recurrence? *J Neurol Neurosurg Psychiatr*. 2021;92(1):22–26.
9. Oderiz CC, von Ellenrieder N, Dubeau F, et al. Association of cortical stimulation–induced seizure with surgical outcome in patients with focal drug-resistant epilepsy. *JAMA Neurol*. 2019;76(9):1070–1078.
10. Motamedi GK, Okunola O, Kalhorn CG, et al. Afterdischarges during cortical stimulation at different frequencies and intensities. *Epilepsy Res*. 2007;77(1):65–69.
11. Chauvel PY, Rey M, Buser P, Bancaud J. What stimulation of the supplementary motor area in humans tells about its functional organization. *Adv Neurol*. 1996;70:199–209.
12. Talairach J, Bancaud J. Lesion," irritative" zone and epileptogenic focus. *Stereotact Funct Neurosurg*. 1966;27(1–3): 91–94.
13. Lee HW, Webber W, Crone N, Miglioretti DL, Lesser RP. When is electrical cortical stimulation more likely to produce afterdischarges? *Clinical Neurophysiol*. 2010;121(1): 14–20.
14. Blume WT, Jones DC, Pathak P. Properties of afterdischarges from cortical electrical stimulation in focal epilepsies. *Clinical Neurophysiol*. 2004;115(4):982–989.
15. Rajasethupathy P, Ferenczi E, Deisseroth K. Targeting neural circuits. *Cell*. 2016;165(3):524–534.
16. Gillinder L, Liegeois-Chauvel C, Chauvel P. What déjà vu and the "dreamy state" tell us about episodic memory networks. *Clin Neurophysiol*. 2022;136:173–181.
17. Chauvel P, Landré E, Trottier S, et al. Electrical stimulation with intracerebral electrodes to evoke seizures. *Adv Neurol*. 1993;63:115–121.
18. Landré E, Turak B, Toussaint D, Trottier S. Intérêt des stimulations électriques intracérébrales en stéréoélectroencéphalographie dans les épilepsies partielles. *Epilepsies*. 2004;16(4):213–225.
19. Wieser H, Bancaud J, Talairach J, Bonis A, Szikla G. Comparative value of spontaneous and chemically and electrically induced seizures in establishing the lateralization of temporal lobe seizures. *Epilepsia*. 1979;20(1): 47–59.
20. Bernier GP, Richer F, Giard N, et al. Electrical stimulation of the human brain in epilepsy. *Epilepsia*. 1990;31(5): 513–520.
21. Chauvel P. The epileptogenic zone: a critical reconstruction. In: Schuele SU, ed. *A Practical Approach to Stereo EEG*. New York, NY: Springer Publishing Company; 2020:105–120.
22. Munari C, Kahane P, Tassi L, et al. Intracerebral low frequency electrical stimulation: a new tool for the definition of the "epileptogenic area"? *Adv Stereotac Funct Neurosurg*. 1993;10:181–185.

CHAPTER 10

# Electrical Stimulation for Functional Mapping During SEEG Exploration

AGNÈS TRÉBUCHON, MD, PHD • DANIEL L. DRANE, PHD, ABPP(CN)

## INTRODUCTION

The challenge in epilepsy surgery is to cure the patient without causing an additional neurological deficit, so the maxim "primum non nocere" should be kept in mind throughout the presurgical investigations, and in particular during SEEG. The goal of the method is to delineate the epileptogenic zone and propose a brain volume for resection without compromising post-operative cognitive, motor, sensory, or socio-emotional brain function (although most emphasis has been on language and motor skills). Functional mapping is therefore, alongside identification of the EZ, a crucial part of the SEEG exploration. The identification of cortical structures essential to cognitive or perceptual function, with great anatomical and physiological precision is challenging. Indeed, it is widely agreed that the human brain is a complex and adaptive system in which a vast range of function arises from coordinated neural activity across diverse spatial and temporal scales.[1] For instance, graph-theoretical investigations have shown that the human brain exhibits a hierarchically modular organization with clusters of nodes (hub, subnetworks) that are densely connected within the cluster, but only sparsely coupled to nodes in other modules.[2] Accordingly, a modern concept of functional mapping needs to take into account this organization and enable the identification of the hub or node essential for function.

The challenge of functional mapping in epilepsy surgery lies in the pathology itself. The lesion underlying drug resistant epilepsy (cortical dysplasia, stroke, cortical malformation, heterotopia) may result in a functional organization that is completely different from that of the healthy subject. In the case of dysplastic tissue, there may be no clear boundaries between the dysplastic and functional networks, as dysplastic cortex is specified prenatally and thus integrated into developing cortical networks. FCD differs from pathologic entities acquired in postnatal life such as tumors, gliosis, and vascular diseases, which often destroy existing networks.[3] Of note, however, research has found surprising consistencies between cortical stimulation mapping results when comparing patients with either early or late onset epilepsy and a third series of patients with new onset, fast growing tumors.[4] Consequently, the clinician assessing language in the epilepsy surgery setting must explore the possibility that language functions may have atypical neural substrates, while being cognizant that for many individuals there may have been no significant reorganization of function (particularly after early epochs of brain development have passed) (see Drane and Pedersen, 2019 for an extended discussion of this topic).[5] Therefore, an individualized and comprehensive assessment should always be done during the presurgical investigation.

Since the early days of presurgical mapping, electrical stimulation was developed to identify essential functional areas.[6] The main principle is simple: electrical stimulation of a specific brain region producing a transient functional impairment might predict which functions will be disturbed if the stimulated cortex were to be removed. For instance, as previously described using ECoG or awake surgery,[7] stimulation is useful to identify essential language cortex in patients undergoing resection of epileptogenic cortex in the specialized language hemisphere.[8–10]

Despite its proven utility, and the fact that functional mapping is commonly performed during SEEG presurgical investigation, stimulation remains challenging and contains pitfalls because of the technical constraints and the requirement to adapt testing at the individual level. Addressing the question of the sensitivity and specificity of the SEEG-stimulation against reference meta-analytic fMRI studies, authors confirmed

The Fundamentals of Stereoelectroencephalography. https://doi.org/10.1016/B978-0-443-10877-8.00001-2

that stimulation can reliably identify contacts with/without language function but may under- detect all language sites.[10] Indeed, the major pitfall with potential clinical consequences for the patient, the failure to identify a specific functional region, is a "false negative stimulation," and has led some to question the validity of this method. Nevertheless, fMRI studies cannot determine which brain areas are essential for function, and it has frequently been shown that such activations may show regional involvement that is not necessarily required for successful task completion.[11]

It should also be noted that "false-positive" errors may also occur in the context of cortical stimulation mapping. The main causes are likely to involve patient fatigue or a lack of appreciation for the effects of after discharges and the extent of electrical spread. These potential problems may be minimized by establishing a baseline performance that is performed at a near perfect level by the patient, making sure that they are not becoming overly fatigued during the mapping session, and carefully attending to the EEG data. In such cases, surgery could be denied, which could have more than likely been safely performed.

The procedure of stimulation during SEEG for eliciting seizures and for functional mapping should be done in conjunction to answer the fundamental question of whether or not there is a spatiotemporal overlap between the epileptogenic and the functional network. Second, to address the question of functional mapping, it is important to know the physiological network organization of the system under exploration. Third, cortical stimulation for functional mapping cannot be unambiguously interpreted in isolation. The integration of physiological rhythms, the presence of a lesion or a cortical malformation must be integrated in the procedure, as well as in the analysis and in the interpretation of the result obtained. Of note, while part and parcel of the traditional French school of SEEG, Americans trained in the "grid and strip" practice of mapping may be less familiar with purposeful seizure induction during intracranial monitoring, and have often been taught that the seizures. occurring through stimulation differ from naturally occurring events (see the following articles for a discussion of eliciting seizures, understanding semiology, and the history of the North American and European schools of stimulation mapping).[12–14] The rise of minimally invasive surgical tools and procedures has seemingly shifted the American programs to replace the grids and strips approach with SEEG. Of note, however, there has been an uneven adoption of European practices and theory, and many American programs are still finding their way.

## WHAT IS THE ROLE OF FUNCTIONAL MAPPING IN AN INDIVIDUAL PATIENT?

### What Do We Need to Know Before Performing Stimulation?

Stimulation for functional mapping cannot be done in isolation of the whole surgical epilepsy exploration. Before addressing the question of function, several factors have to be taken into account.

#### Patient data

A comprehensive clinical assessment should be performed prior to functional mapping by stimulation, in order to determine any pre-existing functional deficits. Some deficits, such as a mild hemiparesis, a proprioceptive deficit, or a quadrantanopia, may be clinically evident, while others, such as a visual agnosia, alexia, prosopagnosia, anomia, or dysexecutive function may only be elicited by detailed neuropsychological assessment, which should be carried out in every patient.

Clinical factors that influence the likelihood of functional reorganization should also be determined, including the age of onset of epilepsy, and the presence and type of any underlying lesion.

#### SEEG data

Knowledge of the precise anatomical position of each electrode contact is crucial to plan the stimulation procedure. First, the testing procedure and the parameters of stimulation must be adapted according to the different physiological system explored. Second, as bipolar stimulations are performed between two adjacent contacts, the exact position of the contact, such as bank of the sulcus, proximity to white matter, orientation in the cortical strip needs to be checked to interpret the effect of the stimulation. For instance, stimulation between two contacts in gray matter may have a different effect to stimulation between one contact in white matter and one in gray matter. It is possible that stimulation within the gray matter may induce more focal dysfunction whereas stimulation within white matter could produce disconnection phenomena. Third, in addition to the anatomical relations of the electrode contacts, their location in relation to an underlying lesion, and the nature of the lesion should be determined. In addition to correlation with neuroimaging, some lesions, such as cortical dysplasia or ischemia may be associated with characteristic patterns of resting SEEG recordings. It is widely accepted that in several types of cortical malformation such as FCD,[3,15] schizencephaly[16] or heterotopia,[17,18] functional connectivity between lesion areas, and regions of normal cortex may occur. It is therefore relevant to note whether signal organization within the supposed lesion is physiological or not. The relationship between each contact and the network organization of spikes, high frequency oscillations and, if already available, the network organization of the seizure, must be considered in stimulation planning.

#### Physiological network

Since the epileptogenic and functional networks may closely overlap, a knowledge of the typical physiological organization of functional networks is essential. Functional connections between two areas, or modular organization of a specific cognitive function are sometimes relevant to the interpretation of a stimulation. We would caution that this is still an evolving area, as the neural circuitry of many functions are complex and not fully understood, and even the cognitive constructs we attempt to measure (e.g., memory, attention, emotion) are undergoing rapid theoretical advancement. Paradigms to employ in stimulation mapping will likewise be expanding over time and a virtuous circle can be created between the research program and clinical activity.[13,19,20]

Even if stimulation is performed in each contact exploring gray matter, choosing the most informative pair of contacts may be complex. Electrophysiological data such as evoked potentials in response to auditory stimuli (pure tones), to visual stimuli (checkerboard, picture, face), to somatosensory stimulation or to cognitive tasks (oddball paradigm, naming, etc.) are useful to guide the selection of the relevant contact in the area explored.

Broad-band high gamma activity, extracted from the SEEG signal, has been shown to be a useful general electrophysiological index of cortical processing, and high gamma responses are consistent across a wide variety of experimental tasks and cortical regions, such as language, vision, and eye movement.[21–24] These data can assist in the selection of testing performed during the procedure. A recent study elegantly demonstrates such an approach before stimulation in SEEG.[25] In addition, Fig. 10.4 illustrates one clinical case in which the recording of gamma activity before stimulation helped to choose the task set, and to understand the underlying processing involved.

### Stimulation Mapping in Clinical Practice

We describe here the general procedure for stimulation, as already reported in a paper[8] and in the expert consensus clinical practice guidelines proposed under the auspices of the French Clinical Neurophysiology Society.[26] Aspects relevant to specific functional networks or cortices will be discussed in more detail in the following chapters. As already outlined in the chapter on stimulation to induce seizures, the stimulation protocol must be adapted, according to the different requirements of individual cases, rather than following a rigid protocol. Stimulation planning must take into account all the data described below.

#### Timing

Stimulation is undertaken during two to five sessions distributed over several days that generally take place after the recording of spontaneous seizures. Distributed sessions should be performed both for patient comfort and for electrophysiological reasons: repetition of stimulation in the same site tends to produce a refractory period and false negative stimulation.[8] The duration of each session should be determined for individual cases, but is usually between 30 and 60 minutes. One important parameter is the time between each stimulation. The physiological state of the tested brain structure before stimulation must be correctly appreciated. It is necessary to have an observation period following each stimulation session, because stimulation may modify the network causing, for example, slowing or after discharges. This is why we propose to space each stimulation by at least 2–3 min and to avoid repeating stimulation of the same structure within a short time frame, to prevent plasticity or summation effects. The EEG should return to its resting state before stimulation is repeated.

Stimulation for functional mapping is often carried out in the context of normal anti-seizure medication (ASM) or very slight reduction. Because it is completely integrated with the SEEG exploration, stimulation can trigger seizures during the procedure.

#### Stimulation parameters

Electrical stimulation between two adjacent contacts of the same electrode (bipolar stimulation) is typically practiced. Fig. 10.1 depicts the different type of parameters used. The charge density delivered is influenced by the position and orientation of the electrode, as well as the type of cortex stimulated.[27] The parameters used in clinical practice are established for platinum–iridium semiflexible multi-contact intracerebral electrodes 0.8 mm diameter and 2 mm long, with contacts at intervals of 1.5 mm. Stimulation is applied between two adjacent contacts utilizing one or both of the following modalities: low frequency pulse stimulation (1Hz) or sustained train of pulses (50Hz or 60 Hz). Pulse width and train frequency generally are kept constant throughout the whole stimulation procedure (0.3–1 ms). Low frequency pulse stimulation consists of a rectangular biphasic single pulse, 2 ms pulse

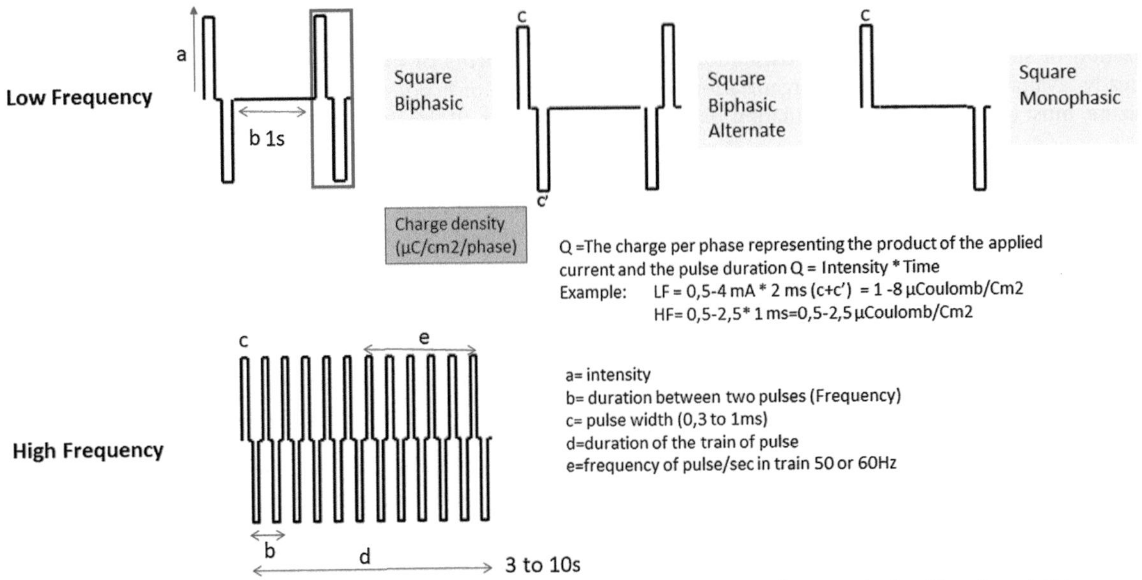


FIG. 10.1 Different parameters of the stimulation between two consecutives contacts. (A) pulse width; (B) time between two single pulse:1s low frequency, 0.02s high frequency; (C) intensity mA.

duration, 0.5 m A to 4 mA delivered every second for a continuous period of up to 40 s. High frequency pulse stimulation consists of a train of rectangular pulses with a 50Hz frequency, 1 ms pulse duration, 0.5–2.5 mA intensity, and 3–5 seconds train duration. These parameters were adjusted to avoid any tissue injury with a charge density per square pulse of <55 μC/cm2.[28] Single pulses have been used for functional mapping, but are less effective in particular to map associative cortex. As a rule, stimulation is begun with low current intensities and gradually increased to reach threshold either for clinical manifestations, such as a positive effect or negative effect of the stimulation or electrophysiological effects such as an afterdischarge or seizure. The initial intensity may vary according to several factors: (i) level of current ASM, (ii) history of generalization (particularly when stimulating lateral premotor or precentral cortex), (iii) whether the area stimulated is proposed to be part of the EZ (as indicated by already recorded spontaneous seizures), (iv) type of cortex stimulated.

To reduce the risk of a false negative stimulation, both the charge density and the duration of the stimulation must be sufficient. Low intensity and inadequate duration of the stimulation have been reported as a cause of false negative stimulations, while in the associative cortices a long lasting stimulation has been shown to increase the occurrence of positive responses.[8]

This stimulation paradigm using adjacent contacts ensures a good spatial specificity with respect to the structures targeted for stimulation. Our choice of bipolar stimulation presumably produces a more focused electrical field thus leading to more accurate anatomical localization of less than 5 mm spatial accuracy, centered around the stimulated dipole.[29] A recent article found that some of the differences in stimulation intensity can be explained by the observation that responses largely depend on the applied charge per phase taking the variable pulse durations into account.[27] According to electrode size (diameter of 0.8 mm, contacts 2 mm long separated by 1.5 mm from one another), the current charge density/cm$^2$/phase, the current density/cm$^2$/second and the total charge density/cm$^2$ can be calculated according to stimulation intensity and train duration (Fig. 10.1). Because the variation of pulse width across center (0.3 or 1 ms), it is preferable to use the total charge density than the intensity in mA to be sure to have an effective stimulation.

### Task used

In functional mapping, selection of the task needs to be tailored to the patient level of functioning and to the site of the stimulation. The choice of tasks performed depends on the functional role of the stimulated regions so knowledge of the physiological network is particularly important. A task which is not relevant to the functional system stimulated, and the absence of behavioral assessment of the patient may result in a false negative stimulation.[8,30] The analysis of the behavioral response of the patient should take into account both the type of errors and the reaction time. Some recent articles on cognitive and socio-emotional mapping with SEEG have included charts of structure-function relationships observed using cortical stimulation mapping in order to help guide task choice.[13]

## LANGUAGE

### Physiological Background

As previously expressed above, stimulation for functional mapping requires knowledge about the physiological network involved in the function. We summarize here some important points about language organization.

It has long been known that the language network is asymmetric between left and right hemisphere: only left hemispheric lesions induce language disturbance in patients with left lateralized language dominance.[31] The idea of a "dominant/major" left hemisphere controlling both language and right hand against a "nondominant/minor" hemisphere was proposed. Thanks to studies of split-brain patients, the specific role of each hemisphere has been described.[32] The left hemisphere hosts linguistic functions, such as phonology and syntax, and the right brain is involved in paralinguistic functions, such as emotional and context processing. The term of "specialized language hemisphere" rather than dominant/nondominant is arguably more appropriate.

Within the left hemisphere the simplistic view of a network between two restricted regions - Broca's and Wernicke's area has been updated. Neuroimaging and electrophysiological data have clearly shown that the language network is widely and mainly distributed around the sylvian fissure. Converging data supported the idea of a dual stream model of organization of language processing with a dorsal stream involving in mapping sound to articulation, and a ventral stream in mapping sound to meaning.[33–35] From the superior temporal gyrus, which is engaged in early cortical stages of speech perception, the system diverges into two processing streams. The dorsal stream, or the "auditory–motor integration," runs dorso-posteriorly through the inferior parietal region and further to motor and prefrontal areas, Broca's area in particular. The posterior–anterior "what" pathway or ventral stream projects laterally to the middle and inferior temporal cortices and serves as a sound-to-meaning interface by mapping sound-based representations of speech to widely distributed conceptual representations.

Within the ventral network, a region localized in the basal temporal region has been described to be included in the language network. The basotemporal language area (BTLA) located 2–9 cm from the tip of the temporal lobe, and surrounding the collateral sulcus (CS) and occipitotemporal sulcus has been described for the first time in the context of epilepsy surgery.[36,37] Since the first description, it is well known today that BTLA is functionally heterogeneous, involving several sub-regions. Visual perceptual processes predominate in the posterior part of the region, which is located relatively near the striate cortex, whereas the territories involved in language processes contributing to lexical retrieval are more anterior.[38] The anterior part is bilaterally involved in multimodal semantic processing and responds to the retrieval of word meaning.[39] Its activation was previously found to be associated with semantic activities focusing on phonological decisions regarding auditorily presented words.[40] Lesions confined to the anterior part of the BTLA are known to impair patients' semantic processing performances.[41] Several parts of this region, in particular the fusiform gyrus, contribute to the language network underlying object naming.

In the context of epilepsy surgery, the cortical network underlying visual object naming should be well understood for two reasons - it is the most prevalent deficit present in patient with epilepsy, and the picture naming task is to the most widely used test during presurgical investigations. Verbal picture naming recruits a widely distributed network of cortical areas, predominantly located in the left hemisphere. The network starts with occipital and ventro-temporal structures. From 200 ms onwards, temporal structures are engaged in lexico-semantic processing (activation of the meaning of the picture and its possible names); later, inferior parietal cortex and posterior temporal lobe are associated with phonological encoding. The left inferior frontal gyrus is thought to resolve conflict among alternative representations, as well as syllabification processes. Finally, bilateral pre-motor and motor areas, as well as the inferior frontal gyri, are engaged for articulatory planning and articulation.[42–44] In addition to this well-defined network some studies have pointed out the specific role of the hippocampus in lexical selection during picture naming.[45,46]

Lesion analysis studies have demonstrated that visual naming can be impaired by surgical lesions occurring nearly anywhere along the ventral visual pathway, with the lateral temporal pole appearing to be more associated with proper noun retrieval.[47–49] Different types of objects appear to be differentially distributed through this visual stream, and in this age of more focal, minimally invasive epilepsy surgical procedures it is common to see both improvements and declines in visual naming resulting from a single destructive procedure in a given patient.[50–52] Despite the aforementioned finding of a possible role of the hippocampus in lexical selection during picture naming, more than one study has demonstrated that visual naming does not decline following the ablation of the left amygdylar-hippocampal complex.[48,53] Of note, the neural substrates of learning naming associations has been less well studied in the setting of neurosurgery.

In summary, the language network is asymmetric, mainly involving the left hemisphere and widely distributed between several temporal regions and the inferior frontal lobe.

## What Can Functional Mapping Tell Us About Language Organization?

So functional mapping in the context of epilepsy surgery must answer two main questions: firstly "what is the language organization in terms of hemispheric specialization?"; secondly "What are the crucial nodes of the network underlying function?"

### *Stimulation and hemispheric organization*

As described above, the left and the right hemisphere have different functions during linguistic processing, but the idea of a simple dichotomy between a homogeneous left hemisphere dedicated to language, and a right hemisphere dedicated to other functions has to be re-examined. First there is a continuum between left and right specialization, and second the hemispheric specialization must be assessed region by region.[54] However three main language representations may be distinguished:

(1) a typical representation consists of principal involvement of the left hemisphere
(2) an atypical organization including a range of configurations between left and right and
(3) an atypical right representation with principal involvement of the right hemisphere.

As we described in the beginning of this chapter, chronic epilepsy or a brain lesion such as stroke or dysplasia may induce a plastic change in language representation, resulting in the higher proportion of atypical language representation that is well recognized in this population.

The issue of hemispheric specialization is usually assessed before SEEG, using several noninvasive tools such as fMRI.[55,56] The techniques of fMRI study have previously shown dissociation between left and right hemispheres, for instance with the left IFG and the right STG involved in a language task.[57,58] Using ECoG, stimulation has already proven to be useful in this type of interhemispheric dissociation, Fig. 10.2.[59]

### *Identification of crucial node for the function*

Because the language network is widely distributed in the left (dominant) hemisphere, and often varies among patients, brain mapping should delineate eloquent areas at the individual level. Stimulations

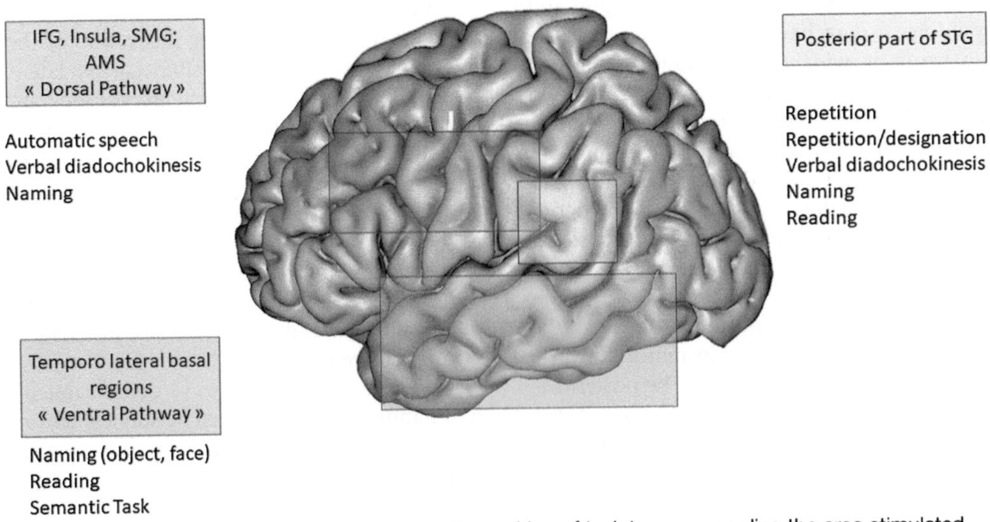


FIG. 10.2 Functional mapping for language. Proposition of task to use according the area stimulated.

have to identify the crucial node for language function. In order to achieve this, as described above, two aspects of the stimulation protocol are critical: (1) to disrupt the language function the stimulation needs to be strong enough to exert a complex effect in a given volume of brain tissue. Stimulation parameters must be carefully chosen to avoid the risk of false negative stimulation. (2) To detect the effect of the stimulation, the task and the analysis of the patient's behavior must be appropriate to the region stimulated.

**Methodological Aspect: An Effective Stimulation.** In associative networks and particularly in the language network, the stimulation needs to be sufficient to apply an effect in the network.

We have found that to prevent the occurrence of false negative effects, stimulation duration around 5 s and intensity up to 1.5 mA are required for language functional mapping in SEEG.[8] Bedos Ulvin and colleagues used the same range of intensity but with a longer duration 5–10 s.[60] The length of the stimulation is clearly an important parameter, a stimulation too short (<4s) may not be enough to disorganize the underlying network. This is in keeping with previous SEEG stimulation studies.[26,61,62]

The recording of an AD or evoked spike AD helps to establish that the effective stimulation threshold of a given structure has been reached. The spatial extent of the AD is important in interpreting the effect of the stimulation. In contrast to local ADs, a remote or regional AD leads to greater complexity in the interpretation of functional effects. The occurrence of an AD depends on the total charge density delivered, but is also dependent on the type of cortex stimulated. For example, ADs are seen more frequently in mesial temporal lobe structures.

Few studies have addressed the question of the effect of an AD on the clinical response. Some studies considered the AD as "pathological" and stimulations producing an after-discharge were excluded from analysis.[61,63,64] On the hand, the majority of studies considered stimulation trials with AD in their analysis.[62,65–67] Conceptually, the presence of an AD can reveal a potentially "nonfocal effect" of a stimulation. As is now well recognized, brain regions are highly interconnected and constitute anatomo-functional networks. The behavioral effects of stimulations critically depend on functional connectivity. Electrode sampling of the area explored and stimulated has an important impact on the ability to capture/observe the whole effect of the stimulation, and should not be underestimated in its interpretation. Finally, a short and focal AD confirms that the threshold of the stimulated structure has been reached. Avoiding false negative effects, it increases the specificity of the technique.

**Methodological Aspect: The Difficult Task Choice.** Within the widespread peri-sylvian language network, different regions have different latencies and linguistic functions.[44] To be effective and avoid false negative stimulation, the patient needs to be engaged in a task adapted to the topography of the testing region.

Practice varies widely across centers as there are no adopted guidelines for cortical stimulation mapping. We list here the tasks usually used in both our centers:

Naming tasks includes a variety of categories of objects, entities (humans and animals), and landmarks, and allows for the evaluation of both common and proper nouns; Automatic speech (counting); repetition of words and sentences; repetition/designation task; tasks include both auditory and visual components, with an effort to examine the same stimuli in different modalities (e.g., the picture of a rooster, the sound of a rooster, and the verbal description of a rooster presented in different modalities); semantic decision tasks; reading aloud of sentences and words; testing in more than one language for bilingual patients; verbal diadochokinesis (the patient is asked to repeat "pataka" 10 times).

The sensitivity of stimulation to produce a functional effect varies according to the task used, as we have previously reported. During automatic speech, stimulation induced fewer positive responses (61% positive/39% negative), compared to reading aloud (78%/22%) or naming (76%/24%), which were more sensitive.[8]

In the posterior part of the left superior temporal gyrus the effect of stimulation is different according to the task and the area stimulated (Fig. 10.3). During a word repetition task hallucinations or illusions are observed when Heschl's gyrus was stimulated without any language deficit, while the stimulation of the planum temporale (PT) induced auditory symptoms along with comprehension deficit. Articulatory or phonological errors are elicited by the stimulation of the left PT during word or pseudo word repetition, presumably due to a difficulty to maintain task-relevant representations in a phonological loop. Lastly, the posterior part of the left superior temporal sulcus (STS) seems involved in more high-level language processes required in naming and reading tasks, because its stimulation did not induce positive auditory symptoms but naming or reading deficits. The reading deficit included graphene decoding, comprehension deficit and graphene to phoneme deficit.[68]

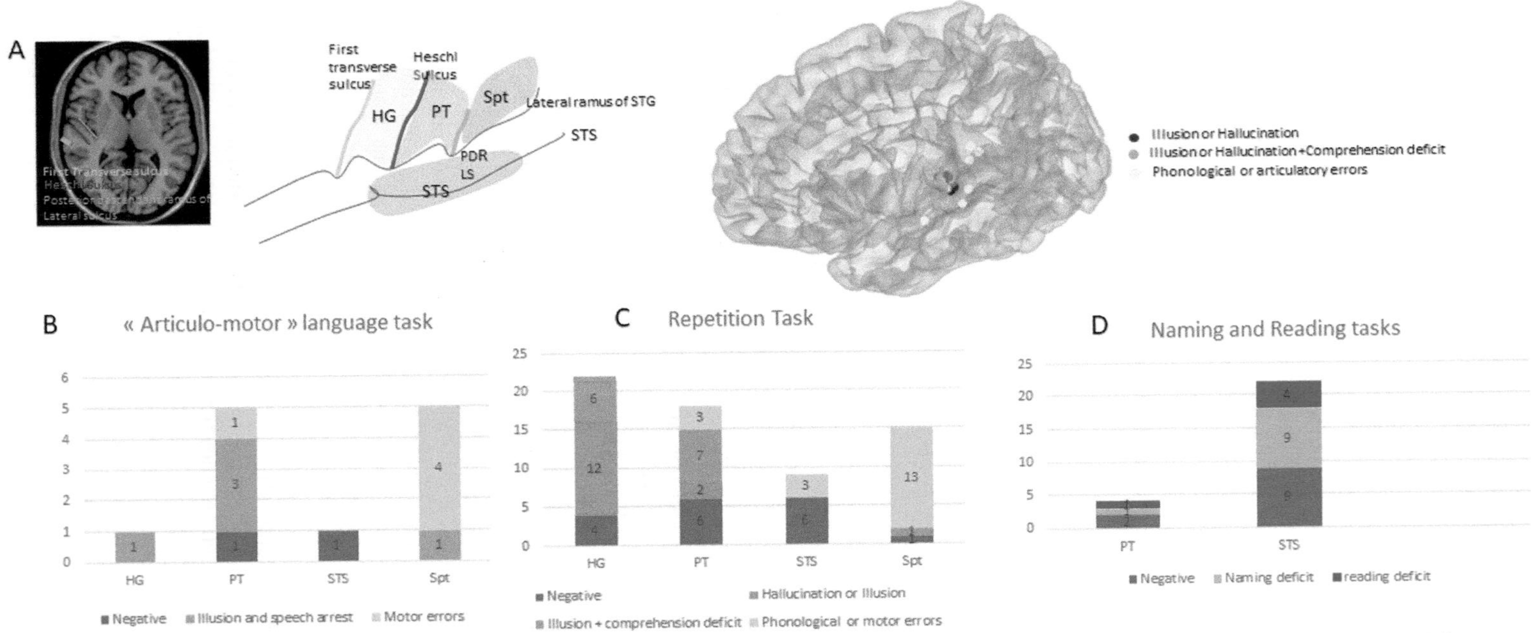


FIG. 10.3 Stimulation of auditory cortex according to the subpart of the auditory cortices during language task (adapt from Trebuchon et al. 2021). A schematic view of the different subparts of posterior STG according to sulcal landmark. B C and D: The Y-axis correspond to the number of stimulations take into account, the color codes to the different type of errors. Each bars graph corresponds to a sub-region (HG, PT, STS and Spt). Each panel corresponds to a specific language task repetition, motor task and reading and naming task on left hemisphere. Hallucinations or illusions only are induced only in HG, whereas stimulation of the PT induced hallucinations/illusion plus comprehension deficit. Stimulation of Spt induce phonological errors and difficulty to maintain in phonological loop. Results obtained during high-level language process such as naming and reading task. The deficit is mainly observed in the posterior part of the STS.

In the medial and basal part of the temporal lobe, the choice of task also produced different results during stimulation. Stimulations performed during naming or reading were more likely to induce a language deficit than during a repetition or automatic speech task. As noted, there can also be differences based upon object or face type (e.g., naming animals vs. objects vs. famous persons or landmarks), and based upon the level of naming specificity (e.g., common vs. proper nouns). In the inferior frontal gyrus or in mesial temporal anterior part (hippocampus, anterior part of the parahippocampal gyrus), the naming task appears to be the most sensitive. In the insula, even with a small sample, we found more elementary speech arrest or slowing in automatic speech than in the inferior frontal gyrus or in anterior temporal lobe.

In the basal temporal region Bedos-Ulvin et al. [60] have demonstrated a disruption during stimulation of a naming task, whereas with the same parameters of stimulation, at the same site, a sematic task such as the semantic picture matching task (picture version of the Pyramids and Palm Trees Test) was perfectly performed.[60] The low sensitivity of certain tasks has also been reported with cortical stimulation performed with grids or during awake craniotomy, in particular the low sensitivity of the automatic speech task.[69]

The importance of task selection should be emphasized because of its clinical and scientific implications. In line with previous reports with subdural grids during presurgical testing, our experience highlights that it is vital to appropriately select the task according to the area explored by the electrode. Fig. 10.3 summarizes the tasks that we propose to be appropriate to different stimulated areas.

**How to Interpret the Effect of the Stimulation.** Outside the methodological pitfalls, language stimulation for functional mapping may be challenging due to other issues inherent to the patient behavior itself. On occasion, the same stimulation with the same parameters does not induce the same effect; sometimes testing must be adjusted to the level of the patient's language ability.

### *Variability of the responses*

Empirically, a language response seems to represent an inhibitory effect of the stimulation due to the temporary inactivation of a local population of neurons (pyramidal cells or interneurons). However, we are far from a perfect understanding of the functional effects of stimulation. When we apply a train of stimulation, we do not know precisely the physiological effect of the stimulation. We regularly observe variability of effect when stimulating the same region, with the same parameters of stimulation. One explanation could be that the "inhibitory effect" of the stimulation induces a rapid plasticity of the system during the minutes following the trial. This is why it is recommended to: (1) verify that the SEEG signal returns to its resting state between stimulations, (2) to space stimulations, and (3) to avoid subsequent stimulation of the same site.

Indeed, since stimulation is disrupting a network, can the effect of stimulation at any given site really be considered as focal? While precise analysis of local effects of stimulation is important, it seems very likely that other effects distant to the stimulation site are involved. A systemic effect of stimulation is an important question to consider for interpretation.

### *How to manage the task according to the level of patient*

In the naming task, another parameter needs to be taken into account, which is the linguistic property of the stimulus used. It is well known that low frequency items such as "penguin" or "hippopotamus" are more difficult to name in term of latencies than the frequently used items "dog" and "cat."

Ideally, the patient should initially be familiarized with all the pictures, to ensure that they can accurately name them. But on the other hand, if we use a limited number of items several times, another issue arises: the fact that the network involved in naming changes according to the number of times that the item has been named.[46,70] Indeed, in a block naming task, in which the same picture is named six times, we have observed a change in the event related potential response after only the second presentation of the same picture. Therefore, it is likely that the network involved in a task repeated two or three times involves the network differently. On the other hand, in patients pre-existing naming difficulties or in left temporal lobe epilepsy, where such difficulties are common, we find a more reliable interpretation is possible when a set of 60 items well known to the patient is used.

### *Values of different types of errors?*

The definition of a positive response to stimulation can be difficult. When the patient stops a naming task and then recovers the name a few seconds later, the result is quite obvious. Other types of errors may be more subtle, e.g., a slightly prolonged latency. In our practice we take into account effects not only occurring immediately during the stimulation, but also 10–20 s later, due to the complex effect of the stimulation, and possible summation of the effect. As we illustrated in Figs. 10.3 and 10.4 the type of errors is important depending which structure is involved. For instance, a naming deficit due to lack of lexical access with

A

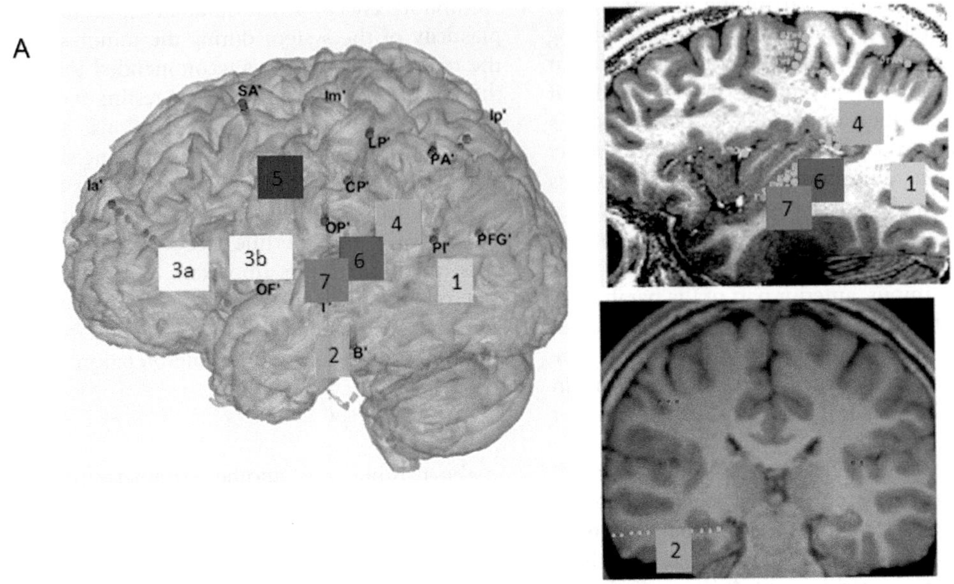


B

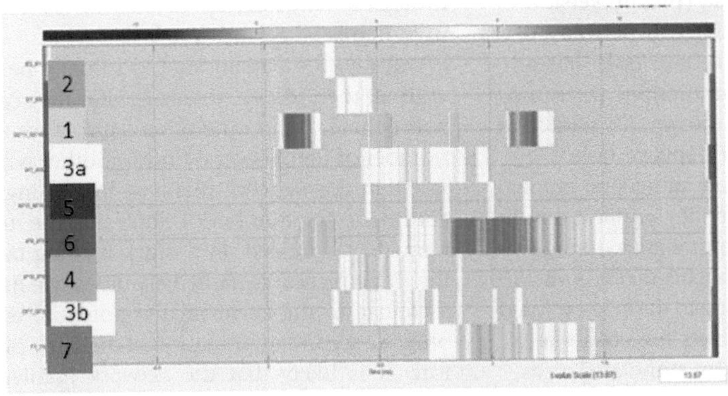


C

| Anatomical | N° | s | mA | AD | Task | |
|---|---|---|---|---|---|---|
| Occipital Lateral | 1 | 5 | 1,5 | 0 | Naming | Visual perceptive deficit of the picture (black form masks the picture) |
| aBTA | 2 | 5 | 1,5 | 0 | Naming | Naming deficit with access to semantic information (gesture of "crab") |
| IFG (PreC) | 3b | 5 | 1,5 | 0 | Naming | No deficit |
| IFG (pars Tri) | 3a | 5 | 1,5 | 0 | Naming | Naming latency >5s to find 'artichoke' |
| sTPJ | 4 | 5 | 1,5 | 0 | Words repetition | Stop repetition, difficulty maintaining phonological loop, "difficult to keep the word in mind" |
| sTPJ | 4 | 5 | 1,2 | 0 | Pataka | Slight slowing of motor aspect |
| Pre Motor | 5 | 5 | 1,5 | 0 | Automatic speech | Counting slow and stops repetitive gesture |
| Auditoty Cortex (PAC) | 6 | 5 | 1 | 0 | Words repetition | No repetition deficit, auditory hallucination |
| Auditoty Cortex (AAC) | 7 | 5 | 1,5 | 0 | Words repetition | Stop repetition, auditory illusion |

FIG. 10.4 Example of language mapping. 17-year-old patient with left temporo-perisylvian epilepsy, MRI negative. (A) Electrode positions, highlighting the 'crucial nodes' of the language network. (B) High frequency gamma (HFG) activity during a naming task (for the method see Dubarry et al.[71]). The time course of

preservation of semantic access (Fig. 10.4, stimulation of aBTLA) allows us to identify "positive" areas as a specific functional sub-unit underlying lexical access.

Conversely, we must keep in mind that the process underling visual naming cannot be treated as a homogenous, unitary phenomenon, but rather a complex, multistep process that involves multiple brain regions.[5,71] This point is particularly well illustrated in the case of the patient in Fig. 10.4, in which we were able to tease apart several steps of the process during a naming task.

## MEMORY

It is well known that successful memory relies on a series of distinct cognitive functions that may be carried out in a distributed manner throughout the brain, in which temporal lobe structures and the hippocampus play a central role. Theta frequency fluctuations of the local field potential recording in the hippocampus have long been implicated in learning and memory. Successful memory is associated both with increased narrow-band theta oscillations and a broad-band tilt of the power spectrum. Theta oscillations specifically support associative memory, whereas the spectral tilt reflects a general index of activation.[72] Hippocampal stimulation may induce memory deficits through disruption of physiological oscillations. Although memory functions are critical in temporal lobe epilepsy surgery, and systematic stimulation studies of the hippocampus pertinent, only a few studies have been performed using depth electrodes. The methodology used in the different studies are relatively varied, and raise the questions of what tasks should be used, when should stimulation be applied, and what type of stimulation is appropriate? Moreover, recent questions have arisen more broadly about how memory should be studied in general, and whether current behavioral testing paradigms actually measure the most meaningful aspects of learning and memory.[13,73]

The verbal memory task used varied from simple paired associative learning task[74] or short word list encoding[75,76] to encoding a list of 16 items or words.[77,78] The interference procedure varied from 10 seconds to 10 minutes. The recollection period was free recall[75,76,79] or a recognition task.[77,78,80] Some studies included a nonverbal memory paradigm.[77,78] Testing must be precisely time-locked to the time of the stimulation and most of the studies used a computer-controlled task.[77–80] The stimulation used was single pulse[77] or a successive train of pulses.[75,76,78–80] The majority used AD subthreshold. Verbal memory tasks consist of 3 phases: encoding phase, distraction phase and recollection phase. Several studies have compared stimulation during the encoding phase and during the recollection phase. According to the results of these studies, the best time to induce a memory deficit is by stimulation in the encoding phase.[77,80]

Recently a study addressed this specific question of the most effective time to stimulate during a verbal memory task.[80] They applied stimulation of the medial temporal lobe during various phases of the task: encoding, distractor, interval, and recall. They found that the disruptive effect of the stimulation of the dominant mesial temporal lobe was timing dependent. Stimulation during the interval between learning and recall most strongly disrupted recall.

As with stimulation of the language functions, stimulation must be of sufficient intensity to exert a disruptive effect on the memory network. Following initial studies which raised the possibility that eliciting an AD might specifically cause a memory deficit, subsequent studies have aimed to avoid such a global effect, by using subthreshold stimulation.

Several studies have shown hemisphere-specific memory deficits induced by stimulation. Left hippocampal stimulation produced word recognition memory deficits, whereas right hippocampal stimulation produced face recognition memory deficits.[78] Conversely, another study suggests that recognition can be processed independently by the hippocampus of either hemisphere.[77] Using the same single pulse

gamma activity illustrates the sequence of processes involved in the language network: 1. occipital lateral: Gamma 80–100 ms after the picture presentation (on response) and activation at 1110 ms (off response) - **perception**; 2. anterior BTLA: Gamma 300–450 ms - **lexical access**; 3. IFG: 450–900 ms - **lexical selection and verbal planning**; 4. sTPJ: 400–700 ms - **phonological loop, dorsal**: 5. Premotor cortex: **Motor planning**; 6. Heschl gyrus and 7. STG: 700–1500 ms - **own voice monitoring.** (C) Result of stimulation. The tasks were chosen according to the site of stimulation and the time course of the observed gamma activity. The types of error are perfectly predicted by the physiological organization of the language network. 1. perceptive deficit during naming task; 2. lexical deficit with preservation of semantic process; 3. lexical selection; 4. phonological loop and dorsal pathway; 5. premotor process; 6. and 7. auditory processing.

stimulation parameters authors described an induction of memory deficits by bilateral hippocampi stimulation only whereas unilateral stimulation did not. Another study showed that stimulation of "pathological" hippocampus, (i.e., included in the epileptogenic zone) failed to induce a verbal memory deficit whereas electrical stimulation of the left hippocampus outside the EZ (right temporal lobe seizure onset) interferes with verbal learning performance.[76]

The paucity of studies of memory mapping reflects the difficulty of functional mapping within the region. Despite the great clinical interest of these procedures, they are rarely used in clinical practice. We routinely perform stimulation of the hippocampus during an associative memory task. However, the results are often difficult to interpret in terms of significance at the individual level, particularly given the range of baseline memory function in this population.

The question of the intensity of the stimulation has also not been resolved. If we consider other studies describing an enhancement of memory function during hippocampal stimulation, we have a long way to go in our understanding of how best to explore memory functions though stimulation. Further studies are needed to reproduce and confirm these results.

Most existing memory stimulation studies were experimental in nature, and did not use the data to predict memory outcome. We recently proposed an "electric Wada," using stimulation from a depth electrode implanted in the left hippocampus in an attempt to determine if a patient could potentially undergo stereotactic laser amygdalohippocampotomy (SLAH) despite failing an intracarotid amobarbital procedure (IAP).[81] The reasoning was that the stimulation of the hippocampus would more accurately simulate the procedure rather than an IAP which would affect the anterior temporal lobe region and not necessarily the entire hippocampus. Stimulation was applied at various intensities and durations while the patient underwent a simulated Wada procedure and a variety of working memory and episodic memory tasks. The patient initially underwent radiofrequency (RF) ablation using the single depth. As there was a brief period of seizure freedom and no apparent cognitive decline on testing, the patient eventually underwent left SLAH, achieved seizure freedom at 1 year, and had a generally positive cognitive and function outcome with no memory decline. Much more work is needed to establish the safety and methodological parameters of such paradigms. It would have been ideal to have stimulated each hippocampus independently, and to sample broader TL regions as well. At present, with stimulation from SEEG, we will not always have the spatial coverage that we may need, and placing extra electrodes would not be without risk to the patient. There are some promising noninvasive techniques that may allow us to conduct such studies in the near future.[82,83]

## OTHER FUNCTIONS

Selimbeyoglu and Parivizi[84] have nicely summarized results based on electrocorticography (ECoG) and SEEG stimulation. Here, we report the main findings published and observed routinely during SEEG.

### Vestibular Symptoms

Two studies have well described vestibular symptoms induced by stimulation of parietal areas. The study by Kahane detailed precisely all the experiences reported.[85] Patients experienced illusions of rotation, translations, or indefinable feelings of body motion. In this study, authors identified a lateral cortical temporo-parietal area called the temporo–peri-sylvian vestibular cortex, from which vestibular symptoms, and above all rotatory sensations, were particularly easily elicited. This area extended above and below the sylvian fissure, mainly inside Brodmann areas 40, 21, and 22. It included the parietal operculum which was particularly sensitive for eliciting pitch plane illusions, and the mid and posterior part of the first and second temporal gyri which preferentially caused yaw plane illusions. In a more recent study, Balestrini and colleagues reviewed stimulation effects in the parietal lobe. The occurrence of vertigo was significantly associated with high frequency electrical stimulation (50 vs. 1Hz) of the posterior cingulum.[61]

### Face Recognition

Stimulation of the right inferior occipital gyrus has induced a transient selective impairment in face recognition (prosopagnosia).[86,87] The region corresponds to the right occipital face area well defined by fMRI. Additionally, stimulation of the ventral visual processing stream of the right TL region has also been associated with deficits in familiar face recognition in the setting of both tumor surgery and epilepsy.[13]

#### *Visual-spatial processing, construction, navigation*

There has been little systematic effort to study these constructs, although the occasional case study or experiment has been completed. Nevertheless, deficits in some of these functions can lead to varying degrees of disability for a given patient. Unilateral spatial neglect tends to occur more often following right-sided lesions, and this function can be mapped with line bisection and cancellation tasks. Limited data have related these functions of spatial neglect and discrimination to the inferior and superior parietal lobules and also portions of the posteriori temporal lobe.[88] Mental rotation tasks have also been used to assess the nondominant parietal lobe in the setting of stimulation mapping.[89,90] Spatial judgment tasks and basic face processing functions have been associated with nondominant parietal lobe stimulation (specifically the parietal-occipital junction) and the posteroinferior frontal lobe.[91] Navigation tasks have also been used in humans, at least for research purposes, but have not routinely made it into clinical use.[92–94] Navigation paradigms have been used extensively in rodents, which has contributed to a discovery of hippocampal place cells, yet there appear to be substantial differences between the rodent and human in this regard.

### Executive control processes

Monitoring of executive functions is particularly important during frontal resections, but it is important to note that executive functions involve more distributed cortico-cortico and cortico-subcortical networks, and deficits in this domain can develop with damage outside the frontal lobes.[95] There has not been a great deal of research completed in this area with stimulation mapping, but there are many tasks which could be explored. For example, Puglisi et al. (2018) employed a Stroop paradigm during stimulation mapping, and noted that sparing the identified subcortical sites in the nondominant frontal lobe region led to preserved executive functions as compared to those who did not receive this evaluation.[96]

### Socio-emotional function

Within the limbic system, the amygdala has been the subject of a large number of studies about its role in emotions. Interestingly, electrical stimulations of right or left amygdala did not induce the same valence in the emotional effect: stimulation of the right amygdala induced negative emotions, especially fear and sadness, whereas stimulations of the left amygdala were able to induce either pleasant (happiness) or unpleasant (fear, anxiety, sadness) emotions.[65] In this study only high frequency stimulation has been reported, and the question of task is not clearly relevant. Well connected to amygdala, stimulation of the insula can induce an anxiety attack.[97]

There are clearly a number of structures implicated in socio-emotional processing, many of which are often involved in the onset zones of various seizure types. These include the amygdalohippocampal complex, the insula, the cingulate cortex, the anterior temporal lobe (e.g., superior temporal pole), select regions of the broader temporal lobe (e.g., the right temporo-parietal junction), select regions of the broader temporal lobe (e.g., the right temporo-parietal junction), the right dorso-medial prefrontal cortex, the bilateral inferior parietal lobules, and the "default mode network."[98–102] We have argued that socio-emotional deficits are more commonplace post-surgical deficits than ever recognized, and have suggested a range of tasks that could be studied as part of a presurgical evaluation.[13] These include functions such as recognizing emotion from facial expression or tone of voice, experiencing emotional valence associated with daily events, aspects of "theory of mind," alterations in level of emotional experience or emotional control, alterations in habits/preferences driven by changes in emotional experience, and secondary effects upon memory (e.g., lack of emotional valence may alter what one attends to in the environment in a detrimental manner, such as diminished fear learning). All of these tasks can be adapted to the SEEG mapping setting, and some work has been completed in this area over the years. As an example, a number of studies have demonstrated that the motor component of an emotional response (e.g., crying, laughing) can be elicited by electrical stimulation without creating the associated emotional valence.[103,104] Our own group found that we could evoke positive affect and anxiolysis from the stimulation of the left dorsal anterior cingulum bundle in four patients, and were able to use this technique to conduct intraoperative cognitive mapping without the sedation of anesthesia.[105] In some cases, inclusion of electrode sites in a surgical procedure which were involved in emotional circuity have resulted in post-surgical deficits. For example, Marincovik et al. (2000) found that destruction of cortical areas that proved sensitive to faces led to post-surgical deficits in emotional face recognition (especially fear).[106] Overall, mapping socio-emotional function may lead to improved functional outcome, but remains in the early stages of development.

## Motor Behaviors

In the central region, shock (pulse) stimulations or a train of short duration is used to induce focal clonic movement.[26] Negative motor responses are seen in the pre-SMA region during testing, whereas SMA proper stimulation induced more elementary positive motor behavior such tonic posturing and or palilalia.[107]

In a recent study, Caruana et al.[108] report a clear functional difference between the subparts of the cingulate gyrus.[108] The pregenual part of the cingulate cortex hosted the majority of emotional, interoceptive and autonomic responses. The anterior midcingulate sector controlled the majority of complex motor behaviors along a ventro-dorsal axis: the whole-body behaviors directed to the extra-personal space were elicited ventrally, close to the corpus callosum, hand actions in the peri-personal space were evoked by the stimulation of the intermediate area, and body-directed actions were induced by the stimulation of the dorsal area of the cingulate sulcus. The caudal part of the midcingulate cortex and the posterior cingulate cortex are mainly devoted to sensory modalities. In addition, the caudal part of the midcingulate cortex hosts the majority of vestibular responses, while the posterior cingulate cortex was the principal recipient of visual effects.

## Sensorimotor System

### *Somato-sensory sensations and pain*

Somato-sensory sensations like anesthesia, paresthesia or thermic dispersion, have been reported mainly during stimulation of the parietal lobe with low and high frequency stimulation.[62,109] The main effect was found in the post central gyrus, but all other parts of the parietal lobe such as the precuneus and posterior cingulum were also involved in the somato-sensory system. Insular stimulation can induce paresthesias and localized warm sensations. Somato-sensory symptoms have been also reported during stimulation of the premotor frontal region especially in the posterior part of the cingulate motor area.[110]

Insular stimulations are well known to elicit painful sensations with high frequency stimulation. Studies suggest that pain is induced preferentially by stimulation of the posterior two thirds of the insula. Painful and nonpainful somesthetic representation in the human insula overlap and both types of responses showed a trend toward a somatotopic organization.[111] Painful sensation has been more frequently described in the nondominant hemisphere.[64]

## Autonomic Nervous System

### *Digestive sensations*

Mulak et al.[63] reported high frequency stimulations eliciting digestive sensation. The temporal pole (BA 38), hippocampus, amygdala and anterior cingulate cortex (ACC; BA 24/BA 32) are the typical anatomical locations connected with epigastric sensations. Retrosternal sensations are preferentially related to the anterior cingulate cortex, while oropharyngeal sensations are mostly related to the suprasylvian opercular cortex and the insula.[63] Authors found a great variability of induced digestive and associated symptoms corresponding to a widely distributed region.

### *Cardiorespiratory response*

Recently, we have gained a deeper understanding of autonomic semiology of seizures using stimulation of limbic system. First stimulation of subcallosal cortex (BA 25) induced a significant systolic hypotensive change because of a reduction in sympathetic drive and a probable reduction in cardiac output rather than bradycardia or peripheral vasodilation–induced hypotension. This effect was not observed after stimulation of the amygdala, hippocampal, insular, orbitofrontal, or temporal cortices.[112]

Secondly, right and left insular stimulations can induce bradycardia or tachycardia.[113] Tachycardia was accompanied by an increase in LF/HF ratio, suggesting an increase in sympathetic tone; while bradycardia tended to be accompanied by an increase in parasympathetic tone reflected by an increase in HF. Authors found mild left/right asymmetry in insular subregions where increased or decreased heart rates were produced after stimulation. Spatial distribution of tachycardia responses predominated in the posterior insula, whereas bradycardia sites were more anterior in the median part of the insula.

Third, stimulation of the amygdala induced a central apnea and oxygen desaturation. This was most frequently observed following stimulation of the medial-most amygdalar contacts located in the central nucleus.[114–117] These studies highlight the role of the amygdala in voluntary respiratory control.

## Visual

One well conducted study reports[87] many visual phenomena evoked electrical stimulations performed with depth electrodes implanted in the occipito-parieto-temporal cortex of 22 epileptic patients. Eighty-five percent of the elementary visual hallucination (spot or a blob) and intermediary hallucinations such as geometric forms (e.g., kaleidoscope, square, triangle, star, diamond) were induced by stimulating the calcarine sulcus, the lingual gyrus, the lateral occipital cortex, the fusiform gyrus and the cuneus/parieto-occipital sulcus. Intermediary hallucinations were evoked at more anterior sites in infra-calcarine occipital structures and in the ventral temporal region than were elementary hallucinations. Most elementary and intermediary hallucinations were colored and moving. Elementary and intermediary hallucinations were all located in the contralateral visual hemifield of the stimulation side, except those elicited by stimulations of the calcarine sulcus, which were in the center of the visual field.

Complex hallucinations defined as meaningful visual hallucinations (e.g., face, landscape, animal, body parts) are less frequently reported, and were induced in more associative cortices. For instance, hallucinations of faces were induced by stimulating the cuneus/parieto-occipital sulcus, the precuneus, and the fusiform gyrus. Visual illusions such as a change of color or spatial modification of the visual background were all elicited by stimulating regions of the right cerebral hemisphere, including the rhinal cortex, parahippocampal gyrus, collateral sulcus, and fusiform gyrus. With the exception of the most posterior cortical sites, the probability of evoking a visual phenomenon was significantly higher in the right than the left hemisphere. Visual perceptive impairments (face recognition) were observed only in two patients. Prosopagnosia was evoked by the stimulation of the right inferior occipital gyrus in one patient and by the stimulation of the right middle fusiform gyrus in the second patient.

The authors observed that the probability of evoking a visual phenomenon decreased substantially from the occipital pole to the most anterior sites of the temporal lobe, and this decrease was more pronounced in the left hemisphere. They hypothesize that greater sensitivity of the right occipito-parieto-temporal regions to intracerebral electrical stimulation to evoke visual phenomena supports the idea of a predominant role of right hemispheric visual areas from perception to recognition of visual forms, regardless of visuospatial and attentional factors.

### Future Directions

As noted throughout, future directions in stimulation mapping with SEEG should involve the continued development of noninvasive methods for mapping that can supplement the SEEG implant scheme,[82,83] the development of methodology to assess memory at the individual subject level, continued development of both active and passive mapping paradigms, and the upgrading of tasks and paradigms to match advances in the theoretical underpinnings of socio-emotional and cognitive processing. The need for more complex test paradigms that mirror the complexity of brain processes and human behavior (e.g., using memory to prospectively plan for the future) are being increasingly recognized. These trends should be supported by the ever-developing nature of technology to allow for paradigmatic studies that were not possible during a prior era (e.g., virtual and augmented reality, machine learning approaches to big data, use of videography/graphic arts).

## SUMMARY

Functional mapping in SEEG is performed to determine whether or not there are overlapping spatio-temporal dynamics between the epileptogenic network and functional networks. Functional mapping procedures cannot be dissociated from the anatomo-electro-clinical correlations seen while carefully analyzing the recorded seizures. The observation of disruptions within functional networks induced by electrical cortical stimulation permits the localization of specific functional sub-units involved in such networks. Functional deficits can be observed during or shortly after seizures. The analysis of these electro-clinical correlations can provide additional information about the functional organization in particular of language and memory. In our practice we combine this electro-clinical data obtained from recorded seizures and stimulation studies with information gathered through different tools such as fMRI, and high gamma activity to support the clinical decision process.

The drive to treat epilepsy through the use of surgery while preserving cognitive function has contributed a substantial wealth of knowledge in our understanding of cognitive function.[5] Stimulation contributes to better understanding of brain functioning in general, in neuroscientific studies, but also on an individual level to enhance the exploration of our patient. What we have learned about brain function representation over the last few years is impressive. However, we have to admit that we have a long way to go in our understanding of the mapping of brain functions. At the bedside, it is sometimes difficult to be confident about the contribution of the area explored to the functional network. Thanks to the increasing body of neuroscience data collected, in future years, the way in which we approach functional mapping may well be very different.

Table 10.1 summarizes the positive stimulation sites according to the cognitive function.

TABLE 10.1
Chart of Positive Neural Stimulation Sites and Specific Neuropsychological Functions (Selected Sample of Representative Studies)

| References | Function Assessed<br>Language<br>Visual Naming | REGION OF STIMULATION<br>Left Hemisphere | <br>Right Hemisphere |
|---|---|---|---|
| Ojemann et al.[118] | Visual naming (General) | Cortical stimulation across language dominant temporal lobe, frontal lobe, and parietal lobe sites (with significant variability across subjects) | N/A |
| Hamberger[119] | Visual naming (objects) | Posterior temporal lobe regions | No effects of stimulation |
| Duffau et al.[120] | Visual naming (objects) | Dorsal PMC and underlying white matter | N/A |
| Bédos Ulvin et al.[60] | Visual naming (objects) | Stimulation of VTC led to naming deficits (particularly the FG and OTS) | Stimulation of VTC led to naming deficits in a single patient with right TL language, but no other subjects |
| Sarubbo et al.[121] | Visual naming (General) | STG, MFG, MFG WM, AG, AG WM, MTG, ITG, STG WM, IFG WM, SMG, insula, lateral FOC, ITG, WM, MTG WM, IFG, SMG WM, lateral FOC WM, FG | AG WM, AG, MTG, WM |
| | **Paraphasic Errors During Stimulation** | **Left Hemisphere** | **Right Hemisphere** |
| Leclercq and Duffau[122] | Phonemic Paraphasic errors during visual naming | AF | No disruption with stimulation |
| Leclercq and Duffau[122] | Semantic Paraphasic errors during visual naming | IFOF | No disruption with stimulation |
| Maldonado et al.[123] | Phonemic Paraphasic errors during visual naming | PostAF (WM) | No disruption with stimulation |
| Miozzo[124] | Semantic Paraphasic errors during visual naming | Mid-middle temporal gyrus | No disruption with stimulation |
| Miozzo[124] | Phonemic Paraphasic errors during visual naming | Middle and posterior STG | No disruption with stimulation |
| | **Auditory Naming (Naming to Description)** | **Left Hemisphere** | **Right Hemisphere** |
| Hamberger | Naming to verbal description (definitions) presented orally | Anterior temporal lobe | No disruption with stimulation |
| | **Transmodal Naming** | **Left Hemisphere** | **Right Hemisphere** |
| Abel et al.[125] | Visual and auditory naming of same semantic concept (e.g., famous person) | Anterior temporal lobe | No disruption with stimulation |
| | **Proper Noun Naming** | **Left Hemisphere** | **Right Hemisphere** |
| Abel et al.[125] | Famous person naming | Anterior temporal lobe/ temporal pole | No disruption with stimulation |
| | **Language Comprehension** | **Left Hemisphere** | **Right Hemisphere** |
| Sarubbo et al.[121] | Comprehension | SPL, STG, insula, SPL WM, SMG WM, MFG WM, STG WM | MFG WM, STG, hippocampus, MFG, STG WM, AG WM, MTG WM, AG, insula, ITG WM, ITG, PostCG, SMFG, MTG |

**TABLE 10.1**
**Chart of Positive Neural Stimulation Sites and Specific Neuropsychological Functions (Selected Sample of Representative Studies)—cont'd**

| References | Function Assessed Language Visual Naming | REGION OF STIMULATION Left Hemisphere | Right Hemisphere |
|---|---|---|---|
| | **Semantic Processing** | **Left Hemisphere** | **Right Hemisphere** |
| Bédos Ulvin et al.[60] | Picture matching (semantically related) | No disruption from stimulation of VTC | No disruption from stimulation of VTC |
| Sarubbo et al.[121] | Semantic processing | MTG WM, insula, MTG, STG, hippocampus, MG WM, ITG, FG, ITG WM, STG WM, MFG, IFG, IFG WM, putamen, lateral FOC, FG WM, SFG, WM | No disruption |
| | **Reading** | **Left Hemisphere** | **Right Hemisphere** |
| Roux et al.[126] | Oral reading | Inferior aspect of pre- and PostCG, SMG, AG, and posterior STG, IFG, MFG, posterior MTG | Inferior aspect of pre- and post CG, IFG |
| Roux et al.[126] | Articulation errors in Oral reading | Inferior aspect of pre- and post CG | Inferior aspect of pre- and post CG |
| Roux et al.[126] | Ocular-induced reading errors | IFG | IFG |
| Sarubbo et al.[121] | Reading | ITG, FG, MTG, IOG, ITG WM, MTG WM, FG WM, IOG WM | ITG, ITG WM |
| Sabsevitz et al.[127] | Reading | Lateral fusiform gyrus (VWFA) | N/A |
| | **Acoustic Responses/ Disruption** | **Left Hemisphere** | **Right Hemisphere** |
| Sarubbo et al.[121] | Acoustic responses | STG, STG WM, MTG | STG, MTG, STG WM, MTG WM |
| Sarubbo et al.[121] | Phonological | ITG, MTG, MTG WM, FG, IFG WM, STG, SPL WM, ITG WM, IFG, MFG, STG WM, AG WM, MFG WM, PostCG WM, SS, PreCG WM, AG, PostCG, SPL, SMG WM, PreCG, SMG, insula | No disruption |
| Duffau et al.[120] | Speech production | Ventral PMC and underlying WM | N/A |
| Sarubbo et al.[121] | Speech production | IFG, IFG WM, PreCG, PreCG WM, MFG, STG, insula, MFG WM, STG WM | PreCG WM, PreCG, MFG, IFG, insula, MFG WM, IFG WM, putamen |
| Sarubbo et al.[121] | Speech articulation | SMG WM, SMG, PostCG, PreCG WM, PostCG WM, PreCG, IFG, MFG, IFG WM, MFG WM, STG, AG WM, AG, insula, SFG WM | SMG, SMG WM, IFG, MFG SFG WM, MFG WM |
| | **Somatosensory** | **Left Hemisphere** | **Right Hemisphere** |
| Maldonado et al.[123] | Somatosensory | PostCG | PostCG |
| Sarubbo et al.[121] | Somatosensory | SPL WM, SPL, PostCG WM, precuneus, PostCG, PreCG, PreCG WM | SPL, PostCG WM, PostCG, SPL WM, SMG, AG, SMG, insula, pre-cuneus, STG, AG WM, PreCG |

*Continued*

TABLE 10.1
Chart of Positive Neural Stimulation Sites and Specific Neuropsychological Functions (Selected Sample of Representative Studies)—cont'd

| References | Function Assessed<br>Language<br>Visual Naming | REGION OF STIMULATION<br>Left Hemisphere | <br>Right Hemisphere |
|---|---|---|---|
| | **Motor Function** | **Left Hemisphere** | **Right Hemisphere** |
| Blanke et al.[128] | Eye movements | Posterior portion of MFG, SFG; no response from IFG or precentral gyrus | Posterior portion of MFG, SFG; no response from IFG or precentral gyrus |
| Sarubbo et al.[121] | Eye movement control | MFG, MFG WM, SFG WM, PreCG, PreCG WM, SFG | MFG, MFG WM, SFG, SFG WM |
| Maldonado et al.[123] | Speech Initiation/Articulation | PO, horizontal portion of the lateral segment of the SLF III. | N/A |
| Sarubbo et al.[121] | Language Initiation and motor planning | CN, SFG WM, SFG, MFG WM, insula, IFG, lateral FOC WM, IFG WM, MFG, putamen, lateral FOC | CN |
| Sarubbo et al.[121] | Motor | PreCG WM, SFG, PreCG, SFG WM, putamen, insula, MFG | preCG WM, SFG, putamen, SFG WM, PreCG, insular, MFG, MFG WM, PostCG, SLF, post CG WM, IFG, IFG WM |
| Sarubbo et al.[121] | Motor control | SFG WM, SFG, MFG WM, MFG, CG, PostCG WM, PostCG, PreCG | SFG, SFG WM, MFG, CG, IFG, IFG WM, insula, MFG WM, putamen, precuneous |
| | **Consciousness/Mental Phenomenology** | **Left Hemisphere** | **Right Hemisphere** |
| Halgren et al.[129] | Déjà vu/"Dreamy state" | Hippocampus and amygdala | Hippocampus and amygdala |
| Gloor[130] | Déjà vu | Lateral TL with spread to medial TL region | Lateral TL with spread to medial TL region |
| Bartolomei et al.[67] | Déjà vu | Enthorhinal cortex, Perirhinal cortex hippocampus, amygdala (while this sensation could occur after stimulation of any of these structures it was much more common after enthorhinal stimulation) | Enthorhinal cortex, Perirhinal cortex hippocampus, amygdala (while this sensation could occur after stimulation of any of these structures it was much more common after enthorhinal stimulation) |
| Bartolomei et al.[67] | Reminiscence of scenes | Perirhinal cortex | Perirhinal cortex |
| Sarubbo et al.[121] | "Mentalizing" | No disruption | MFG WM, IFG, MFG, SFG, IFG WM, SFG WM, CG, CN, insula |
| | **Emotional Responses** | **Left Hemisphere** | **Right Hemisphere** |
| Lanteaume et al.[65] | Experience of negative emotions | Amygdala | Amygdala |
| Lanteaume et al.[65] | Experience of positive emotions | Amygdala | No effect elicited in right hemisphere |
| | **Visual Processing** | **Left Hemisphere** | **Right Hemisphere** |
| Sarubbo et al.[121] | Visual | FG, IOG WM, FG WM, MOG WM, IOG | AG WM, AG, IOG, MTG WM, MOG WM, hippocampus, FG, IOG WM, SPL WM, SOG WM, MOG, MTG, ITG, FG WM, STG WM, SMG WM |

**TABLE 10.1**
**Chart of Positive Neural Stimulation Sites and Specific Neuropsychological Functions (Selected Sample of Representative Studies)—cont'd**

| References | Function Assessed Language Visual Naming | REGION OF STIMULATION Left Hemisphere | Right Hemisphere |
|---|---|---|---|
| | **Visuo-Perceptual/Visual-Spatial** | **Left Hemisphere** | **Right Hemisphere** |
| Vignal[106] | Facial hallucinations | No effect of stimulation | Ventrolateral prefrontal cortex |
| Barbeau et al.[130a] | Famous face recognition | Passive mapping with intracerebral recordings demonstrates early involvement of the FG simultaneously with the IFG, then multiple regions of the ventral visual WM stream, and finally involvement of the hippocampus (much more pronounced in right hemisphere than left) | Passive mapping with intracerebral recordings demonstrates early involvement of the FG simultaneously with the IFG, then multiple regions of the ventral visual WM stream, and finally involvement of the hippocampus (much more pronounced in right hemisphere than left) |
| Fernandez Coello et al.[131] | Recognition of faces and select objects | N/A | Stimulation of ventral visual processing stream (IFOF and ILF) |
| Roux et al.[88] | Spatial neglect | N/A | Posterior part of the right STG and MTG, IPL, and inferior postCG and IFG. SLF II and SOFF |
| Bush et al.[132] | Spatial navigation | Increases in low and high frequency theta power are observed at the onset of movement in the hippocampus and lateral temporal lobe regions | Increases in low and high frequency theta power are observed at the onset of movement in the hippocampus and lateral temporal lobe regions |
| Maidenbaum[133] | Spatial navigation | Enthorhinal theta band activity is related to task performance | Enthorhinal theta band activity is related to task performance |
| Sarubbo et al.[121] | Spatial perception | AG WM, AG | SMG, SMG WM, AG, AG WM, STG, SPL WM STG WM, MFG WM, PostCG WM, SPL, CG, MTG, PreCG WM, MFG |
| | **Arithmetic Skills** | **Left Hemisphere** | **Right Hemisphere** |
| Duffau et al.[134] | Multiplication/Subtraction | AG | N/A |
| Yu et al.[135] | Subtraction – but not multiplication disrupted at right hemisphere sites | N/A | IPL & AG |
| | **Memory Functions** | | |
| Haglund et al.[136]; Ojemann et al.[137] | Veral episodic memory | Disrupted by stimulation of lateral TL cortex | No evidence of disruption from right TL stimulation |
| Coleshill et al.[78] | Verbal episodic memory | Disrupted by stimulation of amygdala and hippocampus | N/A |
| Ezzyat et al.[79] | Verbal episodic memory | Memory was enhanced at some frequencies by stimulation of lateral TL cortex in setting of SEEG | N/A |

*Continued*

TABLE 10.1
Chart of Positive Neural Stimulation Sites and Specific Neuropsychological Functions (Selected Sample of Representative Studies)—cont'd

| References | Function Assessed Language Visual Naming Executive Functions | REGION OF STIMULATION Left Hemisphere | Right Hemisphere |
|---|---|---|---|
| Puglisi et al.[96] | Response Inhibition | No dis | |

*AF*, arcuate fasciculus; *AG*, angular gyrus; *CG*, cingulate gyrus; *FG*, fusiform gyrus; *FOC*, fronts-orbital cortex; *IFG*, inferior frontal gyrus; *IFOF*, inferior frontal occipital fasciculus; *ILF*, inferior longitudinal fasciculus; *IOG*, inferior occipital gyrus; IPL, inferior parietal lobule; *ITG*, inferior temporal gyrus; *MFG*, middle frontal gyrus; *MOG*, middle occipital gyrus; MTGG, middle temporal gyrus; N/A, no assessment was completed; *OTS*, occipital temporal sulcus; *PMC*, pre-motor cortex; *PO*, parietal operculum; *PostAF*, posterior arcuate fasciculus; *PostCG*, postcentral gyrus; *PreCG*, precentral gyrus; *SFG*, superior frontal gyrus; *SLF II/SLF III*, superior longitudinal fasciculus; *SMA*, supplementary motor area; *SMG*, supra marginal gyrus; *SOFF*, superior occipital frontal fasciculus; *SOG*, superior occipital gyrus; *SPL*, superior parietal lobule; *STG*, superior temporal gyrus; *TL*, temporal lobe; *VTC*, ventral temporal cortex; *VWFA*, visual word form area; *WM*, white matter.

## ABBREVIATIONS

| | |
|---|---|
| AD | Afterdischarge |
| AG | Angular gyrus |
| BTLA | Basal temporal language area |
| CS | Collateral sulcus |
| ECoG | Electrocorticography |
| EZ | Epileptogenic Zone |
| FCD | Focal cortical dysplasia |
| fMRI | Functional MRI |
| HGA | High gamma activity |
| IFG | Inferior frontal gyrus |
| pSTG | Posterior part of superior temporal gyrus |
| SEEG | Stereoencephalography |
| SMA | Supplementary motor area |
| STG | Superior temporal gyrus |
| sTPJ | Temporo parietal junction |

## REFERENCES


1. Bassett DS, Bullmore ET. Small-world brain networks Revisited. *Neuroscientist.* 2017:Oct;23(5):499–516. https://doi.org/10.1177/1073858416667720.
2. Bullmore E, OS. Complex brain networks: graph theoretical analysis of structural and functional systems. *Nat Rev Neurosci.* 2009;10(3):186–198. https://doi.org/10.1038/nrn2575.
3. Duchowny M. Clinical, functional, and neurophysiologic assessment of dysplastic cortical networks: Implications for cortical functioning and surgical management. *Epilepsia.* 2009;50(9):19–27. https://doi.org/10.1111/j.1528-1167.2009.02291.x.
4. Corina DP, Loudermilk BC, Detwiler L, Martin RF, Brinkley JF, Ojemann G. Analysis of naming errors during cortical stimulation mapping: Implications for models of language representation. *Brain Lang.* 2010;115(2): 101–112. https://doi.org/10.1016/j.bandl.2010.04.001.
5. Drane DL, Pedersen NP. Knowledge of language function and underlying neural networks gained from focal seizures and epilepsy surgery. *Brain Lang.* 2019; 189(December 2018):20–33. https://doi.org/10.1016/j.bandl.2018.12.007.
6. Ojemann G, Ojemann J, Lettich E, Berger M. Cortical language localization in left, dominant hemisphere. *J Neurosurg.* 2008;108(2):411–421. https://doi.org/10.3171/JNS/2008/108/2/0411.
7. Ojemann GA. The neurobiology of language and verbal memory: Observations from awake neurosurgery. *Int J Psychophysiol.* 2003;48(2):141–146. https://doi.org/10.1016/S0167-8760(03)00051-5.
8. Trébuchon A, Chauvel P. Electrical stimulation for seizure induction and functional mapping in stereoelectroencephalography. *J Clin Neurophysiol.* 2016; 33(6):511–521. https://doi.org/10.1097/WNP.0000000000000313.
9. Young JJ, Coulehan K, Fields MC, et al. Language mapping using electrocorticography versus stereoelectroencephalography: a case series. *Epilepsy Behav.* 2018;84:148–151. https://doi.org/10.1016/j.yebeh.2018.04.032.
10. Arya R, Ervin B, Dudley J, et al. Electrical stimulation mapping of language with stereo-EEG. *Epilepsy Behav.* 2019;99:106395. https://doi.org/10.1016/j.yebeh.2019.06.038.
11. Horak PC, Meisenhelter S, Song Y, et al. Interictal epileptiform discharges impair word recall in multiple brain areas. *Epilepsia.* 2017. https://doi.org/10.1111/epi.13633.
12. Trebuchon A, Racila R, Cardinale F, et al. Electrical stimulation for seizure induction during SEEG exploration: a

useful predictor of postoperative seizure recurrence? *J Neurol Neurosurg Psychiatry*. 2020;92(1):22–26. https://doi.org/10.1136/JNNP-2019-322469.
13. Drane DL, Pedersen NP, Sabsevitz DS, et al. Cognitive and emotional mapping with SEEG. *Front Neurol*. 2021;12:627981. https://doi.org/10.3389/fneur.2021.627981.
14. Chauvel P, Gonzalez-Martinez J, Bulacio J. Presurgical intracranial investigations in epilepsy surgery. *Handb Clin Neurol*. 2019;161:45–71. https://doi.org/10.1016/B978-0-444-64142-7.00040-0.
15. Souci S, Petton M, Jung J, et al. Task-induced gamma band effect in type II focal cortical dysplasia: an exploratory study. *Epilepsy Behav*. 2018;85:76–84. https://doi.org/10.1016/j.yebeh.2018.05.017.
16. Leblanc R, Tampieri D, Robitaille Y, Feindel W, Andermann F, Roberts DW. Surgical treatment of intractable epilepsy associated with schizencephaly. *Neurosurgery*. 1991;29(3):421–429. https://doi.org/10.1227/00006123-199109000-00015.
17. Valton L, Guye M, McGonigal A, et al. Functional interactions in brain networks underlying epileptic seizures in bilateral diffuse periventricular heterotopia. *Clin Neurophysiol*. 2008;119(1):212–223. https://doi.org/10.1016/j.clinph.2007.09.118.
18. Mai R, Tassi L, Cossu M, et al. A neuropathological, stereo-EEG, and MRI study of subcortical band heterotopia. *Neurology*. 2003;60(11):1834–1838. https://doi.org/10.1212/01.WNL.0000065884.61237.24.
19. Bearden DJ, Selawski R, Chern JJ, et al. Intracranial investigation of piriform cortex epilepsy during odor presentation. *Neurocase*. 2023. https://doi.org/10.1080/13554794.2023.2199936.
20. Anders R, Llorens A, Dubarry A-S, Trébuchon A, Liégeois-Chauvel C, Alario F-X. Cortical dynamics of semantic priming and interference during word production: an intracerebral study. *J Cogn Neurosci*. 2019;31(7). https://doi.org/10.1162/jocn_a_01406.
21. Murphy E, Woolnough O, Rollo PS, et al. *Minimal phrase composition revealed by intracranial recordings*. 2022. https://doi.org/10.1523/JNEUROSCI.1575-21.2022.
22. Panzica F, Schiaffi E, Visani E, Franceschetti S, Giovagnoli AR. *Gamma electroencephalographic coherence and theory of mind in healthy subjects*. 2019. https://doi.org/10.1016/j.yebeh.2019.07.036.
23. Völker M, Fiederer LDJ, Berberich S, et al. The dynamics of error processing in the human brain as reflected by high-gamma activity in noninvasive and intracranial EEG. *Neuroimage*. 2018;173:564–579. https://doi.org/10.1016/J.NEUROIMAGE.2018.01.059.
24. Panagiotaropoulos TI, Deco G, Kapoor V, Logothetis NK. Neuronal discharges and gamma oscillations explicitly reflect visual consciousness in the lateral prefrontal cortex. *Neuron*. 2012;74(5):924–935. https://doi.org/10.1016/J.NEURON.2012.04.013.
25. Cuisenier P, Testud B, Minotti L, et al. Relationship between direct cortical stimulation and induced high-frequency activity for language mapping during SEEG recording. *J Neurosurg*. April 2020:1–11. https://doi.org/10.3171/2020.2.jns192751.
26. Landré E, Chipaux M, Maillard L, Szurhaj W, Trébuchon A. Electrophysiological technical procedures. *Neurophysiol Clin*. 2018;48(1):47–52. https://doi.org/10.1016/j.neucli.2017.11.009.
27. Donos C, Mîndrută I, Ciurea J, Mălîia MD, Barborica A. A comparative study of the effects of pulse parameters for intracranial direct electrical stimulation in epilepsy. *Clin Neurophysiol*. 2016;127(1):91–101. https://doi.org/10.1016/j.clinph.2015.02.013.
28. Gordon B, Lesser RP, Rance NE, et al. Parameters for direct cortical electrical stimulation in the human: histopathologic confirmation. *Electroencephalogr Clin Neurophysiol*. 1990;75(5):371–377. https://doi.org/10.1016/0013-4694(90)90082-U.
29. Nathan SS, Sinha SR, Gordon B, Lesser RP, Thakor NV. Determination of current density distributions generated by electrical stimulation of the human cerebral cortex. *Electroencephalogr Clin Neurophysiol*. 1993;86(3):183–192. https://doi.org/10.1016/0013-4694(93)90006-H.
30. Foster BL, Parvizi J. Direct cortical stimulation of human posteromedial cortex. *Neurology*. 2017;88(7):685–691. https://doi.org/10.1212/WNL.0000000000003607.
31. Broca P. Sur le siège de la faculté du langage articulé. *Bull la Société d'anthropologie Paris*. 1865. https://doi.org/10.3406/bmsap.1865.9495.
32. Gazzaniga MS. Cerebral specialization and interhemispheric communication: does the corpus callosum enable the human condition? *Brain*. 2000;123(7):1293–1326. https://doi.org/10.1093/brain/123.7.1293.
33. Démonet J-F, Thierry G, Cardebat D. Renewal of the Neurophysiology of language: functional neuroimaging. *Physiol Rev*. 2005;85(1):49–95. https://doi.org/10.1152/physrev.00049.2003.
34. Poeppel D, Hickok G. Towards a new functional anatomy of language. *Cognition*. 2004;92(1–2):1–12. https://doi.org/10.1016/j.cognition.2003.11.001.
35. Saur D, Kreher BW, Schnell S, et al. Ventral and dorsal pathways for language. *Proc Natl Acad Sci*. 2008;105(46):18035–18040. https://doi.org/10.1073/pnas.0805234105.
36. Luders H, Lesser RP, Hahn J, et al. Basal temporal language area. *Brain*. 1991;114(Pt 2):743–754.
37. Burnstine TH, Lesser RP, Hart J, et al. Characterization of the basal temporal language area in patients with left temporal lobe epilepsy. *Neurology*. 1990;40(6), 966–966.
38. Moore CJ, Price CJ. Three distinct ventral occipitotemporal regions for reading and object naming. *Neuroimage*. 1999;10(2):181–192. https://doi.org/10.1006/nimg.1999.0450.
39. Sharp DJ, Scott SK, Wise RJ. Retrieving meaning after temporal lobe infarction: the role of the basal language area. *Ann Neurol*. 2004;56(6):836–846.
40. Démonet J-F, Chollet F, Ramsay S, et al. The anatomy of phonological and semantic processing in normal

subjects. *Brain.* 1992;115(6):1753–1768. https://doi.org/10.1093/brain/115.6.1753.

41. Schmolck H, Kensinger EA, Corkin S, Squire LR. Semantic knowledge in patient H.M. and other patients with bilateral medial and lateral temporal lobe lesions. *Hippocampus.* 2002;12(4):520–533. https://doi.org/10.1002/hipo.10039.
42. Indefrey P, Levelt WJ. The spatial and temporal signatures of word production components. *Cognition.* 2004;92(1):101–144.
43. Llorens A, Trébuchon A, Liégeois-Chauvel C, Alario F-X. Intra-cranial recordings of brain activity during language production. *Front Psychol.* 2011;2(DEC). https://doi.org/10.3389/fpsyg.2011.00375.
44. Price CJ. A review and synthesis of the first 20years of PET and fMRI studies of heard speech, spoken language and reading. *Neuroimage.* 2012;62(2):816–847. https://doi.org/10.1016/j.neuroimage.2012.04.062.
45. Hamamé CM, Alario FX, Llorens A, Liégeois-Chauvel C, Trébuchon-Da Fonseca A. High frequency gamma activity in the left hippocampus predicts visual object naming performance. *Brain Lang.* 2014;135:104–114. https://doi.org/10.1016/j.bandl.2014.05.007.
46. Llorens A, Dubarry A-S, Trébuchon A, Chauvel P, Alario F-X, Liégeois-Chauvel C. Contextual modulation of hippocampal activity during picture naming. *Brain Lang.* 2016;159:92–101. https://doi.org/10.1016/j.bandl.2016.05.011.
47. Binder JR, Tong JQ, Pillay SB, et al. Temporal lobe regions essential for preserved picture naming after left temporal epilepsy surgery. *Epilepsia.* 2020;61(9):1939–1948. https://doi.org/10.1111/EPI.16643.
48. Drane DL, Loring DW, Voets NL, et al. Better object recognition and naming outcome with MRI-guided stereotactic laser amygdalohippocampotomy for temporal lobe epilepsy. *Epilepsia.* 2015;56(1):101–113. https://doi.org/10.1111/EPI.12860.
49. Kaestner E, Stasenko A, Ben-Haim S, Shih J, Paul BM, McDonald CR. The importance of basal-temporal white matter to pre- and post-surgical naming ability in temporal lobe epilepsy. *NeuroImage Clin.* 2022;34. https://doi.org/10.1016/J.NICL.2022.102963.
50. Drane DL, Ojemann JG, Phatak V, et al. Famous face identification in temporal lobe epilepsy: support for a multimodal integration model of semantic memory. doi:10.1016/j.cortex.2012.08.009.
51. Abel TJ, Rhone AE, Nourski KV, et al. Beta modulation reflects name retrieval in the human anterior temporal lobe: an intracranial recording study. *J Neurophysiol.* 2016;115:3052–3061. https://doi.org/10.1152/jn.00012.2016.-Naming.
52. Drane DL, Ojemann GA, Aylward E, et al. Category-specific naming and recognition deficits in temporal lobe epilepsy surgical patients. *Neuropsychologia.* 2008;46(5):1242–1255. https://doi.org/10.1016/J.NEUROPSYCHOLOGIA.2007.11.034.
53. Donos C, Breier J, Friedman E, et al. Laser ablation for mesial temporal lobe epilepsy: surgical and cognitive outcomes with and without mesial temporal sclerosis. *Epilepsia.* 2018;59:1421–1432. https://doi.org/10.1111/epi.14443.
54. Tzourio-Mazoyer N, Perrone-Bertolotti M, Jobard G, Mazoyer B, Baciu M. Multi-factorial modulation of hemispheric specialization and plasticity for language in healthy and pathological conditions: a review. *Cortex.* 2017;86:314–339. https://doi.org/10.1016/j.cortex.2016.05.013.
55. Janecek JK, Swanson SJ, Sabsevitz DS, et al. Language lateralization by fMRI and Wada testing in 229 patients with epilepsy: rates and predictors of discordance. *Epilepsia.* 2013;54(2):314–322. https://doi.org/10.1111/epi.12068.
56. Szaflarski JP, Gloss D, Binder JR, et al. Practice guideline summary: use of fMRI in the presurgical evaluation of patients with epilepsy. *Neurology.* 2017;88(4):395–402. https://doi.org/10.1212/WNL.0000000000003532.
57. Baciu MV, Watson JM, McDermott KB, et al. Functional MRI reveals an interhemispheric dissociation of frontal and temporal language regions in a patient with focal epilepsy. *Epilepsy Behav.* 2003;4(6):776–780. https://doi.org/10.1016/j.yebeh.2003.08.002.
58. Thivard L, Hombrouck J, Tézenas du Montcel S, et al. Productive and perceptive language reorganization in temporal lobe epilepsy. *Neuroimage.* 2005;24(3):841–851. https://doi.org/10.1016/j.neuroimage.2004.10.001.
59. Creutzfeldt O, Ojemann G, Lettich E. Neuronal activity in the human lateral temporal lobe II. Responses to the subjects own voice. *Exp Brain Res.* 1989;77:476–489.
60. Bédos Ulvin L, Jonas J, Brissart H, et al. Intracerebral stimulation of left and right ventral temporal cortex during object naming. *Brain Lang.* 2017;175(September):71–76. https://doi.org/10.1016/j.bandl.2017.09.003.
61. Balestrini S, Francione S, Mai R, et al. Multimodal responses induced by cortical stimulation of the parietal lobe: a stereo-electroencephalography study. *Brain.* 2015;138(9):2596–2607. https://doi.org/10.1093/brain/awv187.
62. Ostrowsky K, Magnin M, Ryvlin P, Isnard J, Guenot M, Mauguière F. Representation of pain and somatic sensation in the human insula: a study of responses to direct electrical cortical stimulation. *Cereb Cortex.* 2002;12(4):376–385. https://doi.org/10.1093/cercor/12.4.376.
63. Mulak A, Kahane P, Hoffmann D, Minotti L, Bonaz B. Brain mapping of digestive sensations elicited by cortical electrical stimulations. *Neuro Gastroenterol Motil.* 2008;20(6):588–596. https://doi.org/10.1111/j.1365-2982.2007.01066.x.
64. Mazzola L, Isnard J, Peyron R, Guénot M, Mauguière F. Somatotopic organization of pain responses to direct electrical stimulation of the human insular cortex. *Pain.* 2009;146(1–2):99–104. https://doi.org/10.1016/j.pain.2009.07.014.
65. Lanteaume L, Khalfa S, Régis J, Marquis P, Chauvel P, Bartolomei F. Emotion induction after direct intracerebral stimulations of human amygdala. *Cereb Cortex.*

2007;17(6):1307–1313. https://doi.org/10.1093/cercor/bhl041.
66. Vignal JP, Maillard L, McGonigal A, Chauvel P. The dreamy state: hallucinations of autobiographic memory evoked by temporal lobe stimulations and seizures. *Brain.* 2007;130(1):88–99. https://doi.org/10.1093/brain/awl329.
67. Bartolomei F, Barbeau E, Gavaret M, et al. Cortical stimulation study of the role of rhinal cortex in déjà vu and reminiscence of memories. *Neurology.* 2004;63(5):858–864. https://doi.org/10.1212/01.WNL.0000137037.56916.3F.
68. Trébuchon A, Alario F-X, Liégeois-Chauvel C. Functional topography of auditory areas Derived from the combination of electrophysiological recordings and cortical electrical stimulation. *Front Hum Neurosci.* 2021;15:702773. https://doi.org/10.3389/fnhum.2021.702773.
69. Hamberger MJ. Cortical language mapping in epilepsy: a critical review. *Neuropsychol Rev.* 2007;17(4):477–489. https://doi.org/10.1007/s11065-007-9046-6.
70. Llorens A, Trébuchon A, Riès S, Liégeois-Chauvel C, Alario F-X. How familiarization and repetition modulate the picture naming network. *Brain Lang.* 2014;133:47–58. https://doi.org/10.1016/j.bandl.2014.03.010.
71. Dubarry AS, Llorens A, Trébuchon A, et al. Estimating parallel processing in a language task using single-Trial intracerebral electroencephalography. *Psychol Sci.* 2017;28(4):414–426. https://doi.org/10.1177/0956797616681296.
72. Herweg NA, Solomon EA, Kahana MJ. Theta oscillations in human memory. *Trends Cogn Sci.* 2020;24(3):208–227. https://doi.org/10.1016/j.tics.2019.12.006.
73. Bilder RM, Reise SP. Neuropsychological tests of the future: how do we get there from here? *Clin Neuropsychol.* 2019;33(2):220–245. https://doi.org/10.1080/13854046.2018.1521993.
74. Halgren E, Wilson CL. Recall deficits produced by afterdischarges in the human hippocampal formation and amygdala. *Electroencephalogr Clin Neurophysiol.* 1985;61(5):375–380. https://doi.org/10.1016/0013-4694(85)91028-4.
75. Lee GP, Loring DW, Flanigin HF, Smith JR, Meador KJ. Electrical stimulation of the human hippocampus produces verbal intrusions during memory testing. *Neuropsychologia.* 1988;26(4):623–627. https://doi.org/10.1016/0028-3932(88)90118-2.
76. Loring DW, Lee P, Flanigin HF, et al. Verbal memory performance following unilateral electrical stimulation of the human Hippocampus. *Current.* 1988;1(2):79–85.
77. Lacruz ME, Valentín A, Seoane JJG, Morris RG, Selway RP, Alarcón G. Single pulse electrical stimulation of the hippocampus is sufficient to impair human episodic memory. *Neuroscience.* 2010;170(2):623–632. https://doi.org/10.1016/j.neuroscience.2010.06.042.
78. Coleshill SG. Material-specific recognition memory deficits elicited by unilateral hippocampal electrical stimulation. *J Neurosci.* 2004;24(7):1612–1616. https://doi.org/10.1523/JNEUROSCI.4352-03.2004.
79. Ezzyat Y, Kragel JE, Burke JF, et al. Direct brain stimulation modulates encoding states and memory performance in humans. *Curr Biol.* 2017;27(9):1251–1258. https://doi.org/10.1016/j.cub.2017.03.028.
80. Merkow MB, Burke JF, Ramayya AG, Sharan AD, Sperling MR, Kahana MJ. Stimulation of the human medial temporal lobe between learning and recall selectively enhances forgetting. *Brain Stimul.* 2017;10(3):645–650. https://doi.org/10.1016/j.brs.2016.12.011.
81. Kaestner E, Pedersen NP, Hu R, et al. Electrical Wada for pre-surgical memory testing: a case report. *Epileptic Disord.* 2022;24(2):411–416. https://doi.org/10.1684/EPD.2021.1390.
82. Missey F, Rusina E, Acerbo E, et al. Orientation of temporal interference for non-invasive deep brain stimulation in epilepsy. *Front Neurosci.* 2021;15. https://doi.org/10.3389/FNINS.2021.633988.
83. Esmaeilpour Z, Kronberg G, Reato D, Parra LC, Bikson M. Temporal interference stimulation targets deep brain regions by modulating neural oscillations. *Brain Stimul.* 2021;14(1):55–65. https://doi.org/10.1016/j.brs.2020.11.007.
84. Selimbeyoglu A. Electrical stimulation of the human brain: perceptual and behavioral phenomena reported in the old and new literature. *Front Hum Neurosci.* 2010;4. https://doi.org/10.3389/fnhum.2010.00046.
85. Kahane P, Hoffmann D, Minotti L, Berthoz A. Reappraisal of the human vestibular cortex by cortical electrical stimulation study. *Ann Neurol.* 2003;54(5):615–624. https://doi.org/10.1002/ana.10726.
86. Jonas J, Descoins M, Koessler L, et al. Focal electrical intracerebral stimulation of a face-sensitive area causes transient prosopagnosia. *Neuroscience.* 2012;222:281–288. https://doi.org/10.1016/j.neuroscience.2012.07.021.
87. Jonas J, Frismand S, Vignal J-P, et al. Right hemispheric dominance of visual phenomena evoked by intracerebral stimulation of the human visual cortex. *Hum Brain Mapp.* 2014;35(7):3360–3371. https://doi.org/10.1002/hbm.22407.
88. Roux FE, Dufor O, Lauwers-Cances V, et al. Electrostimulation mapping of spatial neglect. *Neurosurgery.* 2011;69(6):1218–1231. https://doi.org/10.1227/NEU.0B013E31822AEFD2.
89. Corballis MC, Badzakova-Trajkov G, Häberling IS. Right hand, left brain: genetic and evolutionary bases of cerebral asymmetries for language and manual action. *Wiley Interdiscip Rev Cogn Sci.* 2012;3(1):1–17. https://doi.org/10.1002/wcs.158.
90. Parsons TD, Larson P, Kratz K, et al. Sex differences in mental rotation and spatial rotation in a virtual environment. *Neuropsychologia.* 2004;42(4):555–562. https://doi.org/10.1016/j.neuropsychologia.2003.08.014.
91. Fried I, Mateer C, Ojemann G, Wohns R, Fedio P. Organization of visuospatial functions in human cortex. Evidence from electrical stimulation. *Brain.* 1982;105(Pt 2):349–371. https://doi.org/10.1093/BRAIN/105.2.349.

92. Miller J, Watrous AJ, Tsitsiklis M, et al. Lateralized hippocampal oscillations underlie distinct aspects of human spatial memory and navigation. *Nat Commun.* 2018; 9(1). https://doi.org/10.1038/S41467-018-04847-9.
93. Chen D, Kunz L, Wang W, et al. Hexadirectional modulation of theta power in human entorhinal cortex during spatial navigation. *Curr Biol.* 2018;28(20):3310–3315. https://doi.org/10.1016/J.CUB.2018.08.029.
94. Aghajan Z M, Schuette P, Fields TA, et al. Theta oscillations in the human medial temporal lobe during real-world ambulatory movement. *Curr Biol.* 2017;27(24): 3743–3751. https://doi.org/10.1016/J.CUB.2017.10.062.
95. Koziol L, Budding D. Subcortical structures and cognition: implications for neuropsychological assessment. https://books.google.fr/books?hl=fr&lr=&id=jS59vnrIbIIC&oi=fnd&pg=PR2&dq=Koziol,+L.F.,+%26+Budding,+D.E.+eds.+(2009).+Subcortical+structures+and+cognition:+Implications+for++neuropsychological+assessment.+Newark,+NJ:+Springer,+2009.+&ots=bUKvE4-D3z&sig=rdkyVWDbcqNJdefozZvNqsy4buE; 2009. Accessed August 11, 2023.
96. Puglisi G, Sciortino T, Rossi M, et al. Preserving executive functions in nondominant frontal lobe glioma surgery: an intraoperative tool. undefined *J Neurosurg*; 2018. thejns.orgG Puglisi, T Sciortino, M Ross A Leonetti, L Fornia, MC Nibali, A Casarotti, F Pessina https://thejns.org/view/journals/j-neurosurg/131/2/article-p474.xml. Accessed August 11, 2023.
97. Afif A, Minotti L, Kahane P, Hoffmann D. Anatomofunctional organization of the insular cortex: a study using intracerebral electrical stimulation in epileptic patients. *Epilepsia.* 2010;51(11):2305–2315. https://doi.org/10.1111/j.1528-1167.2010.02755.x.
98. Raichle ME. Behind the scenes of functional brain imaging: a historical and physiological perspective. *Proc Natl Acad Sci U S A.* 1998;95(3):765–772. https://doi.org/10.1073/PNAS.95.3.765.
99. Raichle ME, MacLeod AM, Snyder AZ, Powers WJ, Gusnard DA, Shulman GL. A default mode of brain function. *Proc Natl Acad Sci U S A.* 2001;98(2): 676–682. https://doi.org/10.1073/PNAS.98.2.676.
100. Schilbach L, Eickhoff SB, Rotarska-Jagiela A, Fink GR, Vogeley K. *Minds at Rest? Social Cognition as the Default Mode of Cognizing and its Putative Relationship to the "Default System" of the Brain.* Elsevier; 2008. https://doi.org/10.1016/j.concog.2008.03.013.
101. Sergerie K, Chochol C, Biobehavioral JA-N. *The Role of the Amygdala in Emotional Processing: A Quantitative Meta-Analysis of Functional Neuroimaging Studies*; 2008. Elsevier https://www.sciencedirect.com/science/article/pii/S0149763408000079. Accessed August 11, 2023.
102. Ju A, Beyeler A. A new player in neural circuits of emotions. *Nat Neurosci.* 2021;24(11):1506–1507. https://doi.org/10.1038/S41593-021-00945-Y.
103. Sperli F, Spinelli L, Pollo C, Epilepsia MS-. Contralateral smile and laughter, but no mirth, induced by electrical stimulation of the cingulate cortex. undefined *Epilepsia.* 2006;47(2):440–443. https://doi.org/10.1111/j.1528-1167.2006.00442.x.
104. Low H, Sayer F, Neurology CH-A of, 2008 undefined. Pathological crying caused by high-frequency stimulation in the region of the caudal internal capsule. jamanetwork.com. https://jamanetwork.com/journals/jamaneurology/article-abstract/795156. Accessed August 11, 2023.
105. Bijanki K, Manns J, et al, CI-TJ of. Cingulum stimulation enhances positive affect and anxiolysis to facilitate awake craniotomy. *J Clin Investig*; 2019. Am Soc Clin InvestigKR Bijanki, JR Manns, CS Inman, KS Choi, S Harati, NP Pedersen, DL Drane, AC WatersThe https://www.jci.org/articles/view/120110. Accessed August 11, 2023.
106. Marinkovic K, Trebon P, Chauvel P, Halgren E. Localised face processing by the human prefrontal cortex: face-selective intracerebral potentials and post-lesion deficits. *Cogn Neuropsychol.* 2000;17(1–3):187–199. https://doi.org/10.1080/026432900380562.
107. Chauvel P, Rey M, Pierre Buser JB. What stimulation of the supplementary motor area in humans tells about its functional organization. *Adv Neurol.* 1996;70:199–209.
108. Caruana F, Gerbella M, Avanzini P, et al. Motor and emotional behaviours elicited by electrical stimulation of the human cingulate cortex. *Brain.* 2018;141(10): 3035–3051. https://doi.org/10.1093/brain/awy219.
109. Mazzola L, Isnard J, Mauguière F. Somatosensory and pain responses to stimulation of the second somatosensory area (SII) in humans. A comparison with SI and insular responses. *Cereb Cortex.* 2006;16(7):960–968. https://doi.org/10.1093/cercor/bhj038.
110. Chassagnon S, Minotti L, Kremer S, Hoffmann D, Kahane P. Somatosensory, motor, and reaching/grasping responses to direct electrical stimulation of the human cingulate motor areas. *J Neurosurg.* 2008;109(4):593–604. https://doi.org/10.3171/JNS/2008/109/10/0593.
111. Pugnaghi M, Meletti S, Castana L, et al. Features of somatosensory manifestations induced by intracranial electrical stimulations of the human insula. *Clin Neurophysiol.* 2011;122(10):2049–2058. https://doi.org/10.1016/j.clinph.2011.03.013.
112. Lacuey N, Hampson JP, Theeranaew W, et al. Cortical structures associated with human blood pressure control. *JAMA Neurol.* 2018;75(2):194–202. https://doi.org/10.1001/jamaneurol.2017.3344.
113. Chouchou F, Mauguière F, Vallayer O, et al. How the insula speaks to the heart: cardiac responses to insular stimulation in humans. *Hum Brain Mapp.* 2019;40(9): 2611–2622. https://doi.org/10.1002/hbm.24548.
114. Nobis WP, Schuele S, Templer JW, et al. Amygdala-stimulation-induced apnea is attention and nasal-breathing dependent. *Ann Neurol.* 2018;83(3):460–471. https://doi.org/10.1002/ana.25178.
115. Dlouhy BJ, Gehlbach BK, Kreple CJ, et al. Breathing inhibited when seizures spread to the amygdala and upon amygdala stimulation. *J Neurosci.* 2015;35(28): 10281–10289. https://doi.org/10.1523/JNEUROSCI.0888-15.2015.
116. Nobis WP, González Otárula KA, Templer JW, et al. The effect of seizure spread to the amygdala on respiration

and onset of ictal central apnea. *J Neurosurg*. 2020; 132(5):1313–1323. https://doi.org/10.3171/2019.1.JNS183157.
117. Lacuey N, Zonjy B, Londono L, Lhatoo SD. Amygdala and hippocampus are symptomatogenic zones for central apneic seizures. *Neurology*. 2017;88(7):701–705. https://doi.org/10.1212/WNL.0000000000003613.
118. Ojemann G, Ojemann J, Lettich E, Berger M. Cortical language localization in left, dominant hemisphere. An electrical stimulation mapping investigation in 117 patients. *J Neurosurg*. 1989;71(3):316–326. https://doi.org/10.3171/JNS.1989.71.3.0316.
119. Hamberger MJ, Drake EB. Cognitive functioning following epilepsy surgery. *Curr Neurol Neurosci Rep*. 2006;6(4):319–326.
120. Duffau H, Capelle L, Denvil D, et al. The role of dominant premotor cortex in language: a study using intraoperative functional mapping in awake patients. *Neuroimage*. 2003;20(4):1903–1914. https://doi.org/10.1016/S1053-8119(03)00203-9.
121. Sarubbo S, Tate M, De Benedictis A, et al. A normalized dataset of 1821 cortical and subcortical functional responses collected during direct electrical stimulation in patients undergoing awake brain surgery. *Data Br*. 2019;28. https://doi.org/10.1016/J.DIB.2019.104892.
122. Leclercq D, Duffau H, Delmaire C, et al. Comparison of diffusion tensor imaging tractography of language tracts and intraoperative subcortical stimulations. *J Neurosurg*. 2010;112(3):503–511. https://doi.org/10.3171/2009.8.JNS09558.
123. Maldonado IL, Moritz-Gasser S, De Champfleur NM, Bertram L, Moulinié G, Duffau H. Surgery for gliomas involving the left inferior parietal lobule: new insights into the functional anatomy provided by stimulation mapping in awake patients. *J Neurosurg*. 2011;115(4):770–779. https://doi.org/10.3171/2011.5.JNS112.
124. Miozzo M, Williams AC, McKhann GM, Hamberger MJ. Topographical gradients of semantics and phonology revealed by temporal lobe stimulation. *Hum Brain Mapp*. 2017;38(2):688–703. https://doi.org/10.1002/HBM.23409.
125. Abel TJ, Rhone XAE, Nourski KV, et al. Direct physiologic evidence of a heteromodal convergence region for proper naming in human left anterior temporal lobe. 2015; 35(4):1513–1520. https://doi.org/10.1523/JNEUROSCI.3387-14.2015.
126. Roux FE, Lubrano V, Lauwers-Cances V, Trémoulet M, Mascott CR, Démonet JF. Intra-operative mapping of cortical areas involved in reading in mono- and bilingual patients. *Brain*. 2004;127(Pt 8):1796–1810. https://doi.org/10.1093/BRAIN/AWH204.
127. Sabsevitz DS, Middlebrooks EH, Tatum W, Grewal SS, Wharen R, Ritaccio AL. Examining the function of the visual word form area with stereo EEG electrical stimulation: a case report of pure alexia. *Cortex*. 2020;129:112–118. https://doi.org/10.1016/J.CORTEX.2020.04.012.
128. Blanke O, Spinelli L, Thut G, et al. Location of the human frontal eye field as defined by electrical cortical stimulation: anatomical, functional and electrophysiological characteristics. *Neuroreport*. 2000;11(9):1907–1913. https://doi.org/10.1097/00001756-200006260-00021.
129. Halgren E, Walter RD, Cherlow DG, Crandall PH. Mental phenomena evoked by electrical stimulation of the human hippocampal formation and amygdala. *Brain*. 1978;101(1):83–115.
130. Gloor P. Experiential phenomena of temporal lobe epilepsy. Facts and hypotheses. *Brain*. 1990;113(6):1673–1694. https://doi.org/10.1093/BRAIN/113.6.1673. Pt 6.
130a. Barbeau EJ, Taylor MJ, Regis J, Marquis P, Chauvel P, Liégeois-Chauvel C. Spatio temporal dynamics of face recognition. *Cerebral Cortex*. 2008 May 1;18(5):997–1009.
131. Coello AF, Duvaux S, De Benedictis A, Matsuda R, Duffau H. Involvement of the right inferior longitudinal fascicle in visual hemiagnosia: a brain stimulation mapping study. *J Neurosurg*. 2013;118(1):202–205. https://doi.org/10.3171/2012.10.JNS12527.
132. Bush D, Bisby JA, Bird CM, et al. Human hippocampal theta power indicates movement onset and distance travelled. *Proc Natl Acad Sci U S A*. 2017;114(46):12297–12302. https://doi.org/10.1073/PNAS.1708716114.
133. Maidenbaum S, Miller J, Stein JM, Jacobs J. Grid-like hexadirectional modulation of human entorhinal theta oscillations. *Proc Natl Acad Sci U S A*. 2018;115(42):10798–10803. https://doi.org/10.1073/PNAS.1805007115.
134. Duffau H, Denvil D, Lopes M, et al. Intraoperative mapping of the cortical areas involved in multiplication and subtraction: an electrostimulation study in a patient with a left parietal glioma. *J Neurol Neurosurg Psychiatry*. 2002;73(6):733–738.
135. Yu X, Chen C, Pu S, et al. Dissociation of subtraction and multiplication in the right parietal cortex: evidence from intraoperative cortical electrostimulation. *Neuropsychologia*. 2011;49(10):2889–2895.
136. Haglund MM, Ojemann GA, Schwartz TW, Lettich E. Neuronal activity in human lateral temporal cortex during serial retrieval from short-term memory. *J Neurosci*. 1994;14(3):1507–1515.
137. Ojemann GA, Creutzfeldt O, Lettich E, Haglund MM. Neuronal activity in human lateral temporal cortex related to short-term verbal memory, naming and reading. *Brain*. 1988;111(6):1383–1403.

## FURTHER READING

1. Sporns O. Contributions and challenges for network models in cognitive neuroscience. *Nat Neurosci*. 2014:May; 17(5):652–660. https://doi.org/10.1038/nn.3690.
2. Rasmussen T, Penfield W. The human sensorimotor cortex as studied by electrical stimulation. *Fed Proc*. 1947;6(1):84.

CHAPTER 11

# The Utility of Stereoelectroencephalography in Lesional Epilepsy

AMMAR KHEDER, MD

## INTRODUCTION

Epilepsy surgery stands as a transformative therapeutic avenue for patients grappling with drug-resistant epilepsy (DRE). The evolution of neuroimaging has heralded a new era in epilepsy surgery, witnessing a notable surge in surgical procedures performed. However, despite this growth, significant enhancements in surgical outcomes have yet to be realized.

Epilepsy surgery started as an acute procedure performed in the operating room with the guidance of the electrocorticography (ECoG). Subsequently, a phase of extraoperative monitoring was implemented thanks to improvements in technology.

Currently, there are two methods for extraoperative recording:

1. Stereoelectroencephalography (SEEG) which was practiced mainly in Europe but has recently become increasingly popular across the globe. SEEG is carried out under the auspice of an anatomo-electro-clinical (AEC) hypothesis driven by the presurgical data. SEEG aims to define the epileptogenic zone and its relation to cortical functions in sampled areas. It guides the therapeutic options, be it resection, ablation or neuromodulation.
2. Subdural grids (SDG) with or without depth electrodes, which was practiced mainly in North America. SDG investigates the cortical surface in a two-dimensional manner.

Both approaches are guided by hypotheses and share the common goal of achieving seizure freedom with minimal or no functional deficit. This objective is typically achieved through either complete resection or disconnection of the epileptogenic zone. However, the two methods diverge in their conceptual approach to defining the epileptogenic zone.

The pioneers of SEEG, Bancaud and Talairach, defined the epileptogenic zone as the "site of the beginning and of the primary organization of the epileptic ictal discharge[1]." Understanding this organization is crucial for interpreting seizure semiology. In essence, SEEG studies the epileptogenic "network," the spatiotemporal dynamics of the epileptic discharges, and how they evolve and spread in three-dimensional fashion, leading to semiology. The spatial and temporal dynamics of the epileptic discharges and their impact on anatomical structures dictate the repertoire of signs and symptoms. These are then deconstructed, when building the AEC hypothesis to define possible anatomic origins.

In contrast, SDG views the epileptogenic zone as "focus" or "The area of cortex that is necessary and sufficient for initiating seizures and whose removal (or disconnection) is necessary for complete abolition of seizures."[2] This is rather a surgical and post hoc definition of "what to remove area." As such, the identification of an epileptogenic lesion or "focus" on imaging became a necessity in the North American school, whereas the advent of neuroimaging did not change the principles of SEEG.

The epileptogenic zone concept is somewhat hypothetical because it cannot be precisely delineated, despite the utility of various methods and interictal data. Achieving high localization accuracy depends on meticulous interpretation of anatomic, clinical, functional, and electrophysiological data. Electrophysiological parameters provide insights into the boundaries of the epileptogenic zone.

## THE THREE-CHANNEL PRECEPT

SEEG exploration provides a three-dimensional insight into brain circuitry, revealing that the epileptogenic

The Fundamentals of Stereoelectroencephalography. https://doi.org/10.1016/B978-0-443-10877-8.00006-1

zone extends beyond a mere lesion. SEEG compartmentalizes the epileptogenic network into three zones: lesional, interictal, and ictal. This categorization prevents biases in localization and aids in accurate interpretation. The lesional zone is characterized by permanent slow background activity, accentuated by postictal slowing. Its spatial dimension is compared with imaging parameters. The irritative zone comprises sites of abnormal interictal paroxysmal activities that spread within cortico-cortical networks. The accuracy of irritative zone as a marker for epileptogenic zone localization is debated due to its complex waveforms and spread. The Epileptogenic Zone represents the primary organization of ictal discharge. It exhibits reproducible frequency spectra and interareal synchronization during seizures, triggered as a whole by stimulation.[3] SEEG precision in Epileptogenic Zone localization ensures optimal electrode placement and identifies multiple epileptogenic zones if conditions are not met. In contrast to the seizure onset zone in other methods, the operational definition of the epileptogenic zone considers early propagation involving the "early spread network," which correlates closely with the semiology.

## THE PREDICAMENT OF LOCALIZATION

In some published series, it has been observed that the presence of a lesion may improve surgical outcomes, but it does not necessarily enhance the localization of the epileptogenic zone.[4,5]

Nevertheless, it will influence the formulation of the presurgical hypothesis. In one study led by Chauvel et al.,[6] the investigators studied the experience of using SEEG in presurgical evaluation in two groups: those with visible lesion on magnetic resonance imaging (MRI), and those with MRI-negative epilepsy. No significant difference in localization was found between lesional and MRI-negative groups. We have replicated those findings in an unpublished series of 27 children studied with SEEG (9 lesional, 18 MRI negative). Overall, Engel class I or II outcome was achieved in 83% and 88% of MRI negative group and lesional groups respectively, with *P*-value of .36.

The localization of the epileptogenic zone can be achieved through a process of indirect inference. This inference is based on studying the semiology, the outward expression of a seizure caused by the interplay between the spatial and temporal evolution of epileptic discharges as they propagate through anatomical structures. While the presence of a lesion identified on MRI may indicate that a specific brain structure plays a role in organizing the epileptogenic zone, the epileptogenic zone itself cannot be solely equated with the lesion.

Lesional zone in SEEG is defined by the presence of continuous or nearly continuous delta activity, along with the disappearance of normal background activity, which can serve as reliable indicators of lesional tissue, particularly in MRI-negative regions.[3]

Analyzing seizure semiology is crucial for localizing the epileptogenic zone, despite inherent limitations and gaps in understanding its generation. It forms the basis for constructing a presurgical anatomo-electro-clinical (AEC) hypothesis, integrating anatomical, electrophysiological, and clinical data. Semiology reflects the intricate interaction between epileptic discharges and cortical and subcortical structures in three-dimensional space and time. As discharges propagate from the seizure onset zone, semiology emerges. Thus, in SEEG, the aim is to sample potential areas or networks capable of producing semiology, regardless of lesion presence. However, it is impractical and unsafe to sample all involved areas, necessitating careful SEEG planning and interpretation within these limitations in mind.

There are essential considerations to take into account when analyzing semiology:

1. The type of the cortex being invaded by the epileptic discharges: the expression of elementary signs or symptoms is related to the activation of primary cortices. However, as the discharges spread to association and multimodal cortices, the manifestations become more elaborate and complex. Equally, the presence of complex behavior at the outset of seizure onset may indicate early involvement of polymodal areas. Emotional and autonomic features may point to contributions from the limbic cortex.
2. The frequency of the discharges: fast discharges in the gamma range typically deactivate normal function, while slow frequency discharges in the theta discharge can mimic physiologic function.[7] For example, low frequency discharges in delta and theta range in the motor area lead to clonic activity, whereas higher frequency in the gamma range can lead to tonic or negative motor phenomenon.
3. Some semiological features can be generated by the synchronization or the desynchronization between anatomically or functionally interconnected structures. Fear, for example can be generated by stimulating the amygdala or by loss of synchrony on the orbitofrontal region.[8] Similarly, ictal humming is generated by increased coherence between the superior temporal gyrus and the inferior frontal gyrus.[9]

Semiologic localization requires sound knowledge of cerebral anatomy and connectivity. Decisions on implantation targets are driven by how functionally or anatomically interconnected regions are assumed to participate in the organization of the epileptic network, and the current understanding of cortical organization, in terms of architecture and connections.

Put simply, cortical zones can be divided into limbic, paralimbic, heteromodal, unimodal and primary areas. Extensive connectivity is typically present between structures within the same zone, and between adjacent zones. Cortical connections can be traced to the concept of dual origin of cortex from two primordial moieties, archicortical (hippocampus) and paleocortical (olfactory cortex), leading to a progressive architectonic trend from periallocortex to proisocortex to isocortex and culminating in pre- and post-Rolandic sensorimotor and association areas.[10] Feedforward connections begin in primary sensory cortices and sequentially terminate in the limbic areas. Conversely, feedback connections are generated from limbic cortices to primary sensory cortices. Inputs and outputs are processed in a serial and parallel fashion in dorsal and ventral streams.

In practical terms, even if a lesion is detected on MRI, an SEEG exploration may still be necessary, depending on its location and the seizure semiology. For example, if the lesion impacts a paralimbic structure like the posterior orbitofrontal area, it might be advisable to explore neighboring paralimbic structures such as the insula, temporal pole, cingulate gyrus, and parahippocampal gyrus during SEEG evaluation. This expanded assessment accounts for the interconnectedness within the paralimbic network, which could influence the epileptogenic zone, regardless of the lesion's location.

Likewise, if a lesion is identified in the posterior fusiform gyrus and the seizure symptoms suggest an early versive head turn, SEEG investigation should encompass both the dorsal and ventral visual streams, with potential sampling of mesial temporal structures. This comprehensive approach is crucial because seizures may engage not only the visual cortex where the lesion is situated in the ventral stream, but also connected regions responsible for visual processing and motor responses in the dorsal stream.

## SEEG IN EPILEPSIES WITH VISIBLE LESION ON IMAGING

A lesion should be considered in relation to the epileptogenic network and other presurgical data.

Lesions do not always indicate where the seizures come from. Indeed, the lesion and the epileptogenic zone do not often overlap. In one study,[11] only one third of patients with focal cortical dysplasia or neurodevelopmental tumor had focal epileptogenic zone, while the other two thirds had a more distributed organization of the epileptogenic network. Thus, as discussed earlier, SEEG should be considered if sufficient localization cannot be accomplished with available presurgical data, regardless of the presence of lesion.

SEEG have been traditionally indicated in MRI negative epilepsy, but there are many other circumstances where it should be considered, even if there is a visible lesion. These are supplemented by a clinical examples in the figures below:

1. The electroclinical data do not correlate with the imaging abnormality. (Fig. 11.1)
2. Bilateral lesions on MRI but the AEC points to a localized epileptogenic network. (Fig. 11.2)
3. The discrepancy between the extent of the epileptogenic network and the size of imaging abnormality. This is the case when the imaging abnormality is relatively small (such as in basal temporal encephalocele) where the epileptogenic network is typically organized around the mesiobasal temporal region. Conversely, only a part of a large lesion (such as in hemispheric polymicrogyria) may contribute to the epileptogenic network. (Fig. 11.3)
4. Temporoperisylvian (or temporal plus) epilepsies, even in the presence of mesial temporal sclerosis. A 16 year old was referred for presurgical evaluation due to ongoing habitual seizures following an anterior temporal lobectomy (ATL) in the setting of mesial temporal sclerosis (MTS). The patient had discrete aura of auditory hallucinations. Exploration with SEEG revealed seizure onset was in the supramarginal gyrus, which was resected and the patient became seizure free (follow up 36 months)
5. Dual pathology such as cortical dysplasia with MTS. The same can be true in the presence of temporal neocortical lesion if there is a concern for a wider epileptogenic network involving mesial temporal structures.
6. The imaging abnormality is not known to generate epileptic electrographic activity such as encephalomalacia or posttraumatic lesions.
7. Surgical failure should prompt a consideration of SEEG exploration rather than extension of prior resection or around prior lesion.
8. Bilateral epilepsy such as bitemporal epilepsy, which can occur even in the presence of unilateral MTS
9. The study of the intrinsic epileptogenicity of certain lesions such as PVNH, polymicrogyria and hypothalamic hamartomas. Nonetheless, studying these deep structures requires a "cortical hypothesis".

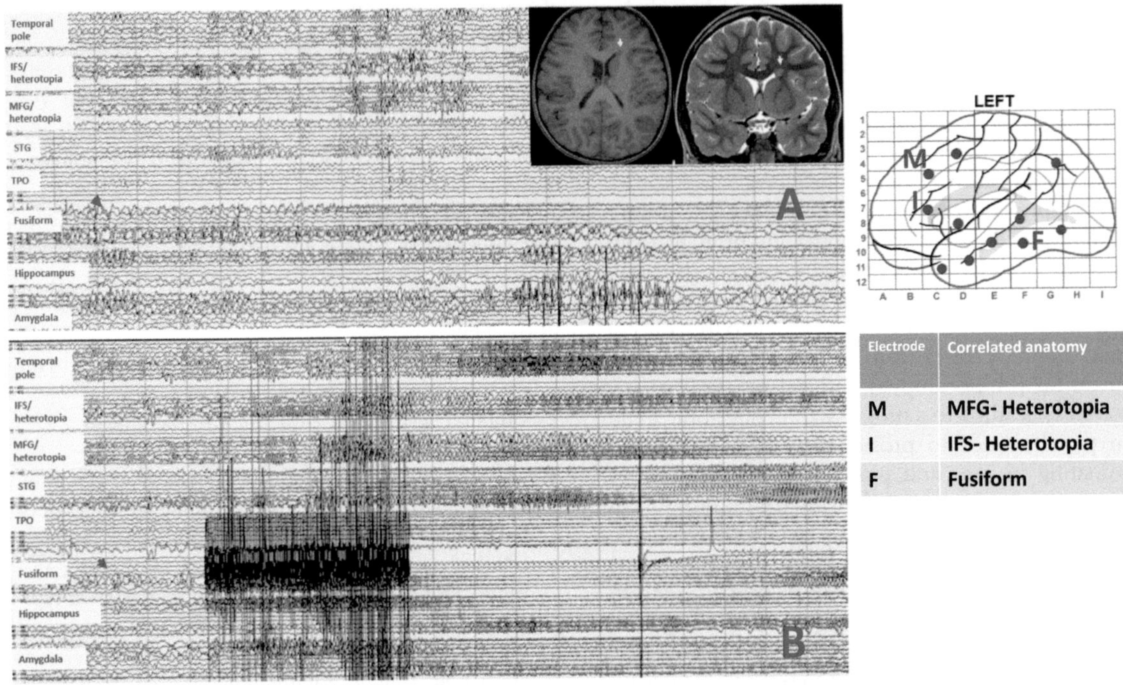


| Electrode | Correlated anatomy |
|---|---|
| **M** | **MFG- Heterotopia** |
| **I** | **IFS- Heterotopia** |
| **F** | **Fusiform** |

FIG. 11.1 A 12-year-old male presented with refractory epilepsy characterized by behavioral arrest, loss of awareness, oral and left hand automatism, and naming difficulties. EEG indicated *left* temporal seizure onset. Concurrently, *left* frontal periventricular heterotopia (PVNH) was observed on MRI (as shown by the *yellow arrow* in (A)). The presence of PVNH in the *left* frontal region was considered an incidental finding unrelated to the patient's epilepsy. The working hypothesis encompassed basal temporal involvement due to naming deficits, along with potential involvement of the temporal pole. SEEG implantation also targeted the PVNH and the inferior frontal gyrus (IFG). Seizure onset was identified on SEEG within the fusiform gyrus (highlighted by the *red arrowhead* in (A)). Cortical stimulation of the fusiform gyrus (depicted in (B)) successfully elicited habitual electroclinical seizures. Following resection of the fusiform gyrus, the patient attained seizure freedom, as evidenced by a 24-month follow-up showing an Engel class I outcome, with no observed functional deficits on neuropsychological evaluation. *IFS*, Inferior frontal sulcus, *MFG*, Middle frontal gyrus, *STG*, Superior temporal gyrus, *TPO*, Temporo-parieto-occipital junction.

## THE PROBLEM WITH "LESION-BASED" EPILEPSY SURGERY

A review of literature suggests that patients who have an identifiable lesion by imaging or/and positive histopathology have a better surgical outcome.[12] It indicated that overall the odds of being seizure-free after surgery were 2.5 times higher in patients with lesions on MRI or histopathology. Not all resections were "lesionectomies" so an explanation could be that an accurate localization can be made easier if presurgical investigation is oriented by an MRI image. On the other hand, it is an argument against "lesion based" epilepsy surgery as many of those who became seizure free needed more tissue to be removed than the lesion itself. There is a need to question the relation of a lesion to a focal epilepsy in general, but to underline that the complexity of their anatomical relation within the epileptogenic zone has certainly been underestimated.

Lesions can be found in about 30% of intractable temporal lobe epilepsy, for example. However, not all lesions detected on MRI are epileptogenic. This has been illustrated in cases of tuberous sclerosis, periventricular nodular heterotopia, and polymicrogyria amongst others.[13–16] Even surgery of likely epileptogenic lesions such as focal cortical dysplasias, when based on imaging only, has heterogeneous and average published outcomes.[17]

In understanding why a lesion identified on MRI might not always be the root cause of epilepsy, several key factors come into play. Firstly, there is the concept

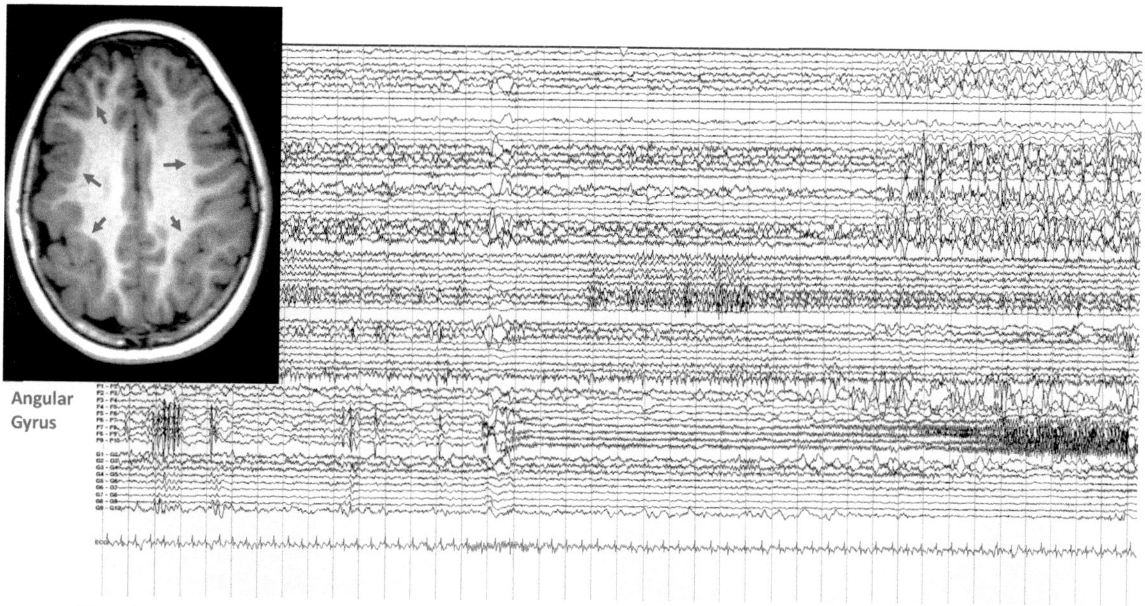


FIG. 11.2 A 16-year-old patient diagnosed with bilateral polymicrogyria (PMG, *red arrows*), impacting the perisylvian region with extensive involvement of the *right* hemisphere, spanning across the temporal, frontal, and parietal cortices, presented with intractable epilepsy marked by numerous daily seizures. The semiology included recurrent episodes of dizziness and vertigo, followed by behavioral arrest, oral and manual automatism, gutteral sounds, and head turning to the *left*. The electroencephalogram (EEG) indicated seizure onset originating from the posterior cortex. SEEG implantation aimed to sampling the bilateral posterior perisylvian cortex, along with the parietal and occipitotemporal regions. Upon SEEG exploration, early organization of the epileptogenic zone was identified within the right angular gyrus. This activity spread early to the right posterior cingulate and right precuneus, then spread to the contralateral hemisphere. These findings align with the clinical suspicion of right posterior cortex epilepsy. Additionally, independent electrographic-only seizures were observed originating from the *left* supramarginal gyrus, without corresponding clinical manifestations. Surgical intervention entailed resection of the angular gyrus. Postoperative assessment revealed no discernible functional deficits, with the patient achieving an Engel class I outcome during the 14-month follow-up period.

of underlying pathology. Some lesions, like those found in conditions such as tuberous sclerosis or periventricular nodular heterotopia, represent developmental abnormalities. Despite their presence, they may not disrupt the brain's normal electrical activity enough to trigger seizures. Additionally, the location of the lesion is crucial. Lesions situated in areas of the brain that are not critical for normal function might not lead to seizures. Furthermore, the state of connectivity matters. An example of a brain lesion that may not cause seizures is a small lacunar infarct. The size and location of the lacunar infarct are crucial factors in determining whether seizures occur. While lacunar infarcts can cause neurological symptoms such as weakness, sensory deficits, or cognitive changes, seizures are not a prominent feature in most cases.

The question then becomes what is a "lesionectomy"? In epilepsy surgery, a "lesion" does not have a simple definition. This is an MRI anomaly. What is the mental representation of such image that generates a rationale leading to a cortical resection susceptible to get to seizure freedom or good outcome in a patient with refractory epilepsy? Is understanding the real (not theoretical) relations between an image and patient's epilepsy quite unnecessary? Is the theoretical model of a "lesion-containing-epilepsy" or of a lesion surrounded by an irritative focus really a sound base for epilepsy surgery? Why a role of brain plasticity in a chronic epilepsy should be denied?

These questions are rather complex. Defining the spatial extent of a lesion by imaging is insufficient to understand its relation to the epileptogenic network

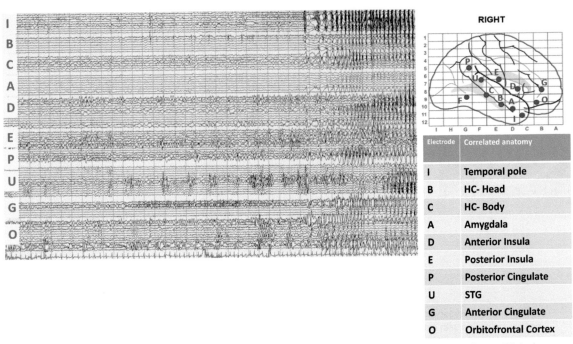

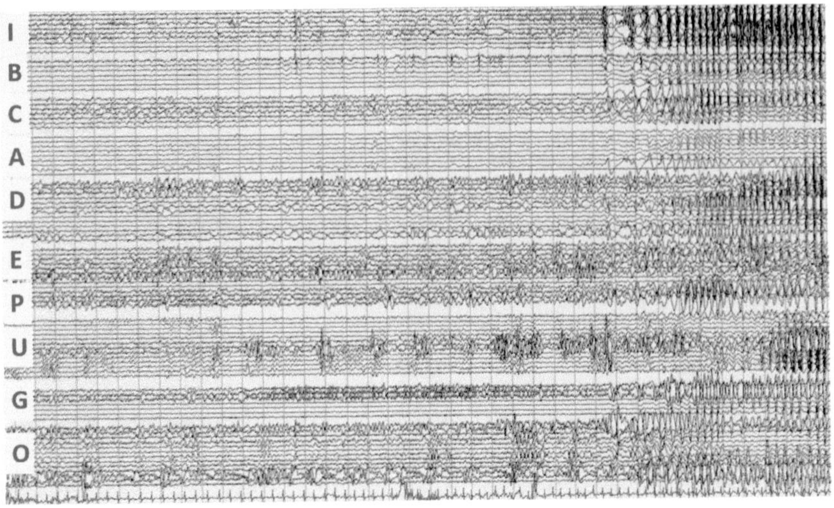


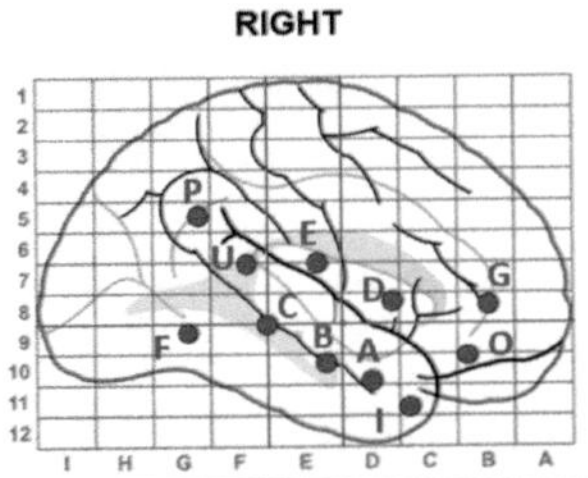


| Electrode | Correlated anatomy |
|---|---|
| **I** | **Temporal pole** |
| **B** | **HC- Head** |
| **C** | **HC- Body** |
| **A** | **Amygdala** |
| **D** | **Anterior Insula** |
| **E** | **Posterior Insula** |
| **P** | **Posterior Cingulate** |
| **U** | **STG** |
| **G** | **Anterior Cingulate** |
| **O** | **Orbitofrontal Cortex** |

FIG. 11.3 A 10-year-old female, with a history of viral encephalitis, presented with refractory epilepsy. Clinical observations during seizures revealed distinctive behaviors, including the patient grasping her ears while vocalizing "it is coming," followed by a sudden scream, behavioral cessation, and subsequent unresponsiveness. EEG findings indicated seizure onset in the right anterior temporal lobe. Magnetic resonance imaging revealed FLAIR changes dispersed throughout the right temporal lobe. In this case, the primary hypothesis centered around the temporoperisylvian region, largely due to the constellation of semiological features observed in the patient, including auditory aura, feelings of fear, vocalization, and stereotyped behavior, all culminating in behavioral arrest. The vocalization aspect of the semiology suggested the potential involvement of key brain regions such as the anterior cingulate cortex (ACC), Supplementary motor area (SMA), and opercular region. However, upon closer examination, it was determined that the observed features were not robust enough to warrant implantation in the SMA region, or wider implantation in the frontal lobe. Given the presence of stereotyped behavior coupled with emotional disturbances, the decision was made to sample mesial temporal structures, orbitofrontal, and anterior cingulate cortex. The auditory aura suggests involvement of the auditory cortex in the superior temporal plane. However, it has also been documented in cases of anterior cingulate epilepsy, likely due to the established connections between the auditory cortex and the mesial frontal region. SEEG exploration, targeting the right perisylvian region alongside the anterior cingulate cortex, unveiled the epileptogenic zone's localization within the right anterior cingulate gyrus. Surgical intervention entailed resection of the right anterior cingulate cortex. Following the procedure, the patient experienced seizure freedom, demonstrated by the absence of seizures throughout the 34-month follow-up period. The surgical pathology was consistent with gliosis. *HC*, Hippocampus, *STG*, Superior temporal gyrus.

producing patient's seizures. Indeed, if lesionectomy was sufficient to cure epilepsy, why do many patients with "lesional epilepsy" continue to have seizures following surgery? There is no single structural, functional or electrographic test that can reliably identify the full extent of all abnormal brain areas involved in a given epilepsy. However, SEEG offers an excellent tool to understand the electroclinical correlation with other data and outline the extent of the epileptogenic network.

Outcomes from the studies of hippocampal sclerosis, focal cortical dysplasia and cavernous malformation have illustrated repeatedly that a limited number of patients become seizure-free following "lesionectomy". The success rate appears to be strongly linked to the underlying etiology or the specific histopathological subtype of the lesion.

In mesial temporal lobe epilepsy with hippocampal sclerosis (MTLE-HS), removing the atrophic medial temporal structures (as done in selective amygdalohippocampectomy (SAH)) has less favorable seizure outcome compared to anterior temporal lobectomy.[18] However, patients who underwent SAH had better neuropsychological outcomes.[19] No single surgical intervention has been proven to be standard of care on MTLE-HS; indeed, an ILAE workshop on MTLE-HS concluded that it denotes several different syndromes.[20] So why does ATL provide better seizure freedom rate than amygdalohippocampectomy in hippocampal sclerosis? This further reinforces the need for careful anatomo-electro-clinical correlation to better understand the epileptogenic network and define the margins of surgical resection. In those who fail temporal lobectomy, the epileptogenic network extends beyond the temporal lobe such as in temporal-frontal or temporo-perisylvian epilepsy.[21] In a published multicenter study on outcomes in mesial temporal lobe epilepsy treated with laser ablation, only 58% of patients achieved seizure freedom. The presence of hippocampal sclerosis did not affect the outcome.[22]

The epileptogenic zone in patients with focal cortical dysplasia (FCD) is better described as an epileptogenic network with possible multilobar organization rather than "focal epilepsy".[11,23] Similarly, epileptogenic network organization in cavernomas is complex and obviously extends beyond the lesion. One study demonstrated that the removal of the hemosiderin ring and surrounding scar is frequently necessary to result in seizure freedom.[24] However, these findings are debatable and should be confirmed in a larger series, particularly in cases when there is a suspicion for a larger epileptogenic network. An SEEG study showed that the relationship between cavernomas and epileptogenic zone is rather complex.[25]

The lack of correlation between the lesion and epileptogenic zone network has also been demonstrated in hypothalamic hamartomas.[26]

## CONSIDERATION IN SEEG PLANNING IN LESIONAL EPILEPSY

Planning SEEG in lesional epilepsy relies on the same principle of a sound AEC hypothesis. The principles remain the same formulating a hypothesis. The following questions should be asked.

- Where is the seizure being generated?
- What are the possible spatiotemporal dynamics of the ictal spread in relation to clinical features? Which is essentially a three dimensional assessment of the epileptogenic network.

Formulating the wrong hypotheses will lead to inadequate sampling, erroneous interpretation and ultimately poor surgical outcome.

Several additional factors should be considered in the presence of a lesion:

1. The presence of a lesion may indicate that it is partially or wholly involved in the organization of the epileptogenic network. Therefore, sampling the lesion or part of a large lesion should be undertaken in alignment with AEC data.
2. The type of lesion can dictate what needs to be sampled. For example, in cavernomas, the perilesional tissue is sampled.
3. The anatomic location of the lesion, as discussed earlier: e.g., a neocortical temporal cortical dysplasia may necessitate sampling of the nearby paralimbic structures.
4. What surgical intervention will likely to take place based on the AEC hypothesis and how can SEEG guide the treatment, by defining resection margins or potential neuromodulatory targets
5. The aforementioned anatomic and connectivity considerations.

## ARE SEEG EXPLORATIONS REQUIRED IN EVERY LESIONAL EPILEPSY?

Lesions are heterogeneous entities. The type of the lesion, the location and possible etiology can help determine if SEEG investigation is needed. Understanding the histopathological correlations of the epileptogenic zone is crucial. Each etiology presents distinct histopathological features that influence the localization and characterization of the epileptogenic zone. For instance, post-TBI epilepsy differs from post-encephalitic epilepsy in terms of underlying brain changes and epileptogenic mechanisms. Similarly, within the spectrum of MCD-related epilepsies, focal cortical dysplasias exhibit diverse histological patterns, which distinguish them from other malformations like periventricular nodular heterotopia or polymicrogyria. Additionally, tuberous sclerosis represents another distinct entity with its unique histopathological characteristics. Recognizing these histopathological differences is essential for guiding clinicians in tailoring treatment strategies based on the specific underlying pathology.

The SEEG method is grounded in the sound principles of AEC hypothesis, and in certain circumstances, the lesion should be viewed from the perspective of the natural history of the epilepsy or epilepsy syndrome. For example, MTS can be a result of recurrent seizures in patients with SCN1A related epilepsies. The study of bilateral MTS in these entities will probably yield very little localization or therapeutic value.

## SUMMARY

The principles of the SEEG method remain the same regardless of the presence (or therefore lack) of a lesion on imaging. The type and location of a lesion may provide further input into potential exploration targets as defined by the AEC hypothesis supported by all the available data and may further influence surgical strategy.

The correlation between a lesion and the epileptogenic zone can be classified into three categories: 1- the lesion is not involved; 2- part of the lesion is involved in a complex epileptogenic network; 3- the lesion is part of a complex epileptogenic network.

In conclusion, it is crucial to recognize that the presence of a lesion does not necessarily equate to epilepsy, and conversely, epilepsy can arise from a range of causes beyond lesions alone. In the contemporary landscape of neuroimaging, the significance of semiology and clinical data is often overshadowed, yet they play a critical role in accurately diagnosing and managing epilepsy.

## ACKNOWLEDGMENTS

The author would like to extend sincere thanks to Professor Chauvel and Professor McGonigal for their insightful comments, and invaluable guidance.

## REFERENCES

1. Talairach J, Bancaud J. Stereotaxic approach to epilepsy. Methodology of anatomo- functional stereotaxic investigations. *Progr Neurol Surg*. 1973;5:297–354.
2. Awad IA, Rosenfeld J, Ahl J, Hahn JF, Lüders H. Intractable epilepsy and structural lesions of the brain: mapping, resection strategies, and seizure outcome. *Epilepsia*. 1991; 32(2):179–186.
3. Chauvel P, Gonzalez-Martinez J, Bulacio J. Presurgical intracranial investigations in epilepsy surgery. *Handb Clin Neurol*. 2019;161:45–71. https://doi.org/10.1016/B978-0-444-64142-7.
4. Vakharia VN, Duncan JS, Witt JA, Elger CE, Staba R, Engel Jr J. Getting the best outcomes from epilepsy surgery. *Ann Neurol*. 2018;83(4):676–690. https://doi.org/10.1002/ana.25205.
5. Schmitt FC, Meencke H. Factors predicting 10-year seizure freedom after temporal lobe resection. *Z für Epileptol*. 2020; 33:50–61.
6. McGonigal A, Bartolomei F, Régis J, et al. Stereoelectroencephalography in presurgical assessment of MRI-negative epilepsy. *Brain*. 2007;130(Pt 12):3169–3183.
7. Chauvel P, McGonigal A. Emergence of semiology in epileptic seizures. *Epilepsy Behav*. 2014;38:94–103.
8. Bartolomei F, Trébuchon A, Gavaret M, Régis J, Wendling F, Chauvel P. Acute alteration of emotional behaviour in epileptic seizures is related to transient desynchrony in emotion-regulation networks. *Clin Neurophysiol*. 2005;116(10):2473–2479.
9. Bartolomei F, Wendling F, Vignal JP, Chauvel P, Liégeois-Chauvel C. Neural networks underlying epileptic humming. *Epilepsia*. 2002;43(9):1001–1012.
10. Yeterian EH, Pandya DN, Tomaiuolo F, Petrides M. The cortical connectivity of the prefrontal cortex in the monkey brain. *Cortex*. 2012;48(1):58–81.
11. Aubert S, Wendling F, Regis J, et al. Local and remote epileptogenicity in focal cortical dysplasias and neurodevelopmental tumours. *Brain*. 2009;132:3072–3086.
12. Téllez-Zenteno JF, Ronquillo LH, Moien-Afshari F, Wiebe S. Surgical outcomes in lesional and non-lesional epilepsy: a systematic review and meta-analysis. *Epilepsy Res*. 2010;89(2–3):310–318.
13. Melikyan AG, Kozlova AB, Vlasov PA, Dorofeeva MY, Shishkina LV, Agrba SB. Epilepsy surgery in children with tuberous sclerosis. *Zh Vopr Neirokhir Im N N Burdenko*. 2023;87(2):5–16.
14. Ostrowsky-Coste K, Neal A, Guenot M, et al. Resective surgery in tuberous sclerosis complex, from Penfield to 2018: a critical review. *Rev Neurol (Paris)*. March 2019;175(3): 163–182.
15. Cossu M, Pelliccia V, Gozzo F, et al. Surgical treatment of polymicrogyria-related epilepsy. *Epilepsia*. December 2016; 57(12):2001–2010.
16. Maillard LG, Tassi L, Bartolomei F, et al. Stereoelectroencephalography and surgical outcome in polymicrogyria-related epilepsy: a multicentric study. *Ann Neurol*. November 2017;82(5):781–794.
17. Rowland NC, Englot DJ, Cage TA, Sughrue ME, Barbaro NM, Chang EF. A meta-analysis of predictors of seizure freedom in the surgical management of focal cortical dysplasia. *J Neurosurg*. May 2012;116(5):1035–1041.
18. Bate H, Eldridge P, Varma T, Wieshmann UC. The seizure outcome after amygdalohippocampectomy and temporal lobectomy. *Eur J Neurol*. 2007;14:90–94.
19. Helmstaedter C, Richter S, Roske S, Oltmanns F, Schramm J, Lehmann TN. Differential effects of temporal pole resection with amygdalohippocampectomy versus selective amygdalohippocampectomy on material-specific memory in patients with mesial temporal lobe epilepsy. *Epilepsia*. 2008;49:88–97.
20. Wieser HG. ILAE commission on neurosurgery of epilepsy. ILAE commission report. Mesial temporal lobe epilepsy with hippocampal sclerosis. *Epilepsia*. 2004;45(6):695–714.

21. Giulioni M, Martinoni M, Marucci G. Temporal plus epilepsy is a major determinant of temporal lobe surgery failures. *Brain*. 2016;139(7).
22. Wu C, Jermakowicz WJ, Chakravorti S, et al. Effects of surgical targeting in laser interstitial thermal therapy for mesial temporal lobe epilepsy: a multicenter study of 234 patients. *Epilepsia*. 2019;60(6):1171–1183.
23. Chassoux F, Devaux B, Landré E, et al. Stereoelectroencephalography in focal cortical dysplasia: a 3D approach to delineating the dysplastic cortex. *Brain*. 2000;123(Pt 8): 1733–1751.
24. Hugelshofer M, Acciarri N, Sure U, et al. Effective surgical treatment of cerebral cavernous malformations: a multicenter study of 79 pediatric patients. *J Neurosurg Pediatr*. 2011;8(5):522–525.
25. Sevy A, Gavaret M, Trebuchon A, et al. Beyond the lesion: the epileptogenic networks around cavernous angiomas. *Epilepsy Res*. 2014;108(4):701–708.
26. Scholly J, Staack AM, Kahane P, et al. Hypothalamic hamartoma: epileptogenesis beyond the lesion? *Epilepsia*. 2017;58(Suppl 2):32–40.

CHAPTER 12

# From SEEG Explorations to Surgical Interventions

GUY M. MCKHANN II, MD • JORGE ÁLVARO GONZÁLEZ-MARTÍNEZ, MD, PHD

## INTRODUCTION

The fundamental objective of SEEG is to facilitate the strategic planning and execution of surgical intervention(s) aimed at cessation of epileptic activity, translated into seizure freedom or at least seizure reduction for the patient. Potentially curative surgery includes the resection, disconnection, or ablation of cortical regions producing epileptogenic activity while ensuring the preservation of essential brain function.[1–10] The decision to undertake either resection or ablation depends upon a comprehensive analysis of SEEG findings, necessitating the collective input of a multidisciplinary cohort comprising neurologists, neurosurgeons, neuroradiologists, and neuropsychologists, united in the pursuit of optimizing patient outcomes.

This chapter will discuss the transition from the interpretive phase of SEEG to the ensuing surgical interventions, which will include resection, ablative procedures, and neuromodulation interventions when curative options are not available.

## GENERAL ASPECTS OF SEEG EXPLORATIONS RELEVANT TO THE FINAL SURGICAL INTERVENTIONS

The foundational precepts governing stereo-electroencephalography (SEEG) investigations play an indispensable role in translating diagnostic insights into efficacious surgical outcomes.[1,6,11–29] This segment details six key facets of SEEG explorations that directly impact ultimate surgical interventions. Regardless of the nature of the surgical modality employed, these six tenets form the basis of subsequent decisions and procedural maneuvers. These principles are:

1. **Deliberate Patient Selection and Scrutiny:** The inaugural principle of SEEG exploration underscores the imperative of meticulous patient selection and evaluation in contemplation of surgical intervention. This process assumes paramount importance as it precludes the engagement of SEEG methodologies in individuals unsuitable for surgical candidacy from inception. The selection criteria (requiring sufficient team expertise to determine this important step) hinge upon a comprehensive clinical assessment encompassing seizure semiology, neuroimaging correlates, and responsiveness to antiepileptic pharmacotherapy. Patients demonstrating unfavorable prognostic indicators for localizable epileptogenic zones (EZs) or evincing reluctance toward curative surgical intervention are deemed unsuitable candidates for SEEG.[30,31]
2. **Rigorous Implantation Strategizing:** The second principle of SEEG exploration revolves around the strategy of SEEG electrode implantation. In the context of resective inquiries, this strategizing necessitates delineation of the EZ localization, anatomical extent, and boundary demarcations. Parameters such as electrode placement, quantity, and orientation must duly encapsulate the suspected EZ, allied functional domains, and the anatomical continuum of prospective treatable regions to inform subsequent surgical interventions.[32,33]
The SEEG exploratory process provides multiple converging opportunities to delineate and confirm the EZ. The approach is based on sampling sets of connected brain structures (networks) rather than attempting to achieve "coverage". Direct electrical stimulation is an essential step in evaluating the EZ.
3. **Functional Elucidation:** SEEG allows interrogation of functional cerebral substrates, inclusive of eloquent cortical territories and white matter tracts, with the aim of mitigating the postoperative risk of neurological compromise. Functional exploration mandates the identification of structures

The Fundamentals of Stereoelectroencephalography. https://doi.org/10.1016/B978-0-443-10877-8.00007-3

necessitating preservation during forthcoming surgical endeavors.[16,32,34–38]

4. **Anatomical and Functional Constraints:** Knowledge of anatomical and functional constraints assumes primacy in shaping the contours of final surgical intervention. This entails the delineation of safe surgical trajectories, circumvention of eloquent cortical territories, and the surgical strategy of complete EZ resection or ablation while safeguarding essential neurological functionalities.
5. **Multidisciplinary Synergy:** SEEG inquiries and subsequent surgical undertakings necessitate good communication and teamwork among neurologists, neurosurgeons, neuroradiologists, neuropsychologists, and allied specialists. Multifaceted deliberations engender a comprehensive evaluative milieu conducive to optimized surgical planning.
6. **Ethical Deliberations:** Ethical considerations, foregrounding patient autonomy, beneficence, and nonmaleficence, are paramount in the context of SEEG investigations and ensuing surgical modalities. Prerequisites such as informed consent, deference to patient preferences, and circumspect evaluation of potential risks vis-à-vis benefits, emerge as axiomatic imperatives.[39]

In summation, the foundational tenets underpinning SEEG explorations also guide final surgical interventions for epilepsy patients. The combination of careful patient selection, implantation planning, functional elucidation, anatomical and functional constraints, multidisciplinary collaboration, and ethical probity collectively help determine surgical outcomes after SEEG-guided interventions.

## DIFFERENT TYPES OF SEEG-GUIDED INTERVENTIONS

Several surgical techniques may be deployed for cortical and subcortical interventions subsequent to SEEG evaluation:

1. **Asleep Resections/Disconnections:** This approach entails the excision (or disconnection) of epileptogenic tissue utilizing conventional microsurgical methodologies with patients under general anesthesia. The surgical execution adheres rigorously to the predefined plan, ensuring comprehensive removal/disconnection of the targeted tissue while safeguarding vital surrounding brain tissue and arteries and veins. Notably, functional assessment is largely completed during the SEEG evaluation, obviating the need for supplementary functional information to ensure the safety of the resection. However, asleep sensorimotor mapping can be used in anatomically relevant surgeries under general anesthesia as needed.[40]
2. **Awake Resections:** In instances where the resection implicates eloquent cortical territories, an awake craniotomy may be warranted. This modality enables real-time mapping of functional cerebral areas, thereby ensuring the preservation of eloquent cortex during the resection, while complementing the functional insights garnered during the extra-operative SEEG evaluation.
3. **Minimally Invasive Techniques:** In select clinical scenarios, minimally invasive modalities such as laser interstitial thermal therapy (LITT) or radiofrequency thermocoagulation (RFTC) may be employed to ablate epileptogenic foci. These techniques confer the advantage of minimal collateral damage to surrounding brain parenchyma coupled with expedited patient recovery.[9,19,23,24,41]
4. **SEEG-Guided Neuromodulation:** When curative resections are precluded either due to inadequate localization or the inherent risk of neurological sequelae, neuro-modulatory interventions emerge as a palliative recourse. In certain contexts, SEEG data may inform the deployment of neuromodulation modalities such as deep brain stimulation (DBS) or responsive neurostimulation (RNS) although how best to choose DBS target and protocol at the individual patient level remains an area of active clinical research.[42–51] In bilateral mesial temporal epilepsy, bilateral amygdalo-hippocampal depth electrode placement tethered to either an open-loop (DBS) or closed-loop (RNS) configuration may be contemplated. RNS is the preferred modality in the United States, as DBS of bilateral hippocampi is not FDA approved; while hippocampal DBS is preferred in many other parts of the world, where RNS is not yet an option. Of course, we recognize that some world regions do not have any access to intracranial DBS after SEEG. In cases where the EZ spans beyond the mesial temporal compartment, involving adjacent neocortical territories bilaterally, the indications and outcomes of SEEG-guided neuromodulation are less well known and more research is needed.

## DETERMINANT FACTORS RELATED TO SEEG-GUIDED INTERVENTION STRATEGIES SELECTION

SEEG-guided interventions are adapted to individual patients, contingent upon the comprehensive outcomes and interpretations derived from that patient's evaluation. Enumerated below are delineations concerning the determinants governing the judicious selection of SEEG-guided procedures:

1. **Location and Volume of the Epileptogenic Zone (EZ):** In neocortical epilepsies, the treatment modality post-SEEG evaluation is markedly influenced by the dimensions and morphological complexities of the EZ. Robustly sized EZs ($>2\ cm^3$) or those evincing intricate contours typically necessitate direct resection or disconnection, affording superior outcomes vis-à-vis minimally invasive modalities such as laser interstitial thermal therapy (LITT). Microsurgical interventions proffer heightened precision in anatomical resections, particularly advantageous for extensive EZs, which may pose geometrical challenges for laser-based therapies. Conversely, in instances where the EZ is restricted to deep-seated cortical locations with smaller volume, SEEG-guided LITT is a minimally invasive promising alternative to open surgery.[1,52,53]
   In neocortical epilepsy, LITT may be particularly beneficial for patients harboring deep-seated, focal, and compact EZs, such as the insular-opercular, mid to posterior cingulate, and mesial temporal regions. In the insula, particularly the posterior superior part, open surgical resection carries the risk of stroke of one of the small deep perforating arteries off the middle cerebral artery M3 branches located within the insular sulci. A very small infarction in the corona radiata in this region can result in a clinically significant patient deficit. Use of LITT to ablate insular opercular epilepsy is gaining traction in the epilepsy community. Existing data underscore notable rates of seizure freedom, ranging from 53% to 69%,[54–62] following resection or ablative interventions targeting insulo-opercular regions, predominantly observed in cases accompanied by associated lesions. However, specific data pertaining to seizure outcomes in nonlesional insulo-opercular epilepsy remain scant. Nonlesional pure insular epilepsies are less common. Most of these patients have a combined insulo-opercular EZ revealed by SEEG that then must be subsequently treated by resection or ablation.
   If SEEG identifies the EZ as restricted to the motor or posterior cingulate, many epilepsy centers are now using LITT. The motor cingulate requires surgical resection along the medial bank of the hemisphere, below the leg Rolandic cortex, while the posterior cingulate can be quite deep within the medial brain, below the precuneus. These areas are surgically accessible but pose some increased risk due to their specific locations and associated venous anatomy abutting the sagittal sinus. LITT is being used more as a tool to carry out corpus callosotomy, and similar strategies are being applied to the cingulate region, just above the corpus callosum.
   In scenarios where the EZ is confined to mesial temporal structures, microsurgical selective amygdalohippocampectomy is the time-tested surgical strategy, but LITT also warrants consideration. Whether to use open surgical resection, LITT, or brain stimulation to treat a mesial temporal EZ depends on several factors including cerebral dominance, MRI findings (mesial temporal sclerosis, low grade epilepsy associated tumor, MRI normal), patient neuropsychological function/risk of worsening, and surgeon experience.
2. **Proximity to Eloquent Cortex:** The adjacency between the EZ and functionally vital areas delineated by SEEG constitutes a key determinant in the selection of surgical interventions post-SEEG assessment. Instances of close spatial juxtaposition often necessitate surgical resection guided by intraoperative functional mapping, with awake procedures frequently warranted for enhanced assessment of language-associated cortical and subcortical domains. Furthermore, intraoperative neuromonitoring techniques, encompassing somatosensory evoked potentials, motor evoked responses, and direct cortical and subcortical stimulation, can help in evaluating sensory and motor function integrity. Awake patient testing during SEEG-guided LITT procedures is challenging and rarely attempted, as the patient needs to hold perfectly still within the MRI scanner during the procedure. In clinical scenarios where there is considerable overlap between the EZ and functionally important territories, invasive monitoring modalities such as responsive neurostimulation (RNS) or deep brain stimulation (DBS), should be considered as palliative interventions.
3. **Patient Expectations:** The consideration of patient expectations and aspirations assumes paramount significance in delineating the post-SEEG surgical treatment modality. While the attainment of sustained seizure freedom remains the primary objective, proximity between the EZ and functional territories may result in unacceptable risk of neurological compromise with surgical resection or ablation. In such scenarios, patients may opt for palliative modalities such as RNS or DBS (if available) to assuage seizure burden while minimizing the prospect of significant functional deficits. A

comprehensive elucidation of risks and benefits is imperative in tailoring the treatment paradigm in consonance with the individualized needs and risk tolerance of the patient.

## THE TALAIRACH SPACE AND THE TRANSLATION TO THE THREE-DIMENSIONAL SURGICAL ANATOMY

The conceptual framework of Talairach space, delineated by coordinates derived from the anterior and posterior commissures along with the midsagittal plane, has revolutionized neurosurgical precision by facilitating the precise targeting of discrete cerebral regions for therapeutic interventions. This pivotal innovation has not only heralded a paradigm shift in neurosurgical planning and execution but also constitutes a fundamental cornerstone in translating SEEG interpretations into actionable surgical strategies[63–67] (Fig. 12.1). To ensure a seamless transition, consideration of three critical aspects is imperative:

1. **Effective Communication Between Epileptologist and Neurosurgeon:** Central to this translational process is the cross-disciplinary exchange between

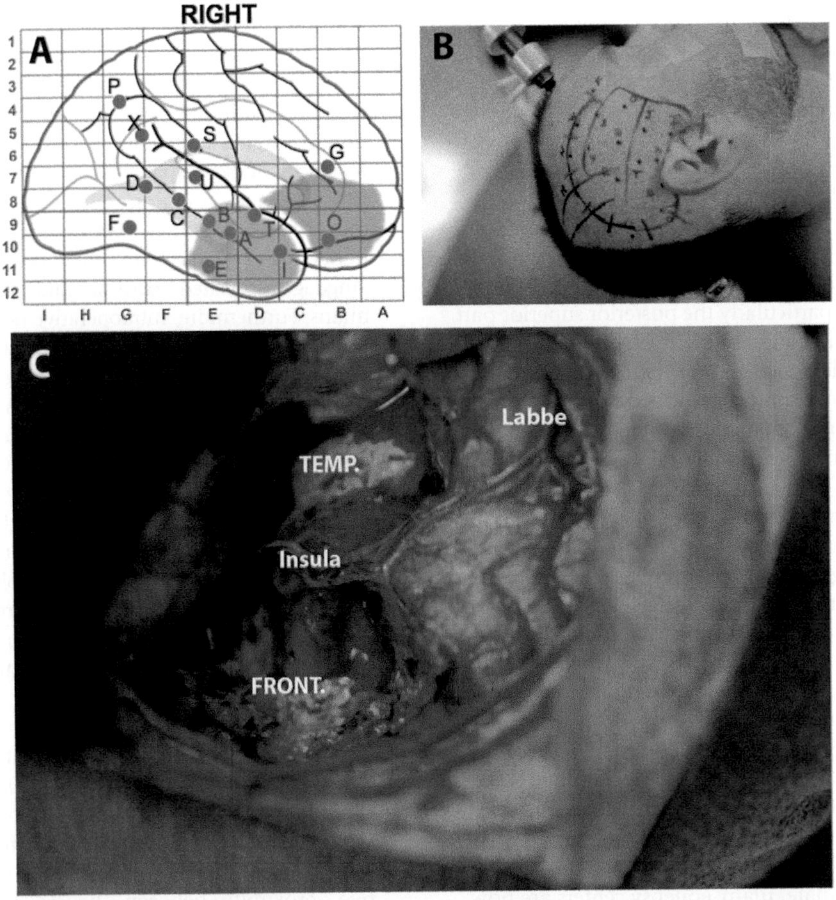


FIG. 12.1 The Talairach stereotaxic space and guided resection. Panel A depicts the SEEG electrode implantation schema, representing orthogonally placed electrodes as blue circles. The plan of resection, which is highlighted in blue, include perisylvian areas in the anterior temporal and frontal neocortex. Panel B depicts the translation of the SEEG implanted electrode entry points (demarcated by the presence of the implantation scar and by neuronavigation) into the intraoperative environment. Note the representations of the sylvian fissure and the Rolandic motor and sensory areas. Panel C demonstrated the final aspect of the resection, after the removal of the temporal and frontal areas and the preservation of the insula cortex. Note the presence of the vein of Labbe and the superficial sylvian veins, which were preserved. (With courtesy Dr. Aung.)

epileptologists and neurosurgeons, both preoperatively and intraoperatively. This collaborative dialog necessitates a comprehensive discourse encompassing the localization and volumetrics of resection, potential overlaps with functional cortical and subcortical territories, and a holistic understanding of patient expectations. The synthesis of complementary expertise spanning clinical semiology, electrophysiology, and structural and functional neuroanatomy is indispensable in formulating a precise tailored resection plan that optimizes both efficacy and safety.

2. **Cognizance of Anatomical and Functional Variables:** A nuanced understanding of anatomical and functional variables that may impede the comprehensive resection of the epileptogenic zone or necessitate procedural modifications is imperative. For instance, careful attention to vascular structures during temporal lobe resections is paramount to avoid inadvertent compromise of critical structures.
3. **Intraoperative Recognition of Electrode Positions:** Accurate localization of electrode positions relative to cortical anatomy is fundamental in ensuring the efficacy and safety of SEEG-guided procedures. Using advanced imaging modalities and computer-assisted software, neurosurgeons can construct detailed patient-specific anatomical models, enabling precise intraoperative navigation. Failure to rigorously plan electrode positions during the intraoperative phase may compromise the precision of prior localization efforts, leading to unpredictable neurological deficits and procedural failures. Following the completion and interpretation of SEEG-guided procedures, the electrodes are typically removed, necessitating a reliable method for precisely localizing the explored cortical and subcortical areas. Various intraoperative techniques for recognizing SEEG-recorded cortical regions exist, contingent upon the availability of specific imaging technologies, surgeon preferences, and the surgical site (Fig. 12.2). These methods, whether employed individually or in combination, serve to enhance localization accuracy. Here, we delineate several such approaches:
   A. **Recognition of Superficial Cortical and Vascular Anatomy:** Via fusion of pre-operative MRIs with SEEG post-operative CTs, surgeons can discern cortical regions and associated sulci patterns, facilitating intraoperative identification. This analysis enables visualization of the SEEG-recorded areas within the context of unique anatomical configurations. Additionally, recognition of cortical veins, particularly major branches, provides further localization cues, while arteries, though more subtle, may also serve as fiducial markers.
   B. **Recognition of SEEG Electrode Entry-Point Sites:** Among the most precise methods of intraoperative electrode localization is the recognition of electrode entry points in conjunction with superficial cortical and vascular anatomy. Electrode scars, unaffected by brain shifts during surgical manipulations, serve as precise markers of prior electrode positions. Through careful intraoperative comparison with cortical landmarks, these scars facilitate the identification of explored cortical areas and regions slated for treatment. This method extends beyond superficial cortical regions to encompass deep cortical territories, contingent upon electrode orientation and patient positioning.
   C. **Application of Intraoperative Neuronavigational Devices:** Neuronavigation, integrated with visualization techniques such as cortical anatomy and residual electrode markers, provides a robust method for intraoperative localization. By digitally fusing post-SEEG implanted CT images with pre-resection structural MRIs, surgeons can readily identify prior electrode placements. However, reliance solely on neuronavigation may be limited by tissue displacement during craniotomy and errors in registration, necessitating caution to mitigate potential complications.
   D. **Intraoperative Confirmation of Extraoperative Functional Mapping:** Intraoperative confirmation of extraoperative functional mapping through direct electrical stimulation offers precise validation of cortical localization and treatable areas. Despite its precision, this method is susceptible to variations in anesthesia levels, body temperature, and probe positioning. Moreover, its efficacy hinges on the combined expertise of clinical neurophysiologists and the operating surgical team and necessitates integration with complementary nonelectrophysiological methods to optimize outcomes.

## SEEG-GUIDED RESECTIONS IN SPECIFIC CLINICAL SCENARIOS

SEEG-guided resections in specific clinical scenarios represent a nuanced and tailored approach to epilepsy surgery, necessitating consideration of

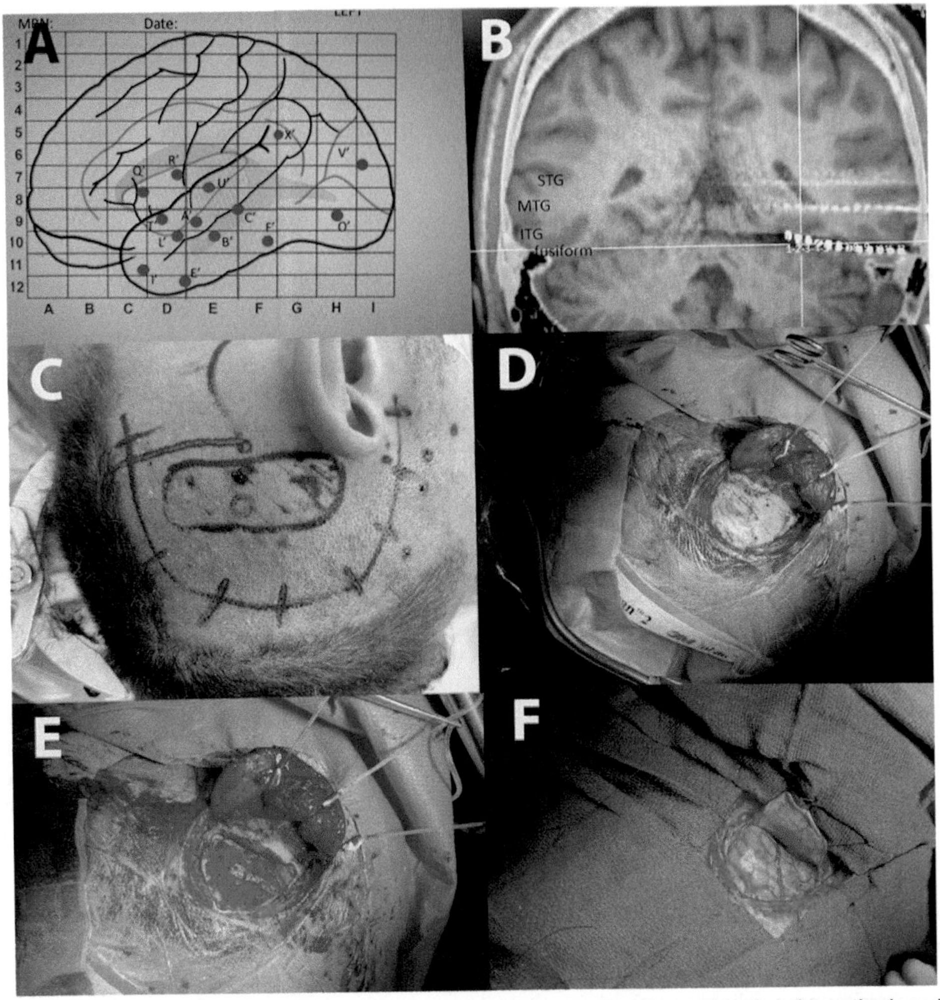


FIG. 12.2 Method of intraoperative recognition of SEEG electrodes. The figure describes the method used by the authors to recognize the anatomical position of previous SEEG electrodes in order to guide SEEG resections. Panel A depicts the SEEG implantation schema of an exploration in the dominant temporo-occipital areas. Here, the SEEG evaluation reviewed the location of a restricted EZ located at the basal surface of the temporo-occipital areas, at the vicinity of electrode F′ and O′. Panel B illustrate the position of electrode F′, with the anatomical localization of the EZ in the fusiform gyrus. Panel C illustrate the skin incision planning as well as the areas of resection based on the superficial scar markers left by the SEEG electrode orthogonal implantations. Panel D depicts the exposure of the temporo-occipital bone structures. Note the presence of the pinholes from the previous SEEG electrode implantation, demarcating the subsequent craniotomy. Panel E and F illustrate the exposure of the dura and the adjacent cortical areas related to the electrodes of interest.

patient-specific factors.[32,68–72] Below, we discuss the application of SEEG-guided resections in distinctive clinical scenarios:

The **"nonlesional"** scenario epitomizes focal epilepsy cases where noninvasive electroclinical data suggest a unifocal spatially restricted cerebral organization of seizures, but where conventional imaging fails to reveal identifiable lesions. In Fig. 12.3, we illustrate the case of a 35-year-old right-handed man afflicted with medically refractory epilepsy, marked by auditory auras progressing to language impairment and tonic-clonic seizures. SEEG exploration was pursued to validate the suspicion of left neocortical temporal lobe epilepsy, and the epileptogenic zone was shown to be intricately intertwined with primary auditory and posterior language areas.

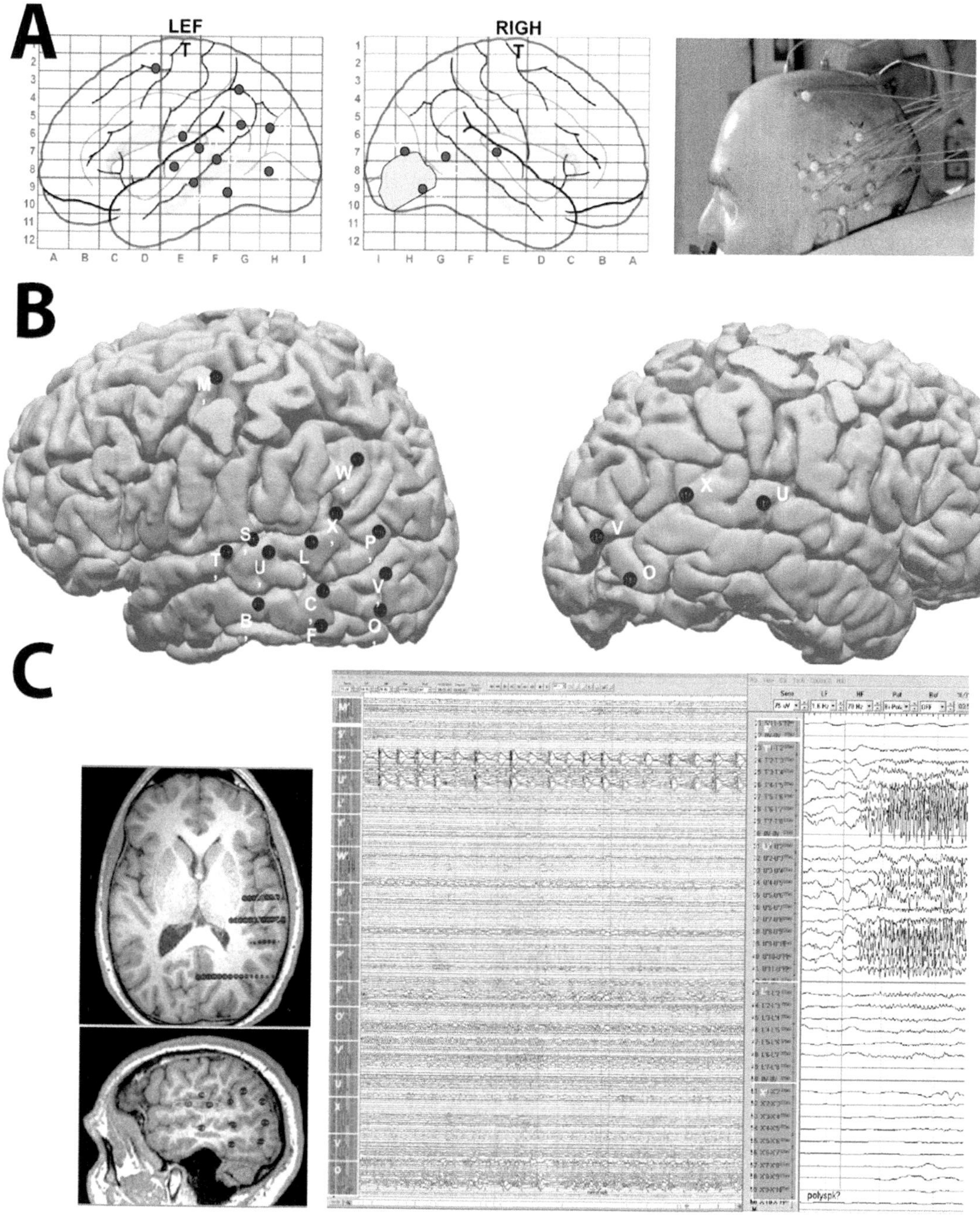


FIG. 12.3 SEEG exploration in nonlesional and dominant hemisphere scenario in young adult presenting with auditory aura followed by generalized tonic-clonic seizures. (A) Schema of implantation centered in the left posterior perisylvian and occipital parietal areas. Right panel depicts the final aspect of the implantation. (B) demonstrates cortical rendering in relation to the entry point of the orthogonally placed electrodes. (C) illustrates an interictal and ictal sample of SEEG recordings. The ictal sample onset is time locked with the emerging of the clinical semiology (not shown). The EZ is located in the planum temporale, at the vicinity of Heschl gyrus, in the dominant temporal lobe (left panel). (With courtesy of Drs Najm, Wang and Bulacio.)

In our illustrative case, SEEG ictal recordings, correlated with clinical and anatomical data, pinpointed the epileptogenic zone to the superior temporal gyrus, specifically the lateral aspects of Heschl's gyrus (contacts T′) and the planum temporale (contacts U′). Notably, electrical stimulation of these contacts elicited speech impairment, validating their significance. Guided by SEEG findings, the patient underwent a tailored SEEG-guided resection of the lateral portions of the planum temporale, augmented by intraoperative EcoG and awake speech mapping (Fig. 12.4). During surgery, mild speech difficulties were encountered during the resection of the caudal portions of the planum temporale, aligning with the pre-planned resection based on SEEG analysis.

Post-operatively, the patient experienced transient and mild language disturbances, which resolved within 2 weeks, with complete cessation of seizures. Surgical pathology revealed focal cortical dysplasia (FCD) type II, affirming the precision of the SEEG-guided resection.

This case exemplifies the successful outcome achievable in some MRI based "nonlesional" neocortical epilepsy cases. Many subtle FCD lesions can be missed by high resolution MRI scans, despite expert neuroradiology input and multidisciplinary epilepsy team review. In investigating nonlesional epilepsies, correlative analysis of semiological features with scalp EEG and anatomical characteristics are imperative. The SEEG findings in our case delineated the EZ within the superior temporal gyrus, necessitating precise delineation of resection margins. Notably, the absence of involvement of adjacent electrodes and early spread of ictal activity were helpful in defining the extent of resection.

Implantations may occasionally exhibit incomplete cortical sampling, necessitating adaptation strategies during resection planning. The application of anatomo-electro-correlations and intraoperative EcoG aids in overcoming sampling limitations, ensuring a safe and efficient resection. Additionally, intraoperative confirmation through EcoG validates resection strategies, further enhancing surgical precision. We present

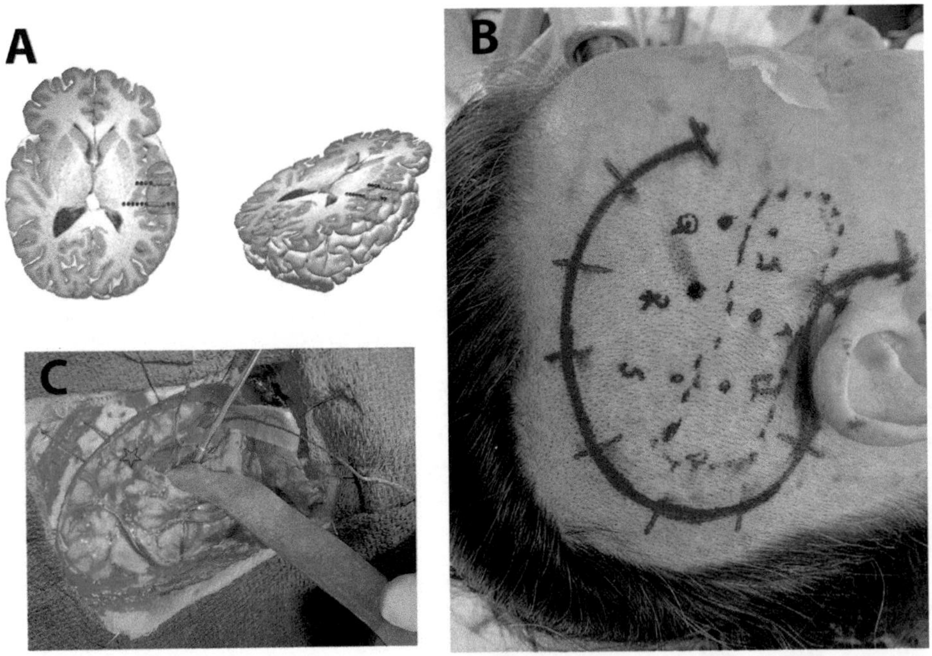


FIG. 12.4 SEEG-guided resection from the case example illustrated in figure 2. (A) Panel depicts the anatomical translation of the SEEG clinical-electrophysiological correlation to the patient's anatomy. The EZ location and extension is highlighted by the blue transparent shape, in the planum temporale, involving portions of the lateral Heschl's gyrus, center at the electrodes T′ and U'. (B) Illustration of the intraoperative aspect during the resection phase. The entry points of the previously implanted electrodes are highlighted in blue and the area of resection is outlined with doted lines. (C) Panel illustrates the intraoperative visualization of the posterior perisylvian cortex with the exposure of the planum temporale and polare. The blue star indicated the tip of Heschl's gyrus (not resected). (With courtesy of Drs Wang and Liegeois-Chauvel.)

another illustrative case in Fig. 12.5, detailing the application of SEEG-guided resections in a young patient with EZ located in the dominant basal temporo-occipital cortex, further corroborating the efficacy of SEEG-guided interventions in nonlesional clinical scenarios.

The **"lesional"** scenario in epilepsy surgery underscores the role of imaging, particularly MRI, in shaping hypotheses regarding the localization of the epileptogenic zone (EZ) and guiding subsequent investigations. The same principles of careful assessment of electroclinical data and all other noninvasive data apply, when deciding about the need or not for SEEG in a given patient's presurgical evaluation. If noninvasive investigations do not allow for sufficient clinical probability of a likely role for the lesion in EZ, and/or if questions of functional risks are present, then SEEG may be indicated in order to carry out further invasive inquiries. Termed "questions addressed to SEEG", these inquiries—distinct from the EZ hypothesis itself—orient SEEG exploration and resection strategies toward three key questions: (1) Do the anatomical boundaries of the lesion partially or fully coincide with those of the EZ? (2) Is the lesion implicated in epilepsy but is not the region of seizure onset? (3) Is the lesion perhaps even completely unrelated to the epilepsy? While the discovery of a lesion statistically correlates with operability and potential cure, this relationship may stem from a heuristic guidance for epileptologists in the absence of definitive hypotheses.

The assertion that an MRI-identifiable lesion alone is sufficient for defining a surgical strategy in patients with focal epilepsy is oversimplified and potentially perilous if applied as a general rule rather other on a case by case basis. Three primary reasons advocate against "stand-alone" MRI-guided lesionectomies: Firstly, the EZ may not invariably align with the lesion's location. Secondly, even if the EZ centers around the lesion, this information may inadequately delineate the EZ's limits and, consequently, the requisite extent of surgery. Thirdly, evidence of EZ organization around the lesion does not preclude involvement of distant cortical or subcortical structures in epilepsy. This crucial consideration is exemplified in Fig. 12.6, where SEEG exploration and subsequent resection revealed an extended EZ encompassing not only the anterior insula cortex but also portions of the orbitofrontal cortex.

To translate SEEG findings into the operative suite, a thoughtful strategy is imperative. In the illustrated case, initial exposure of the frontal and temporal cortex facilitated SEEG electrode implantation, followed by intraoperative EcoG recording. Subsequent resection of the orbitofrontal cortex, guided by SEEG conclusions, permitted clear visualization and *en bloc* resection of the anterior insula while preserving adjacent structures. Post-resection EcoG confirmed the absence of epileptiform activity, validating the efficacy of the tailored surgical approach.

Furthermore, the nature of the lesion profoundly influences SEEG-guided resection strategy. Lesion type significantly modulates the lesion's localizing power, with Type IIa and Taylor-type IIb FCD more closely associated with EZ topology compared to other lesions such as Type I FCD and chronic epilepsy associated cavernomas. Discrete abnormal gyration patterns may serve as EZ markers; however, caution is warranted to differentiate them from epileptogenic lesions and normal sulcal variations. For instance, encephaloclastic lesions like perinatal infarcts or post-traumatic lesions may not always correlate with epileptogenicity, necessitating nuanced evaluation.

In summary, the "lesional" scenario underscores the multifaceted considerations guiding SEEG-guided resections, emphasizing the critical interplay between imaging, electroclinical correlation, and surgical strategy optimization.

## REPORTS OF OUTCOME AND COMPLICATIONS IN SEEG-GUIDED RESECTIONS

Evaluating the outcomes of SEEG-guided resections entails scrutiny of diverse parameters including seizure freedom rates, postoperative neurological deficits and other complications, quality of life metrics, and long-term prognoses. The synthesis of outcome reports from various clinical studies furnishes a comprehensive panorama of SEEG-guided resections' therapeutic efficacy across diverse patient cohorts and epilepsy etiologies. These reports serve as benchmarks for comparative analysis and ultimately for development of guidelines, enabling clinicians to discern optimal treatment modalities and refine surgical strategies based on empirical evidence and clinical experience. Objective documentation and analysis of complications arising from SEEG-guided resections highlight potential procedural pitfalls, underscore safety considerations, and inform risk mitigation strategies.

The assessment of outcomes and complications associated with SEEG-guided resections presents a complex yet indispensable facet of contemporary epilepsy surgery. However, it is imperative to approach these reports with discernment, recognizing their role as general reference points rather than absolute determinants for

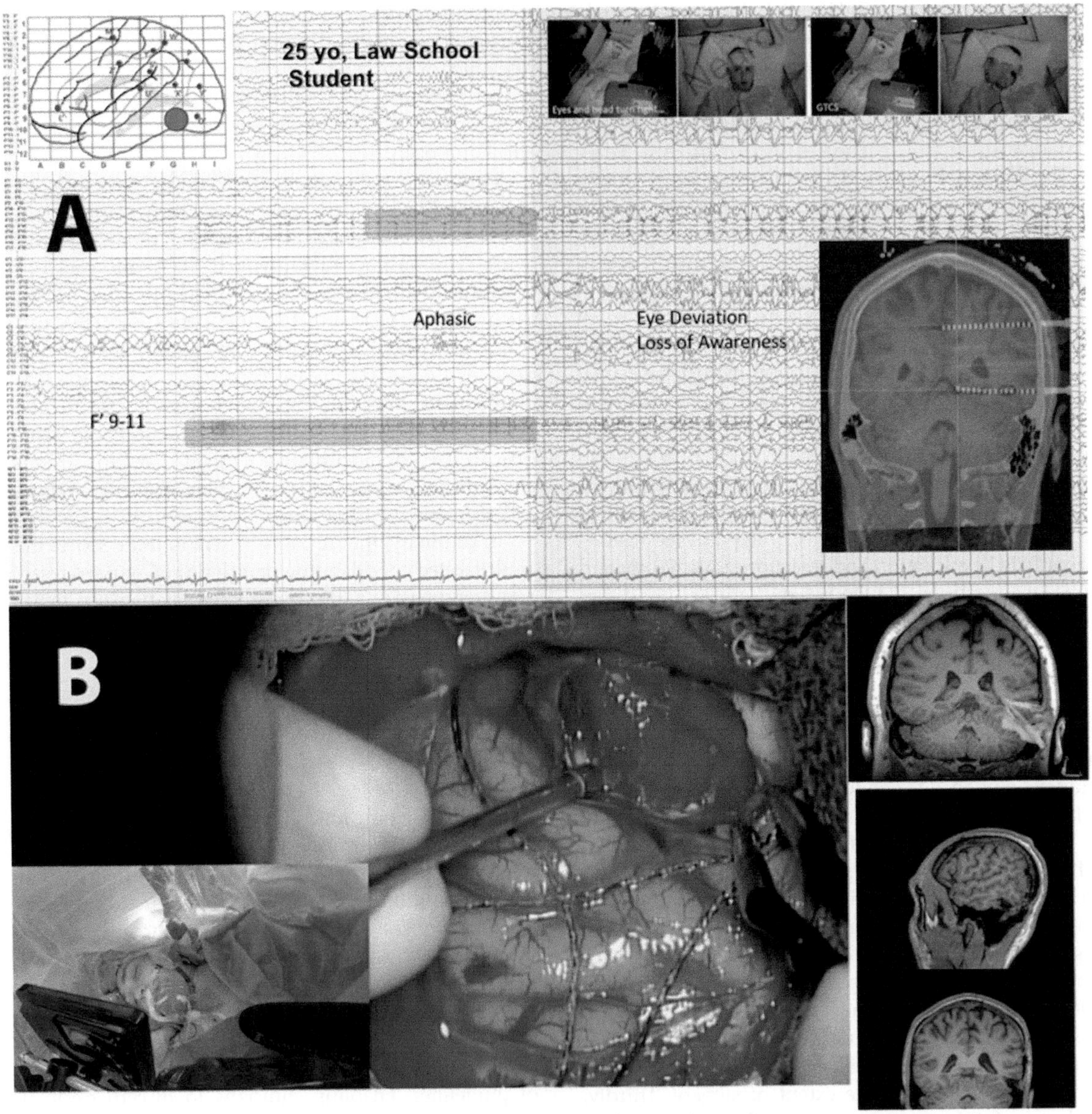


FIG. 12.5 SEEG guided resection in a 25-year-old law school student with medically refractory epilepsy characterized by visual and language disturbances, conjugate eye deviation to the right and loss of conscious. (A) Panel depicts the anatomical translation of the SEEG clinical-electrophysiological correlation to the patient's anatomy. The EZ location and extension is highlighted by the red circle, located at the depts of the temporo-occipital sulcus on the left side, at the basal temporo-occipital transition. (B) Illustration of the intraoperative aspect during the resection phase, with the patient under awake condition. As shown at the top subpanel on the right, the resection areas were in close proximity with the terminations of the arcuate fascicle subtle picture recognition deficits were observed during the resection, which completely subsided in the post-operative period. Patient remains seizure free after 2 years. (With courtesy of Drs Chauvel, Aung and Mahon.)

surgical decision-making and prognostication. Optimal interpretation of SEEG recordings and formulation of resection strategies demand individualized consideration, underpinned by the expertise and collective experience of the clinical team. Moreover, the option of nonoperative management should not be overlooked, particularly in cases where SEEG findings exhibit inconsistencies or fail to elucidate the underlying pathophysiology of the patient's symptoms through anatomo-electro-clinical correlations. Put simply, the validity of results depends to a great degree on the experience of the team as well as cohort size, with a learning curve for every individual practitioner and team.

A recent study by the authors[28] scrutinized a cohort of 200 patients who underwent a total of 2663 SEEG electrode implantations for invasive intracranial EEG monitoring, guided by tailored pre-implantation hypotheses aimed at delineating and characterizing the epileptogenic zone (EZ). Focal cortical dysplasia type I emerged as the most prevalent pathological diagnosis in this cohort (55 patients, 61.1%). Despite the cohort's complexity, with a notable proportion of patients having undergone prior surgical interventions for medically refractory epilepsy, SEEG successfully confirmed the EZ in 154 patients (77.0%).

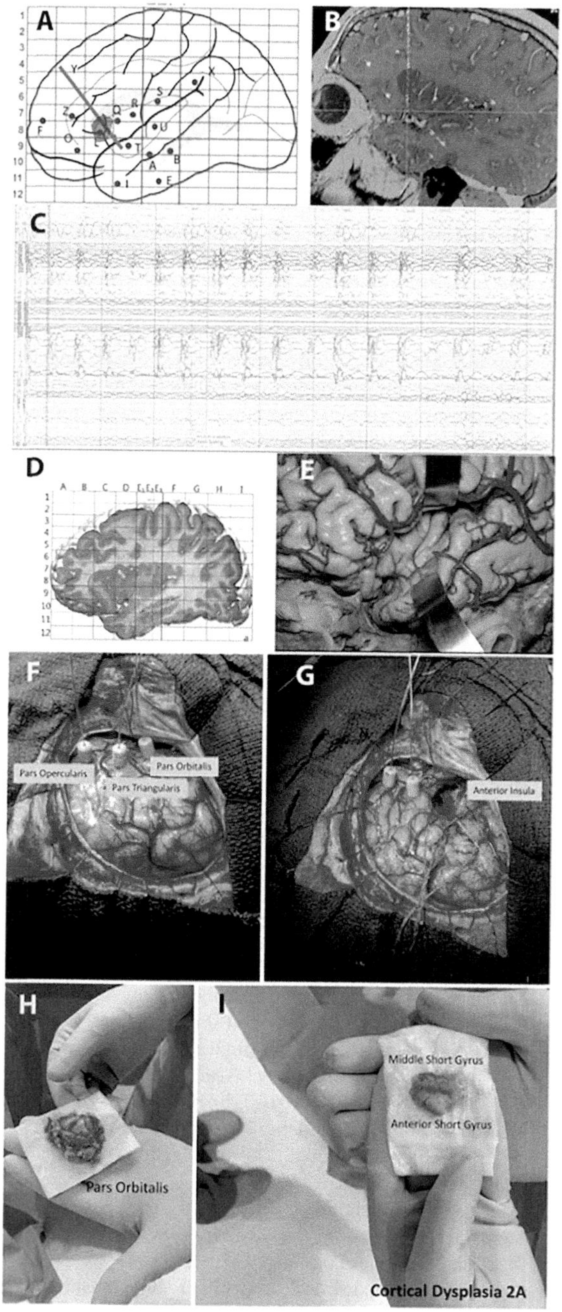


FIG. 12.6 SEEG-guided resection in a 12-year-old child with medically refractory epilepsy characterized by episodes of nausea and vomiting followed by loss of conscious and generalization. Pre-operative data reviewed interictal and ictal activity predominantly on the left frontal-parietal regions and MRI revealing a possible lesion (increase in thickness of cortical areas in the anterior limitans sulcus of the insula associated with increased signal on T2-FLAIR images in the same region). After discussion at PMC, decision was made to further evaluate with an SEEG exploration. Panel A depicts the implantation schema, with mostly orthogonal electrodes exploring the perisylvian cortical areas, including the insula cortex, anterior temporal lobe areas and orbito-frontal/frontal polar areas. An additional oblique electrode was placed in the anterior insular areas, exploring the MRI visible lesion in the anterior limitans sulcus of the insula. Panel B depicts the correlation of MRI and post implantation CT images, showing the region of the oblique electrode (Y′) and orthogonal electrode (L′) in relation with the identified lesion (*red circle*). C panel demonstrates sample of interictal SEEG recordings with continuous polyspike wave complexes located in the anterior insula and orbito-frontal cortical regions. Panel D depicts the plan of resection highlighted with blue shape, including the anterior portions of the insula and the posterior aspect of the orbito-frontal cortex. Panel E depicts an anatomical specimen of left hemisphere with the exposure of the anterior insula and posterior orbito-frontal areas, to better illustrate the anatomical complexity of the region of interest. Panels F and G depicts intra-operative pictures during the resection phase. Panel F depicts the implantation of depth electrodes in the frontal operculum and insula during ECOG and panel G shows the final aspect of resection, after the removal of the orbito-frontal areas and insula. Panels H and I show the resection specimens. (With courtesy of Drs Patterson and Welsh.)

Subsequently, 134 patients (87.0%) underwent SEEG-guided craniotomy, with 67.8% achieving seizure freedom (Engel I outcome) during a minimum post-operative follow-up period of 12 months. Notably, the incidence of complications was minimal, with a total morbidity rate of 2.5%.

These findings align with previous studies in the literature, reflecting both the efficacy and safety of SEEG-guided resections. Munari et al. reported on a cohort of 70 patients, where individualized surgical resections were performed in 85.7% of cases, with a low morbidity rate of 1.4%.[13] Similarly, Guenot et al. observed favorable outcomes in 84% of cases, with complications occurring in 5% of cases, including one mortality.[73] Additional studies by Cossu et al.,[20] and Cardinale et al.[74] corroborate these findings, underscoring the overall safety and efficacy of SEEG-guided resections, with complication rates consistently below 5%.[74]

In summation, the collective evidence underscores the favorable seizure outcomes and low complication rates associated with SEEG-guided resections, reaffirming its role as a safe and efficacious therapeutic modality for patients with challenging-to-localize focal epilepsies. As an evolving field, ongoing research endeavors and interdisciplinary collaborations will continue to refine surgical techniques, enhance patient care protocols, and optimize outcomes in epilepsy surgery.

## CONCLUSIONS

As we stand on the threshold of a new era propelled by emerging technologies like augmented reality and artificial intelligence, the transition from the conventional Talairach space to three-dimensional surgical anatomy represents a transformative milestone in neurosurgery. This journey epitomizes the fusion of classical stereotaxic principles pioneered by Talairach with the latest advancements in imaging modalities and surgical techniques. Within this landscape of innovation, SEEG-guided treatment methods help redefine the boundaries of surgical precision and patient care.

## REFERENCES


1. Aung T, Grinenko O, Li J, Mosher JC, Chauvel P, Gonzalez-Martinez J. Stereoelectroencephalography-guided laser ablation in neocortical epilepsy: electrophysiological correlations and outcome. *Epilepsia*. November 2023; 64(11):2993–3012. https://doi.org/10.1111/epi.17739.
2. de Souza J, Mullin J, Wathen C, et al. The usefulness of stereo-electroencephalography (SEEG) in the surgical management of focal epilepsy associated with "hidden" temporal pole encephalocele: a case report and literature review. *Neurosurg Rev*. January 2018;41(1):347–354. https://doi.org/10.1007/s10143-017-0922-0.
3. Enatsu R, Bulacio J, Najm I, et al. Combining stereo-electroencephalography and subdural electrodes in the diagnosis and treatment of medically intractable epilepsy. *J Clin Neurosci*. August 2014;21(8):1441–1445. https://doi.org/10.1016/j.jocn.2013.12.014.
4. Fallah A, Rodgers SD, Weil AG, et al. Resective epilepsy surgery for tuberous sclerosis in children: determining predictors of seizure outcomes in a multicenter retrospective cohort study. *Neurosurgery*. October 2015;77(4):517–524. https://doi.org/10.1227/NEU.0000000000000875.
5. Gonzalez-Martinez J. Convergence of stereotactic surgery and epilepsy: the stereoelectroencephalography method. *Neurosurgery*. August 2015;62(Suppl 1):117–122. https://doi.org/10.1227/NEU.0000000000000787.
6. Gonzalez-Martinez J, Lachhwani D. Stereoelectroencephalography in children with cortical dysplasia: technique and results. *Childs Nerv Syst*. November 2014;30(11): 1853–1857. https://doi.org/10.1007/s00381-014-2499-z.
7. Gonzalez-Martinez J, Vadera S, Mullin J, et al. Robot-assisted stereotactic laser ablation in medically intractable epilepsy: operative technique. *Neurosurgery*. June 2014; 10(Suppl 2):167–172. https://doi.org/10.1227/NEU.0000000000000286.
8. Gonzalez-Martinez JA, Abou-Al-Shaar H, Mallela AN, et al. The endoscopic anterior transmaxillary temporal pole approach for mesial temporal lobe epilepsies: a feasibility study. *J Neurosurg*. April 1, 2023;138(4):992–1001. https://doi.org/10.3171/2022.7.JNS221062.
9. Ross L, Naduvil AM, Bulacio JC, Najm IM, Gonzalez-Martinez JA. Stereoelectroencephalography-guided laser ablations in patients with neocortical pharmacoresistant focal epilepsy: concept and operative technique. *Oper Neurosurg (Hagerstown)*. December 1, 2018;15(6):656–663. https://doi.org/10.1093/ons/opy022.
10. Vadera S, Burgess R, Gonzalez-Martinez J. Concomitant use of stereoelectroencephalography (SEEG) and magnetoencephalographic (MEG) in the surgical treatment of refractory focal epilepsy. *Clin Neurol Neurosurg*. July 2014;122: 9–11. https://doi.org/10.1016/j.clineuro.2014.04.002.
11. Bancaud J. Surgery of epilepsy based on stereotactic investigations–the plan of the SEEG investigation. *Acta Neurochir Suppl*. 1980;30:25–34.
12. Bancaud J, Angelergues R, Bernouilli C, et al. Functional stereotaxic exploration (SEEG) of epilepsy. *Electroencephalogr Clin Neurophysiol*. January 1970;28(1):85–86.
13. Munari C, Giallonardo AT, Brunet P, Broglin D, Bancaud J. Stereotactic investigations in frontal lobe epilepsies. *Acta Neurochir Suppl*. 1989;46:9–12. https://doi.org/10.1007/978-3-7091-9029-6_2.
14. Talairach J, Bancaud J, Bonis A, et al. Surgical therapy for frontal epilepsies. *Adv Neurol*. 1992;57:707–732.
15. Alomar S, Jones J, Maldonado A, Gonzalez-Martinez J. The stereo-electroencephalography methodology. *Neurosurg Clin N Am*. January 2016;27(1):83–95. https://doi.org/10.1016/j.nec.2015.08.003.

16. Antony AR, Alexopoulos AV, Gonzalez-Martinez JA, et al. Functional connectivity estimated from intracranial EEG predicts surgical outcome in intractable temporal lobe epilepsy. *PLoS One*. 2013;8(10):e77916. https://doi.org/10.1371/journal.pone.0077916.
17. Aung T, Mallela A, Ho J, Tang LW, Abou-Al-Shaar H, Gonzalez Martinez J. Challenging cortical explorations in difficult-to-localize seizures: the rationale and usefulness of perisylvian paralimbic explorations with orthogonal stereoelectroencephalography depth electrodes. *Neurosurgery*. December 4, 2023. https://doi.org/10.1227/neu.0000000000002787.
18. Cardinale F, Rizzi M, Vignati E, et al. Stereoelectroencephalography: retrospective analysis of 742 procedures in a single centre. *Brain*. September 1, 2019;142(9):2688–2704. https://doi.org/10.1093/brain/awz196.
19. Cossu M, Cardinale F, Casaceli G, et al. Stereo-EEG-guided radiofrequency thermocoagulations. *Epilepsia*. April 2017;58(Suppl 1):66–72. https://doi.org/10.1111/epi.13687.
20. Cossu M, Cardinale F, Castana L, et al. Stereoelectroencephalography in the presurgical evaluation of focal epilepsy: a retrospective analysis of 215 procedures. *Neurosurgery*. October 2005;57(4):706–718.
21. Cossu M, Cardinale F, Colombo N, et al. Stereoelectroencephalography in the presurgical evaluation of children with drug-resistant focal epilepsy. *J Neurosurg*. October 2005;103(4 Suppl):333–343. https://doi.org/10.3171/ped.2005.103.4.0333.
22. Cossu M, d'Orio P, Barba C, et al. Focal cortical dysplasia IIIa in hippocampal sclerosis-associated epilepsy: anatomo-electro-clinical profile and surgical results from a multicentric retrospective study. *Neurosurgery*. January 13, 2021;88(2):384–393. https://doi.org/10.1093/neuros/nyaa369.
23. Cossu M, Fuschillo D, Cardinale F, et al. Stereo-EEG-guided radio-frequency thermocoagulations of epileptogenic grey-matter nodular heterotopy. *J Neurol Neurosurg Psychiatry*. June 2014;85(6):611–617. https://doi.org/10.1136/jnnp-2013-305514.
24. Cossu M, Fuschillo D, Casaceli G, et al. Stereo electroencephalography-guided radiofrequency thermocoagulation in the epileptogenic zone: a retrospective study on 89 cases. *J Neurosurg*. December 2015;123(6):1358–1367. https://doi.org/10.3171/2014.12.JNS141968.
25. Cossu M, Lo Russo G, Francione S, et al. Epilepsy surgery in children: results and predictors of outcome on seizures. *Epilepsia*. January 2008;49(1):65–72. https://doi.org/10.1111/j.1528-1167.2007.01207.x.
26. Cossu M, Pelliccia V, Gozzo F, et al. Surgical treatment of polymicrogyria-related epilepsy. *Epilepsia*. December 2016;57(12):2001–2010. https://doi.org/10.1111/epi.13589.
27. Gonzalez-Martinez J, Bulacio J, Alexopoulos A, Jehi L, Bingaman W, Najm I. Stereoelectroencephalography in the "difficult to localize" refractory focal epilepsy: early experience from a North American epilepsy center. *Epilepsia*. February 2013;54(2):323–330. https://doi.org/10.1111/j.1528-1167.2012.03672.x.
28. Serletis D, Bulacio J, Bingaman W, Najm I, Gonzalez-Martinez J. The stereotactic approach for mapping epileptic networks: a prospective study of 200 patients. *J Neurosurg*. November 2014;121(5):1239–1246. https://doi.org/10.3171/2014.7.JNS132306.
29. Tassi L, Colombo N, Garbelli R, et al. Focal cortical dysplasia: neuropathological subtypes, EEG, neuroimaging and surgical outcome. *Brain*. August 2002;125(Pt 8):1719–1732. https://doi.org/10.1093/brain/awf175.
30. Gonzalez-Martinez J, Najm IM. Indications and selection criteria for invasive monitoring in children with cortical dysplasia. *Childs Nerv Syst*. November 2014;30(11):1823–1829. https://doi.org/10.1007/s00381-014-2497-1.
31. Miserocchi A, Cascardo B, Piroddi C, et al. Surgery for temporal lobe epilepsy in children: relevance of presurgical evaluation and analysis of outcome. *J Neurosurg Pediatr*. March 2013;11(3):256–267. https://doi.org/10.3171/2012.12.PEDS12334.
32. Chauvel P, Gonzalez-Martinez J, Bulacio J. Presurgical intracranial investigations in epilepsy surgery. *Handb Clin Neurol*. 2019;161:45–71. https://doi.org/10.1016/B978-0-444-64142-7.00040-0.
33. Steriade C, Martins W, Bulacio J, et al. Localization yield and seizure outcome in patients undergoing bilateral SEEG exploration. *Epilepsia*. January 2019;60(1):107–120. https://doi.org/10.1111/epi.14624.
34. Abarrategui B, Mariani V, Rizzi M, et al. Language lateralization mapping (reversibly) masked by non-dominant focal epilepsy: a case report. *Front Hum Neurosci*. 2023;17:1254779. https://doi.org/10.3389/fnhum.2023.1254779.
35. Arnulfo G, Wang SH, Myrov V, et al. Long-range phase synchronization of high-frequency oscillations in human cortex. *Nat Commun*. October 23, 2020;11(1):5363. https://doi.org/10.1038/s41467-020-18975-8.
36. Balestrini S, Francione S, Mai R, et al. Multimodal responses induced by cortical stimulation of the parietal lobe: a stereo-electroencephalography study. *Brain*. September 2015;138(Pt 9):2596–2607. https://doi.org/10.1093/brain/awv187.
37. Bancaud J, Talairach J. [Functional organization of the supplementary motor area. Data obtained by stereo-E.E.G]. *Neurochirurgie*. May-Jun 1967;13(3):343–356.
38. Breault MS, Sacre P, Gonzalez-Martinez J, Gale JT, Sarma SV. An exploratory data analysis method for identifying brain regions and frequencies of interest from large-scale neural recordings. *J Comput Neurosci*. February 2019;46(1):3–17. https://doi.org/10.1007/s10827-018-0705-9.
39. Consejo YCC, Gonzalez-Martinez JF. [Ethics and methodology: the importance of promoting, evaluating and implementing education and humanities research in health]. *Rev Med Inst Mex Seguro Soc*. Jul-Aug 2017;55(4):412–415.
40. Rizzi M, Revay M, d'Orio P, et al. Tailored multilobar disconnective epilepsy surgery in the posterior quadrant. *J Neurosurg*. April 26, 2019;132(5):1345–1357. https://doi.org/10.3171/2019.1.JNS183103.

41. Mirandola L, Mai RF, Francione S, et al. Stereo-EEG: diagnostic and therapeutic tool for periventricular nodular heterotopia epilepsies. *Epilepsia*. November 2017;58(11): 1962–1971. https://doi.org/10.1111/epi.13895.
42. Dolezalova I, Kunst J, Kojan M, Chrastina J, Balaz M, Brazdil M. Anterior thalamic deep brain stimulation in epilepsy and persistent psychiatric side effects following discontinuation. *Epilepsy Behav Rep*. 2019;12:100344. https://doi.org/10.1016/j.ebr.2019.100344.
43. Gross RE, Fisher RS, Sperling MR, Giftakis JE, Stypulkowski PH. Analysis of deep brain stimulation lead targeting in the stimulation of anterior nucleus of the thalamus for epilepsy clinical trial. *Neurosurgery*. August 16, 2021;89(3):406–412. https://doi.org/10.1093/neuros/nyab186.
44. Halpern CH, Samadani U, Litt B, Jaggi JL, Baltuch GH. Deep brain stimulation for epilepsy. *Neurotherapeutics*. January 2008;5(1):59–67. https://doi.org/10.1016/j.nurt.2007.10.065.
45. Hamani C, Andrade D, Hodaie M, Wennberg R, Lozano A. Deep brain stimulation for the treatment of epilepsy. *Int J Neural Syst*. June 2009;19(3):213–226. https://doi.org/10.1142/S0129065709001975.
46. Hamani C, Dubiela FP, Soares JC, et al. Anterior thalamus deep brain stimulation at high current impairs memory in rats. *Exp Neurol*. September 2010;225(1):154–162. https://doi.org/10.1016/j.expneurol.2010.06.007.
47. Jones N. Epilepsy: DBS reduces seizure frequency in refractory epilepsy. *Nat Rev Neurol*. May 2010;6(5):238. https://doi.org/10.1038/nrneurol.2010.40.
48. Lozano AM, Hamani C. The future of deep brain stimulation. *J Clin Neurophysiol*. Jan-Feb 2004;21(1): 68–69. https://doi.org/10.1097/00004691-200401000-00008.
49. Ryvlin P, Jehi LE. Neuromodulation for refractory epilepsy. *Epilepsy Curr*. Jan-Feb 2022;22(1):11–17. https://doi.org/10.1177/15357597211065587.
50. Ryvlin P, Rheims S, Hirsch LJ, Sokolov A, Jehi L. Neuromodulation in epilepsy: state-of-the-art approved therapies. *Lancet Neurol*. December 2021;20(12):1038–1047. https://doi.org/10.1016/S1474-4422(21)00300-8.
51. Salanova V. Deep brain stimulation for epilepsy. *Epilepsy Behav*. November 2018;88S:21–24. https://doi.org/10.1016/j.yebeh.2018.06.041.
52. Barot N, Batra K, Zhang J, et al. Surgical outcomes between temporal, extratemporal epilepsies and hypothalamic hamartoma: systematic review and meta-analysis of MRI-guided laser interstitial thermal therapy for drug-resistant epilepsy. *J Neurol Neurosurg Psychiatry*. February 2022; 93(2):133–143. https://doi.org/10.1136/jnnp-2021-326185.
53. Gupta K, Dickey AS, Hu R, Faught E, Willie JT. Robot assisted MRI-guided LITT of the anterior, lateral, and medial temporal lobe for temporal lobe epilepsy. *Front Neurol*. 2020;11:572334. https://doi.org/10.3389/fneur.2020.572334.
54. Aum DJ, Reynolds RA, McEvoy S, et al. Surgical outcomes of open and laser interstitial thermal therapy approaches for corpus callosotomy in pediatric epilepsy. *Epilepsia*. September 2023;64(9):2274–2285. https://doi.org/10.1111/epi.17679.
55. Drane DL. MRI-Guided stereotactic laser ablation for epilepsy surgery: promising preliminary results for cognitive outcome. *Epilepsy Res*. May 2018;142:170–175. https://doi.org/10.1016/j.eplepsyres.2017.09.016.
56. Tao JX, Wu S, Lacy M, et al. Stereotactic EEG-guided laser interstitial thermal therapy for mesial temporal lobe epilepsy. *J Neurol Neurosurg Psychiatry*. May 2018;89(5): 542–548. https://doi.org/10.1136/jnnp-2017-316833.
57. Whiting AC, Bingaman JR, Catapano JS, et al. Laser interstitial thermal therapy for epileptogenic periventricular nodular heterotopia. *World Neurosurg*. June 2020;138: e892–e897. https://doi.org/10.1016/j.wneu.2020.03.133.
58. Wicks RT, Jermakowicz WJ, Jagid JR, et al. Laser interstitial thermal therapy for mesial temporal lobe epilepsy. *Neurosurgery*. December 2016;79(Suppl 1):S83–S91. https://doi.org/10.1227/NEU.0000000000001439.
59. Wong GM, McCray A, Hom K, et al. Outcomes of stereoelectroencephalography following failed epilepsy surgery in children. *Childs Nerv Syst*. April 23, 2024 https://doi.org/10.1007/s00381-024-06420-w.
60. Youngerman BE, Oh JY, Anbarasan D, et al. Laser ablation is effective for temporal lobe epilepsy with and without mesial temporal sclerosis if hippocampal seizure onsets are localized by stereoelectroencephalography. *Epilepsia*. March 2018;59(3):595–606. https://doi.org/10.1111/epi.14004.
61. Zemmar A, Nelson BJ, Neimat JS. Laser thermal therapy for epilepsy surgery: current standing and future perspectives. *Int J Hyperthermia*. July 2020;37(2):77–83. https://doi.org/10.1080/02656736.2020.1788175.
62. Zheng B, Abdulrazeq H, Shao B, et al. Seizure and anatomical outcomes of repeat laser amygdalohippocampotomy for temporal lobe epilepsy: a single-institution case series. *Epilepsy Behav*. September 2023;146:109365. https://doi.org/10.1016/j.yebeh.2023.109365.
63. Talairach J. [Stereotaxic radiologic explorations]. *Rev Neurol (Paris)*. 1954;90(5):556–584.
64. Talairach J, Bancaud J, Bonis A, Tournoux P, Szikla G, Morel P. [Functional stereotaxic investigations in epilepsy. Methodological remarks concerning a case]. *Rev Neurol (Paris)*. August 1961;105:119–130.
65. Talairach J, Bancaud J, Szikla G, Bonis A, Geier S, Vedrenne C. [New approach to the neurosurgery of epilepsy. Stereotaxic methodology and therapeutic results. 1. Introduction and history]. *Neurochirurgie*. June 1974; 20(Suppl 1):1–240.
66. Talairach J, David M, Fischgold H, Metzger J. [Radiography, encephalography, and angiography in lipoma of the corpus callosum]. *Rev Neurol (Paris)*. 1951;85(6): 511–517.
67. Talairach J, Tournoux P, Musolino A, Missir O. Stereotaxic exploration in frontal epilepsy. *Adv Neurol*. 1992;57: 651–688.
68. Chauvel P, Buser P, Badier JM, Liegeois-Chauvel C, Marquis P, Bancaud J. [The "epileptogenic zone" in

humans: representation of intercritical events by spatio-temporal maps]. *Rev Neurol (Paris)*. 1987;143(5):443–450.

69. Chauvel P, Kliemann F, Vignal JP, Chodkiewicz JP, Talairach J, Bancaud J. The clinical signs and symptoms of frontal lobe seizures. Phenomenology and classification. *Adv Neurol*. 1995;66:115–125.
70. Gonzalez-Martinez JA, Chauvel PY. Letter to the Editor. The importance of orthogonal implantation in SEEG: historical considerations. *J Neurosurg*. February 5, 2021; 135(1):332–333. https://doi.org/10.3171/2020.10.JNS203393.
71. Grappe A, Sarma SV, Sacre P, Gonzalez-Martinez J, Liegeois-Chauvel C, Alario FX. An intracerebral exploration of functional connectivity during word production. *J Comput Neurosci*. February 2019;46(1):125–140. https://doi.org/10.1007/s10827-018-0699-3.
72. Grinenko O, Li J, Mosher JC, et al. A fingerprint of the epileptogenic zone in human epilepsies. *Brain*. January 1, 2018;141(1):117–131. https://doi.org/10.1093/brain/awx306.
73. Catenoix H, Bourdillon P, Guenot M, Isnard J. The combination of stereo-EEG and radiofrequency ablation. *Epilepsy Res*. May 2018;142:117–120. https://doi.org/10.1016/j.eplepsyres.2018.01.012.
74. Cardinale F, Cossu M, Castana L, et al. Stereoelectroencephalography: surgical methodology, safety, and stereotactic application accuracy in 500 procedures. *Neurosurgery*. March 2013;72(3):353–366. https://doi.org/10.1227/NEU.0b013e31827d1161.

# Index



'*Note:* Page numbers followed by "f" indicate figures.'

9780443108778